Best of Five MCQs for the MRCP Part 1

Volume 3

Best of Five MCQs for the MRCP Part 1

Volume 3

Edited by

Iqbal Khan

Consultant Gastroenterologist and Associate Director of Undergraduate Education, Northampton General Hospital, Northampton, UK

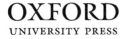

OXFORD
UNIVERSITY PRESS

OXFORD
UNIVERSITY PRESS

Great Clarendon Street, Oxford, OX2 6DP,
United Kingdom

Oxford University Press is a department of the University of Oxford.
It furthers the University's objective of excellence in research, scholarship,
and education by publishing worldwide. Oxford is a registered trade mark of
Oxford University Press in the UK and in certain other countries

First Edition published in 2017

Impression: 5

Published in the United States of America by Oxford University Press
198 Madison Avenue, New York, NY 10016, United States of America

British Library Cataloguing in Publication Data

Data available

Library of Congress Control Number: 201694 122

Set ISBN 978–0–19–878792–1
Volume 1 978–0–19–874672–0
Volume 2 978–0–19–874716–1
Volume 3 978–0–19–874717–8

Printed in Great Britain by
Clays Ltd, Elcograf S.p.A.

PREFACE

The Membership of the Royal College of Physicians (MRCP) is a mandatory exam for trainees in the UK intending to enter a career in a medical speciality. The MRCP exam has three parts: MRCP Part 1 (written paper); MRCP Part 2 (written paper); and MRCP Part 2 Clinical Examination (PACES).

The MRCP (UK) Part 1 Examination is designed to assess a candidate's knowledge and understanding of the clinical sciences relevant to medical practice and of common or important disorders to a level appropriate for entry to specialist training. Candidates must sit two papers, each of which is three hours in duration and contains 100 multiple choice questions in 'best of five' format. These are designed to test candidates' core knowledge, the ability to interpret information, and clinical problem solving. The MRCP Part 1 requires a huge breadth of information to be revised.

Whilst books and resources are available, there is a huge variation in the number and quality of practice questions available. Online revision websites can be very expensive and impractical for busy junior doctors in clinical posts. These three volumes have been written with these busy junior doctors in mind and are designed to be studied one volume at a time. The three volumes together cover the full syllabus of the MRCP part 1 exam, and the number of questions per speciality is proportional to that seen in the exam. It is suggested that doctors preparing for the exam should carry one of the books into work each day and use every opportunity to study, even if it is for brief intervals. When time permits a more detailed review of the subject should take place to ensure full understanding of each topic.

The questions have been written and reviewed by experts in their respective fields and I would like to use this opportunity to thank each and every one of them for their excellent contributions.

Iqbal Khan

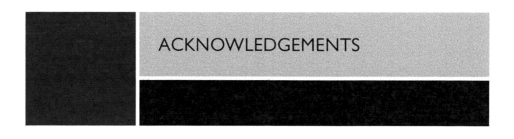

ACKNOWLEDGEMENTS

A small selection of questions have been kindly reproduced from *Oxford Assess and progress: Psychiatry*, edited by Jill Myers and Melissa Gardner, with series Editors Kathy Boursicot and David Sales, © Oxford University Press 2014.

CONTENTS

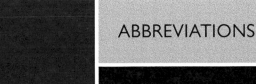

ABBREVIATIONS

μmol/L	micromoles per litre
A&E	Accident and Emergency
AAFB	acid-alcohol fast bacilli
ABG	arterial blood gas
ABPA	allergic bronchopulmonary aspergillosis
ACE	angiotensin-converting enzyme
AChR	acetylcholine receptor
ACR	American College of Rheumatology
ACTH	adrenocorticotropic hormone
ADEM	acute disseminated encephalomyelitis
ADH	antidiuretic hormone
AF	atrial fibrillation
AIDP	acute inflammatory demyelinating polyradiculoneuropathy
AIDS	autoimmune deficiency syndrome
Alb	albumin
ALP	alkaline phosphatase
ALT	alanine aminotransferase
AMTS	abbreviated mental test score
ANA	antinuclear antibodies
ANCA	antineutrophil cytoplasmic antibodies
APKD	adult polycystic kidney disease
APTT	activated partial thromboplastin time
ARA	American Rheumatism Association
ARDS	acute respiratory distress syndrome
AST	aspartate amino transferase
BCG	bacille Calmette–Guérin
BD	bis in die
BIPAP	bilevel positive airway pressure
BM	blood glucose monitoring

BMD	bone mineral density
BMI	body mass index
BNF	British National Formulary
BODE	body mass index, airflow obstruction, dyspnea and exercise
BP	blood pressure
BPAD	bipolar affective disorder
bpm	beats per minute
BTS	British Thoracic Society
Ca_2	calcium
CAH	chronic active hepatitis
CAM	Confusion Assessment Method
c-ANCA	cytoplasmic antineutrophil cytoplasmic antibodies
CAPD	continuous ambulatory peritoneal dialysis
CCP	cyclic citrullinated peptide
CF	cystic fibrosis
CFTR	cystic fibrosis transmembrane conductance regulator
CIDP	chronic inflammatory demyelinating radiculoneuropathy
CJD	Creutzfeld–Jakob disease
CMT	Charcot–Marie–Tooth
Cl	chlorine
CK	creatine kinase
CKD	chronic kidney disease
CLOX 1	clock drawing test
CMV	cytomegalovirus
CN	cranial nerves
CNS	central nervous system
CO_2	carbon dioxide
COPD	chronic obstructive pulmonary disease
CPAP	continuous positive airway pressure
CPP	calcium pyrophosphate
CPPD	CPP deposition
CPR	cardiopulmonary resuscitation
Cr	creatinine
CRAB	hypercalcemia, renal dysfunction, anaemia, and lytic bone lesions
CRP	C-Reactive Protein
CSF	cerebrospinal fluid

CT	computed tomography
CTG	cardiotocograph
CTPA	CT pulmonary angiography
CVST	cerebral venous sinus thrombosis
CXR	chest X-ray
DAS	disease activity score
DKA	diabetic ketoacidosis
DLCO	diffusion lung capacity for CO
DMD	Duchenne muscular dystrophy
DVLA	Driver and Vehicle Licensing Agency
DVT	deep vein thrombosis
DXA	dual energy x-ray absorptiometry
EBV	Epstein–Barr virus
ECG	electrocardiogram
ED	Emergency department
EEG	electroencephalogram
EGFR	epidermal growth factor receptor.
EMG	electromyogram
ENT	ear, nose, and throat
ESPS-2	European Stroke Prevention Study 2
ESR	erythrocyte sedimentation rate
FAST	Fast Alcohol Screening Test
FBC	full blood count
FDG-PET	fluorodeoxyglucose positron emission tomography
FEV	forced expiratory volume
FEV	forced expiratory volume in one second
FFP	fresh frozen plasma
FRS	first-rank symptoms
FSH	follicle stimulating hormone
FVC	forced vital capacity
GAA	glucosidase, alpha, acid
GABA	gamma-aminobutyric acid
GBM	glioblastoma multiforme
GBS	Guillain-Barré syndrome
GCS	Glasgow Coma Scale/Score
g/dL	grammes per decilitre

GDS	Geriatric Depression Score
GI	gastrointestinal
GN	glomerulonephritis
GORD	gastro-oesophageal reflux disease
GP	general practitioner
Hb	haemoglobin
HCO_3	bicarbonate
HDU	high dependency unit
HIV	human immunodeficiency virus
HONK	hyperosmolar non-ketotic coma
HPO(A)	hypertrophic pulmonary osteoarthropathy
HPOA	hypertrophic pulmonary osteoarthropathy
HRCT	high-resolution computed tomography
HSV-2	Herpes simplex virus-2
HUS	haemolytic uremic syndrome
IBD	inflammatory bowel disease
ICS	inhaled corticosteroids
ICU	intensive care unit
IgA	immunoglobulin A
IgD	immunoglobulin D
IgE	immunoglobulin E
IgG	immunoglobulin class G
IgM	immunoglublin class M
IIH	idiopathic intracranial hypertension
IM	intramuscular
INO	internuclear ophthalmoplegia
IPF	Idiopathic pulmonary fibrosis
IQ	intelligence quotient
INR	international normalized ratio
IP	intraperitoneal
IQCODE	Informant Questionnaire on Cognitive Decline in the Elderly
ITU	intensive treatment unit
IU/L	international unites per litre
IU/ml	international units per millimetre
IV	intravenous
IVIg	intravenous immunoglobulin

JC virus	John Cunningham virus
JVP	jugular venous pressure
K	potassium
kg	kilogram
kPa	kilo Pascal
LABA	long-acting beta agonist
LAMA	long-acting muscarininc antagonist
LFT	liver function test
LH	luteinizing hormone
LMN	lower motor neurone
LTOT	long-term oxygen therapy
LV	left ventricle
MAPK	mitogen-activated protein kinase
MAU	Medical Assessment Unit
mcg/l	microgram per litre
MCTD	mixed connective tissue disease
mg	milligramme
MG	myasthenia gravis
MHA	Mental Health Act
micromole/l	micromoles per litre
MLF	medial longitudinal fasciculus
mmol	millimols per litre
MMSE	Mini Mental State Examination
MND	motor neurone disease
mOsmol/kg	milliosmols per kg
MR	magnetic resonance; modified release
MRA	magnetic resonance angiography
MRC	Medical Research Council
MRI	magnetic resonance imaging
MRV	magnetic resonance venography
MS	multiple sclerosis
ms	milliseconds
MSU	mid-stream urine
MTP	metatarsalphalangeal
MU	million units
NA	sodium

NDMA	N-methyl-d-aspartate
NFI	Neurofibromatosis type 1
NIV	non-invasive mechanical ventilation
NMO	neuromyelitis optica
NMS	neuroleptic malignant syndrome
NNT	number needed to treat
NPH	Neutral Protamine Hagedorn; normal pressure hydrocephalus
NSAID	nonsteroidal anti-inflammatory drug
NSCLC	non-small cell lung cancer
NSIP	non-specific interstitial pneumonitis
NSTEMI	non-ST-elevation myocardial infarction
O_2	oxygen
OA	osteoarthritis
od	omni die
OPD	outpatient department
OSA	obstructive sleep apnoea
$PaCO_2$	potential carbon dioxide
PACS	partial anterior circulation stroke
PAN	polyarteritis nodosa
pANCA	perinuclear anti-neutrophil cytoplasmic antibodies
PaO_2	potential oxygen
PCR	polymerase chain reaction
PD	personality disorder
PDGF	platelet derived growth factor
PEF	peak expiratory flow
PEFR	peak expiratory flow rate
PFO	patent foramen ovale
pH	potential hydrogen
PML	progressive multifocal leukoencephalopathy
PO	per mouth
pO_2	potential oxygen
PO_4	phosphorus
POCS	posterior circulation stroke
PRN	pro re nata
PSA	prostate specific antigen
PSP	progressive supranuclear palsy

PT	prothrombin time
PTH	parathyroid hormone
RA	rheumatoid arthritis
RAPD	relative afferent pupillary defect
RAST	RadioAllergoSorbent Testing
RCP	Royal College of Physicians
REM	rapid eye movement
RF	rheumatoid factor
rINN	recommended International Non-Proprietary Name
RIOTT	Randomised Injectable Opiate Treatment Trial
RNA	ribonucleic acid
RTA	road traffic accident
SABA	short-acting B-agonist
SAH	subarachnoid haemorrhage
SCLE	subacute cutaneous lupus erythematosus
SHO	senior house officer
SIADH	syndrome of inappropriate antidiuretic hormone
SLE	systemic lupus erythematosus
SpO_2	peripheral capillary oxygen saturation
SS	Sjögren's syndrome
SSRI	selective serotonin reuptake inhibitor
SUNCT	short-lasting unilateral neuralgiform headache attacks with conjunctival injection and tearing
TA	temporal arteritis
TAC	trigeminal autonomic cephalalgia
TACS	total anterior circulation stroke
TB	tuberculosis
TDS	ter die sumendum
TENS	transcutaneous electrical nerve stimulation
TGA	transient global amnesia
TIA	transient ischaemic attack
TIPs	transjugular intrahepatic portosystemic shunt
TLCO	transfer factor of the lung for carbon monoxide
TNF	tumour necrosis factor
TOE	trans-oesophageal echocardiography
tPA	tissue plasminogen activator
TSH	thyroid stimulating hormone

TTP	thrombotic thrombocytopenic purpura
U&E	urea and electrolytes
UEC	uterine endometrial carcinoma
U/l	units per litre
UMN	upper motor neuron
USS	ultrasound scan
UTI	urinary tract infection
VEGF	vascular endothelial growth factor
VF	ventricular fibrillation
VGCC	voltage-gated calcium channel antibodies
VGKC	voltage-gated potassium channel antibodies
VGNC	voltage-gated sodium channel antibodies
VGHC	voltage-gated hydrogen channel antibodies
VIP	vasoactive intestinal peptide
VQ	ventilation/perfusion scan
vWf	von Willebrand factor
VZV	varicella zoster virus.
WBC	white blood cell count
WCC	white cell count
WFNS	World Federation of Neurological Surgeons

1. **What is the prevalence of Alport's syndrome?**
   A. 1 in 10000
   B. 1 in 5000
   C. 1 in 2500
   D. 1 in 1000000
   E. 1 in 100000

2. **A 62-year-old man on chronic haemodialysis for the management of end-stage renal failure secondary to polycystic kidneys is seen for review. His current medication include alfacalcidol, simvastatin, lanthanum carbonate, and felodipine. X-ray of his hands shows changes of osteitis fibrosa cystica. His blood tests show: serum calcium 2.6 mmol/l, serum phosphate 1.7 mmol/l, alkaline phosphatase 321 IU/l, PTH 86 pmol/l (normal range 1–9 mmol/l). What is the most appropriate treatment for his hypercalcaemia?**
   A. Stop alfacalcidol
   B. Discontinue lanthanum carbonate
   C. Start cinacalcet
   D. Refer for parathyroidectomy
   E. Increase alfacalcidol

3. **A 63-year-old man sustained a myocardial infarct. Echocardiography showed poor left ventricular function and he was started on perindopril, furosemide in addition to aspirin and simvastatin. His serum creatinine on admission to the coronary care unit was 134 micromol/l. He was seen in follow-up two weeks post discharge as he had felt unwell. Routine blood tests showed a serum creatinine of 356 micromol/l and serum potassium was 5.9 mmol/l. What is the next most appropriate investigation to determine the aetiology of his deteriorating renal function?**
    A. Coronary angiography
    B. Echocardiography
    C. Renal arteriography
    D. Renal ultrasound
    E. Renal biopsy

4. **What is the commonest form of glomerulonephritis in adults worldwide?**
    A. Minimal change nephropathy
    B. Focal segmental glomerosclerosis
    C. Mesangiocapillary glomerulonephritis
    D. IgA nephropathy
    E. Antiglomerular basement membrane disease

5. **A 38-year-old diabetic with type I diabetes (diagnosis at the age of 12) presents with right loin pain and investigations reveal urea 32 mmol/l and serum creatinine 521 micromol/l with a serum potassium of 6.7 mmol/l. She had previously had a left nephrectomy following trauma. She was catheterized and found to be anuric. A plain abdominal X-ray showed no urolithiasis. What is the cause of her renal failure?**
    A. Bladder tumour
    B. Diabetic nephropathy
    C. Papillary necrosis
    D. Renal vein thrombosis
    E. Retroperitoneal fibrosis

6. **You have been asked to see a 43-year-old man because of electrolyte disturbance. He had a past history of multiple sclerosis and suffered from ataxia, numbness of his left leg, and trigeminal neuralgia. Investigations: serum sodium 121 mmol/l, serum potassium 3.7 mmol/l, urea 2.9 mmol/l, serum creatinine 99 micromol/l. What is the cause of his electrolyte disturbance?**
    A. Adrenal insufficiency
    B. Psychogenic polydipsia
    C. Renal tubular acidosis
    D. Salt depletion
    E. Syndrome of inappropriate secretion of antidiuretic hormone

7. **A 32-year-old woman who is being managed by her GP for joint pains and lethargy comes to the renal clinic. On examination she is hypertensive at 165/90 and looks pale. Investigations: haemoglobin 10.2 g/dl (11.5–16.5), white cell count 12.3 x 10⁹/l (4–11), platelets 151 x 10⁹/l (150–400), serum sodium 139 mmol/l (135–146), serum potassium 4.9 mmol/l (3.5–5), creatinine 154 micromol/l (79–118); urine: blood ++, protein +; renal biopsy: positive staining for complement, IgM, and IgG. Which of the following is the most likely diagnosis?**

A. IgA nephropathy

B. Minimal change disease

C. Post streptococcal glomerulonephritis

D. Systemic lupus erythematosis

E. Wegener's granulomatosis

8. **A 35-year-old man presents with hypertension, but is otherwise well. His father died of a cerebral bleed at the age of 46 but his mother is alive and well on no medication. Investigations: urea 12 mmol/l, serum creatinine 231 micromol/l, and haemoglobin 14.4 mg/l. What is the likely cause of his renal impairment and hypertension?**

A. Adult polycystic kidney disease.

B. Focal segmental glomerulosclerosis

C. IgA nephropathy

D. Reflux nephropathy

E. Tuberose sclerosis

9. **A 70-year-old man has multiple medical problems including epilepsy, atrial fibrillation, and left ventricular failure. He is admitted after an acute diarrhoeal illness and has a rapid rise in his creatinine to 220 micromol/l. The protein binding of which of the following drugs is likely to be significantly altered?**

A. Bisoprolol

B. Phenytoin

C. Felodipine

D. Indapamide

E. Atorvastatin

10. You are asked to see a 71-year-old man who has a history of benign prostatic hypertrophy and was admitted 24 hours previously with a urinary tract infection. He also has a history of type 2 diabetes and takes a range of medication including gliclazide, pioglitazone, ramipril, and amlodipine. He is initially treated with gentamycin and you are asked to review his renal status. His BP on examination is 105/63, his pulse is 88 and regular. Investigations: Hb 11.7 g/dl, WCC 14.3 x10^9/l, PLT 232 x10^9/l, Na$^+$ 138 mmol/l, K$^+$ 5.4 mmol/l, creatinine 262 micromol/l (151 some 3 weeks earlier), urinary sodium 7, glucose 10.4 mmol/l, trough gentamicin level 2.6 mg/l. Which of the following is the most likely cause of her renal impairment?

    A. Acute tubular necrosis
    B. Interstitial nephritis
    C. Renal vein thrombosis
    D. Pre-renal failure
    E. Post-renal failure

11. A 75-year-old man has a productive cough with specks of blood in the sputum. Chest X-ray reveals a mass lesion in the L lower zone. Na 110 mmol/l (137–144), K 4.0 mmol/l (3.5–4.9), bicarbonate 24 mmol/l (20–28), U 3.0 mmol/l (2.5–7.5), Cr 80 micromol/l (60–110). Which of the following suggests a diagnosis of syndrome of inappropriate anti-diuretic hormone (SIADH)?

    A. Presence of ascites
    B. Plasma osmolality 236 mOsm/kg (278–305)
    C. Urine flow rate 20 ml/h
    D. Urine osmolality 250 mOsm/kg (350–1000)
    E. Urine sodium 110 mmol/l

12. A 22-year-old man presents to the emergency department complaining of left loin pain. He tells you his GP has recently started investigating him for hypertension and that his father has chronic renal failure. On examination he has obvious bilateral renal masses, pain on the left-hand side to palpation and a raised BP of 155/90. Investigations: haemoglobin 10.9 g/dl (13.5–17.7), white cell count 8.0 x 10^9/l (4–11), platelets 222 x 10^9/l (150–400), serum sodium 142 mmol/l (135–146), serum potassium 4.7 mmol/l (3.5–5), creatinine 139 micromol/l (79–118), urine: haematuria ++. Which of the following is the most likely cause of his pain?

    A. Renal artery embolus
    B. Renal vein thrombosis
    C. Haemorrhage into a renal cyst
    D. Interstitial nephritis
    E. Acute tubular necrosis

13. **A 52-year-old man is receiving cisplatin-based chemotherapy for colonic carcinoma with hepatic metastases. He has begun to feel rather tired and has been suffering from increasing muscle cramps and palpitations. Bloods reveal a mild anaemia with a haemoglobin of 9.9 g/dl, but his routine U&E are normal. Which one of the following deficiencies is most likely to be responsible for his symptoms?**
    A. Magnesium
    B. Sodium
    C. Chloride
    D. Phosphate
    E. Thyroxine

14. **A 33-year-old man who is under investigation by his GP for a chronic cough comes to the clinic for review because he is developing pitting oedema of both lower limbs, he also feels increasingly nauseous. On examination his BP is elevated at 155/92, his pulse is 80 and regular. There are fine crackles on auscultation of the chest, splenomegaly, and bilateral pitting oedema. Investigations: haemoglobin 12.5 g/dl (13.5–17.7), white cell count 9.0 x 10^9/l (4–11), platelets 181 x 10^9/l (150–400), serum sodium 140 mmol/l (135–146), serum potassium 4.6 mmol/l (3.5–5), creatinine 130 micromol/l (79–118), calcium 3.1 mmol/l (2.2–2.6); ultrasound: two normal-sized kidneys; CXR: interstitial fibrosis; 24-hour urinary protein 2.5 g (<300 mg). Which of the following is the most likely cause of his proteinuria?**
    A. Minimal change disease
    B. Membranous nephropathy
    C. Crescenteric glomerulonephritis
    D. Sarcoidosis
    E. Wegener's granulomatosis

15. **A 72-year-old man is admitted to the hospital with acute urinary retention. He has a history of previous inferior myocardial infarction and hypertension but is otherwise well. On examination he has a BP of 155/92, a pulse of 90 regular, and is in some pain. He has a large bladder on palpation of his abdomen and a smoothly enlarged prostate on PR. Investigations: Hb 12.9, WCC 8.9, PLT 203, Na 139, K 5.4, Cr 192. He is catheterized. Which of the following is the most appropriate next step?**
    A. Early transurethral prostatectomy
    B. Initiation of alpha blockade
    C. Initiation of anti-androgen therapy
    D. Removal of catheter after three days
    E. Teaching on managing a permanent catheter

16. **Which one of the following statements is true with respect to renal carcinoma?**
    A. It often presents with haematuria
    B. More than 25% of patients present with the classic triad of haematuria, flank pain, and a palpable abdominal mass
    C. Anaemia is observed in up to 20% of patients at presentation
    D. It is commonly associated with secondary amyloidosis
    E. Patients with von Hippel–Lindau syndrome, tuberous sclerosis or Peutz–Jeghers syndrome are at increased risk of renal cell carcinoma

17. **A patient with hepatitis B develops nephrotic syndrome. He has a renal biopsy, which reports thickening of the glomerular capillary wall, and subepithelial immune complex deposition. Which of the following conditions fits best with this picture?**
    A. Minimal change glomerulonephritis (GN)
    B. Mesangiocapillary GN
    C. Medullary sponge kidney
    D. Membranous GN
    E. IgA nephropathy

18. **You are reviewing a 71-year-old man with CKD stage 5 who has suffered an inferior myocardial infarction. You are reviewing his cardiovascular drugs. His BP is 155/92, his total cholesterol is 7.1. You decide to start additional medication for blood pressure and cholesterol lowering. Which of the following drugs is used at potentially submaximal dose in CKD-5, but need not be avoided completely?**
    A. Atorvastatin
    B. Pravastatin
    C. Simvastatin
    D. Rosuvastatin
    E. Doxasosin

19. **A 62-year-old man with chronic renal failure comes to the clinic for review. He has type 1 diabetes and has been under the management of the renal physicians for the past four years. Current symptoms include nausea and lethargy. On examination his BP is 155/82, pulse is 78 and regular. Chest is clear and abdomen is soft and non-tender. Investigations: Hb 11.0, WCC 7.0, PLT 181, Na 137, K 5.3, Cr 220, Ca 2.25, PO_4 1.9. Which of the following is the most appropriate treatment to reduce his phosphate?**
    A. Sevelamer
    B. Risedronate
    C. Resonium
    D. Cinacalcet
    E. Calcium carbonate

20. When assessing patients with renal stones which of the following abnormalities are regarded as protective against renal stone formation?

A. Hypercalcaemia
B. Hypercalciuria
C. Hyperuricaemia
D. Hypercitraturia
E. Hyperuricosuria

21. A 39-year-old woman who has been treated for heavy proteinuria secondary to idiopathic membranous glomerulonephritis presented with right flank pain and haematuria. The renal function was mildly impaired. While in hospital she developed acute shortness of breath and haemoptysis. The most likely cause of the respiratory complaint is?

A. Pulmonary embolism
B. Primary bronchial carcinoma
C. Idiopathic pulmonary haemosiderosis
D. Pulmonary tuberculosis
E. Staphylococcus pneumonia

22. Struvite kidney stones are invariably associated with urinary tract infections, specifically urease-producing bacteria. Which of the following bacteria is often implicated?

A. *Proteus*
B. *Escherichia coli*
C. *Streptococci*
D. *Enterococci*
E. *Citrobacter*

23. A man has developed end-stage renal failure at the age of 30. He is also found to have sensorineural deafness. The ophthalmologist detected a regular conical protrusion on the anterior aspect of the lens on slit lamp examination. What is the likely diagnosis?

A. Ehler's Danlos syndrome
B. Marfan's syndrome
C. Polycystic kidney disease
D. von Hippel–Lindau syndrome
E. Alport's syndrome

24. **A 47-year-old man with a long-standing history of severe back pain and stiffness presents with ankle swelling. Investigations are: urea 8.8 mmol/l, serum creatinine 143 micromol/l, total protein 47 g/l, albumin 21 g/l, other liver function tests normal. What is the cause of his hypoalbuminaemia?**
   A. Amyloidosis
   B. Coeliac disease
   C. Membranous glomerulonephritis
   D. Myeloma
   E. Protein-losing enteropathy

25. **A man has developed end-stage renal failure at the age of 30. He is also found to have sensorineural deafness. The ophthalmologist detected regular conical protrusion on the anterior aspect of the lens on slit lamp examination. Which type of collagen does the genetic mutation affect?**
   A. Type I
   B. Type II
   C. Type III
   D. Type IV
   E. Type V

26. **A 24-year-old man is seen in the renal clinic for resistant hypertension. He is currently managed with an ACE inhibitor, indapamide, and felodipine. His BP in the clinic is 159/92. There are bilateral ballotable masses on palpation of the abdomen. His creatinine is elevated at 184 micromol/l and there is haematuria ++ on dipstick testing. Which of the following conditions may also be seen in the presence of his renal diagnosis?**
   A. Pancreatitis
   B. Cirrhosis
   C. Diabetes mellitus
   D. Mitral valve prolapse
   E. Aortic regurgitation

27. **A 35-year-old woman with chronic renal failure related to diabetic nephropathy from long-standing type 1 diabetes comes to the clinic for review and possible intervention for her anaemia. A most recent Hb was 9.8 g/dl and creatinine 187 micromol/l. According to NICE guidelines on anaemia management, which of the following is?**
   A. Maintain Hb in the 11–13 range
   B. Consider another cause for anaemia if the GFR is >60 ml/min
   C. Prescribe concomitant vitamin C. for treatment of anaemia
   D. Measure Epo levels as a marker of successful treatment
   E. Blood transfusion is an important option in those who may undergo a renal transplant

28. **A 67-year-old man with known amyloidosis (secondary to ankylosing spondylitis) presents with severe left loin pain. Investigations reveal: urea 15.4 mmol/l, serum creatinine 212 micromol/l, serum albumin 18 g/l. What is the likely cause for his pain?**

    A. Acute pyelitis
    B. Perinephric haematoma
    C. Renal amyloidosis
    D. Renal artery thrombosis
    E. Renal vein thrombosis

29. **A 78-year-old woman is admitted after being found on the floor by her home help. She has apparently been lying there for a number of hours after suffering a stroke. On admission she is drowsy, with obvious evidence of a left-sided hemiparesis. She has bilateral basal crackles on auscultation of the chest. Investigations: Hb 12.3g/dl (11.5–16.0), WCC 12.5 x10⁹/l (4–10), PLT 233 x 10⁹/l (150–400), sodium 142 mmol/l (134–143), potassium 5.9 mmol/l (3.5–5), creatinine 237 micromol/l (60–120), urine blood +++. Chest X-ray reveals some evidence of fluid accumulation, although this is not particularly marked. Which of the following is the best initial way to treat her renal impairment?**

    A. Alkaline diuresis
    B. Furosemide
    C. Normal saline
    D. Haemofiltration
    E. Haemodialysis

30. **A 51-year-old publican with alcoholic liver disease comes to the clinic with a deterioration, suffering from increasing nausea over the past few days. He is currently managed with high-dose propranolol for portal hypertension and spironolactone for ascites. On examination his BP is 100/60, his pulse is 85 and regular. He has extensive ascites and multiple signs consistent with chronic liver disease. Investigations: haemoglobin 10.1 g/dl (13.5–18), white cell count 7.2 x 10⁹/l (4–10), platelets 104 x 10⁹/l (150–400), sodium 141 mmol/l (134–143), potassium 5.3 mmol/l (3.5–5), creatinine 182 micromol/l (60–120). He is catheterized but only passes 80 ml of urine over the course of four hours. Urine sodium is <10 mmol/l. Which of the following is the most likely diagnosis?**

    A. Hepatorenal syndrome
    B. Spontaneous bacterial peritonitis
    C. Acute GI haemorrhage
    D. Acute tubular necrosis
    E. Renal tubular acidosis

31. **A man has developed end-stage renal failure at the age of 30. He is also found to have sensorineural deafness. The ophthalmologist detected regular conical protrusion on the anterior aspect of the lens on slit lamp examination. Which is the commonest form of genetic inheritance for this condition?**
    A. Autosomal dominant
    B. Autosomal recessive
    C. X-linked
    D. Autosomal codominant
    E. Due to sporadic mutations

32. **A 17-year-old girl who works in a children's nursery comes to the emergency room with diarrhoea and increasingly severe lethargy, and nausea and dull abdominal pain. She became unwell a few days earlier and thinks it may have been due to finishing off some beef burgers that were left by the children. On examination her BP is elevated at 155/88. She has a soft abdomen but it is generally tender. Investigations: haemoglobin 9.7 g/dl (11.5–16.5), white cell count 12.2 x 10⁹/l (4–11), platelets 87 x 10⁹/l (150–400), serum sodium 141 mmol/l (135–146), serum potassium 5.7 mmol/l (3.5–5), creatinine 230 micromol/l (79–118), PT 18.2 seconds (12–16). Which of the following measures is most likely to be reduced significantly?**
    A. APTT
    B. Bleeding time
    C. ADAMTS 13
    D. Von Willebrand factor
    E. Complement activity

33. **A 35-year-old man who undergoes regular haemodialysis comes to the clinic very worried as his right forearm dialysis site, partially constructed using a dacron graft, is swollen, erythematous, and painful. On examination his BP is 155/100, his pulse is 80 and regular, but you cannot feel a pulse through the dialysis site and it appears thrombosed. Which of the following is the most appropriate initial therapy?**
    A.   Intravenous unfractionated heparin
    B. Subcutaneous low molecular weight heparin
    C. Locally delivered tPA
    D. Angioplasty
    E. Surgical revision

34. **A 76-year-old man who is known to have CKD 3 presents to the emergency department with severe nausea, vomiting, and diarrhoea after eating a take-away meal. He has not been able to keep food down for the past few days, but has maintained intake of his medications which include ramipril, spironolactone, and indapamide. Investigations reveal a creatinine of 390 micromol/L, a urea of 24 mmol/L and a potassium of 7.6 mmol/L. ECG reveals QRS widening. Which of the following is the most appropriate next intervention?**

    A. IV calcium gluconate
    B. IV salbutamol
    C. IV insulin and dextrose
    D. Oral calcium resonium
    E. IV sodium hydroxide

35. **A 52-year-old man who has a tunnelled catheter for haemodialysis presents to his routine clinic appointment complaining that he has been feeling increasingly unwell with fevers and sweats over the past few days. On examination he is pyrexial 39.2°C. His chest is clear and there are no murmurs on auscultation. Investigations: Hb 10.3 g/dl, WCC 11.9 x10^9/l, PLT 169 x10^9/l, Na$^+$ 141 mmol/l, K$^+$ 5.1 mmol/l, creatinine 730 micromol/l (pre-dialysis), CRP 102 mg/l, urine analysis unremarkable. He may have a line infection. Which of the following organisms is most likely to be responsible?**

    A. *S. aureus*
    B. *S. epidermidis*
    C. *K. pneumoniae*
    D. *P. aeruginosa*
    E. *C. albicans*

36. **A 62-year-old man comes to the clinic for review. He has a history of chronic renal failure related to diabetes mellitus. He takes a number of medications including BD mixed insulin, ramipril, and indapamide. Over the past few months he has been complaining of non-specific bony aches and pains. On examination in the clinic he looks a little pale. His BP is mildly elevated at 155/88. Investigations: haemoglobin 11.0 g/dl (13.5–17.7), white cells 7.1 x 10^9/l (4–11), platelets 190 x 10^9/l (150–400), sodium 140 mmol/l (135–146), potassium 4.3 mmol/l (3.5–5), creatinine 187 micromol/l (79–118), phosphate 1.7 mmol/l (0.8–1.5), calcium 2.1 mmol/l (2.2–2.67), glucose 9.8 mmol/l (<7.0), PTH 2.2 times the upper limit of normal. Which of the following is the most appropriate intervention?**

    A. Calcium tablets
    B. Daily 1-alpha calcidol supplementation
    C. Weekly 1-alpha calcidol supplementation
    D. Cinacalcet
    E. Sevelamer

37. **A 64-year-old woman moves GP, and has some routine blood tests done. They are all normal, apart from calcium which is elevated at 2.84. She is completely well and there are no suspicious signs or symptoms to suggest underlying malignancy. Her bone mineral density is normal, but at the lower end of the range, and PTH is at the upper limit of the normal range. Which of the following is the most appropriate course of action?**

    A. Phosphate supplementation
    B. Calcium and vitamin D therapy.
    C. Neck scan to explore the possibility of hyperparathyroidism
    D. Start hormone replacement therapy
    E. Observe

38. **A 48-year-old man had some blood tests as part of a medical for his life insurance. Corrected calcium was 2.95 mmol/l (2.20–2.60). His doctor therefore added some more blood tests. PTH 1.2 pmol/l (0.9–5.4), serum ACE 30 U/l (25–82), urinary calcium to creatinine clearance ratio <0.01 indicating relative hypocalciuria. Which is the most likely diagnosis?**

    A. Malignancy
    B. Sarcoidosis
    C. Paget's disease
    D. Primary hyperparathyroidism
    E. Familial hypocalciuric hypercalcaemia (FHH)

39. **A 71-year-old man is found unconscious by his home help. He is known to suffer from COPD for which he takes a tiotropium inhaler, and has been unwell for the past few days with a severe cough. On examination in the emergency room he is unconscious. He is pyrexial 37.8°C, his BP is 100/60, and his pulse is 95. There are signs of a right-sided pneumonia. Investigations: haemoglobin 11.6 g/dl (13.5–17.7), white cell count 13.1 x 10^9/l (4–11), platelets 199 x 10^9/l (150–400), serum sodium 112 mmol/l (135–146), serum potassium 3.9 mmol/l (3.5–5), creatinine 99 micromol/l (79–118). He unfortunately suffers a grand mal seizure whilst you are reviewing his investigations. Which of the following is the maximal rise in mmol/l of sodium that you wish to target in the first 24 hours?**

    A. 5 mmol/l
    B. 7 mmol/l
    C. 10 mmol/l
    D. 15 mmol/l
    E. 20 mmol/l

40. **The father of an 18-year-old girl with sensorineural deafness and haematuria comes to the clinic with his new partner. They are keen to start a new family and she wants to know about the risks that he will pass on a defective gene to their new children. He tells you that males are more severely affected than females, and some have even required renal replacement before the age of 30. What is the likely mode of inheritance?**

A. X-linked recessive

B. Autosomal dominant

C. Autosomal recessive

D. X-linked dominant

E. Polysomal

41. **A 32-year old-man with type 1 diabetes and advanced diabetic nephropathy comes to the renal clinic for review. He is taking ramipril, amlodipine, indapamide, and doxazosin for control of blood pressure. It is stable at 115/72, pulse is 72 and regular. HbA1c is stable at 7.2%, creatinine has risen to 350 micromol/L from 320 micromol/L. What would you do next?**

A. Stop his ACE inhibitor

B. Reduce the dose of his ACE inhibitor

C. Keep his BP medication the same

D. Stop his indapamide

E. Arrange an urgent renal USS

42. **A 63-year-old woman with a history of chronic renal failure presents to the emergency room because one of her CAPD exchange bags has become cloudy. In addition she has suffered from dull abdominal pain, nausea, and night sweats over the past two days. On examination her BP is 145/88, her temperature is 37.9 °C., and her abdomen is diffusely tender but soft. Investigations: haemoglobin 11.4 g/dl (11.5–16.5), white cells 14.2 x 10⁹/l (4–11), platelets 201 x 10⁹/l (150–400), sodium 139 mmol/l (135–146), potassium 5.9 mmol/l (3.5–5), creatinine 409 micromol/l (79–118), 200 cells per mm³ on analysis of the peritoneal fluid. Which of the following organisms is most likely to be responsible?**

A. *S. epidermidis*

B. *S. aureus*

C. *S. viridans*

D. *Proteus*

E. *Klebsiella*

43. A 24-year-old woman presents to the emergency department with dysuria and supra-pubic pain over the past 48 hours. She has a previous history of a urinary tract infection some two years earlier, but nil else of note. She has a stable sexual partner. Her only medication is the oral contraceptive pill. On examination her BP is 110/70, pulse is 92 and regular, temperature is 38.0°C. There is supra-pubic tenderness on abdominal palpation. Bloods reveal a white count just above the upper limit of normal with a neutrophilia, and normal urea and electrolytes. Which of the following is the most appropriate treatment?

    A. Oral trimethoprim
    B. Oral amoxycillin
    C. Oral ciprofloxacin
    D. IV ciprofloxacin
    E. IV co-amoxiclav

44. A 40-year-old woman with a history of Crohn's disease presents to the emergency department with left renal colic. This is her second episode over the course of the last three months. She has undergone extensive small bowel resections in four different operations over the past four years and has progressively lost weight. On examination her BP is 155/72, pulse is 85 and regular. She has severe left renal angle tenderness. Her BMI is 18.5. Which of the following is the most likely constituent of any renal stones?

    A. Calcium carbonate
    B. Calcium oxalate
    C. Calcium pyrophosphate
    D. Ammonium magnesium phosphate
    E. Calcium urate

45. A 40-year-old Caucasian man presents with severe acute right-sided flank/loin pain. This is the first time he has ever had such severe pain. He has no past medical history of cardiovascular or renal disease, although the nurse at the GP's has been monitoring his BP for the past few months. His brother died suddenly of a stroke. On examination his blood pressure is 169/92 mmHg, pulse 89 bpm and regular. His JVP is not raised, heart sounds are normal and his chest is clear. His liver is not palpable but he has a right sided mass. The mass is bimanually palpable and you can get above it. Investigations: Na+ 138 mmol/L, K+ 4.1 mmol/L, urea 13.0 mmol/L, creatinine 223 μmol/L, Hb 15.2 g/dL, WCC 4.9 x 10^9/L, MCV 82 fl, platelets 248 x 10^9/L, ESR 12 mm/hr, urine dipstick blood +++, protein +. Which of the following is the most likely diagnosis?

    A. Renal carcinoma
    B. Polycystic kidney disease
    C. IgA nephropathy
    D. Membranous nephritis
    E. Transitional cell carcinoma

46. **What is contained within the fluid found in a standard CAPD bag?**
    A. Amino acids
    B. Icodextrin
    C. Bicarbonate
    D. Dextrose
    E. Lactate

47. **A 58-year-old man who has been using peritoneal dialysis for diabetes-related end-stage renal failure comes to the emergency department with abdominal pain, distension, and a cloudy bag. On examination his temperature is 38.5°C, BP is 110/60 and he looks unwell. His abdomen is distended but soft, and is generally tender. Bowel sounds are quiet but present. You suspect he has CAPD-related peritonitis. Which of the following is the most appropriate empirical antibiotic therapy?**
    A. Vancomycin and gentamicin in combination delivered intraperitoneally
    B. Vancomycin intraperitoneally and oral ciprofloxacin
    C. Oral ciprofloxacin and IV gentamicin
    D. IV vancomycin and oral ciprofloxacin
    E. IV gentamicin and intraperitoneal vancomycin

48. **A 72-year-old woman presents for follow-up after four episodes of uncomplicated urinary tract infection and one of fever, right loin, and supra-pubic pain during the past 18 months. The latter three of these have been identified as *Proteus* infections. A left-sided stag horn calculus is identified on plain abdominal X-ray. Her creatinine is mildly elevated at 142 micromol/l. What is the calculus most likely to be composed of?**
    A. Calcium oxalate
    B. Calcium urate
    C. Calcium carbonate
    D. Cystine
    E. Ammonium magnesium phosphate

49. **A 62-year-old woman with a history of nephrotic syndrome and multiple other medical problems comes to the clinic for review. A recent albumin was measured at 21, and her creatinine was measured at 123. Out of her medication list, use of which of the following is most likely to be associated with toxicity?**
    A. Ramipril
    B. Gliclazide
    C. Phenytoin
    D. Omeprazole
    E. Digoxin

50. **A 27-year-old woman comes to the emergency room with severe nausea and lethargy. She spent the weekend on an outward bound course for her friend's pre-wedding party and as part of that they had to cook food they found in the wild. This included a range of field mushrooms which they picked. She says on the Sunday afternoon she suffered from very severe vomiting, but had recovered. It is now four days later. Her blood pressure is 170/92, and her pulse is 87. Investigations: haemoglobin 11.4 g/dl (11.5–16.5), white cells 8.3 x10⁹/l (4–11), platelets 203 x10⁹/l (150–400), sodium 138 mmol/l (135–146), potassium 6.1 mmol/l (3.5–5), creatinine 715 micromol/l (79–118). Which of the following is the most likely type of mushroom ingested?**

    A. Inocybe
    B. Coprinus
    C. Liberty cap
    D. Cortinarius
    E. Amanita phalloides

51. **A 72-year-old man comes to the emergency department with acute abdominal pain, diarrhoea, and vomiting. He feels this is due to an undercooked roast chicken. He has a past history of lower back pain which his GP has put down to osteoporotic collapse and prescribed non-steroidals for pain relief. On examination his BP is 110/70, his pulse is 90, and he has a postural drop of 20 mmHg. Investigations: haemoglobin 9.0 g/dl (11.5–16.5), white cell count 8.3 x 10⁹/l (4–11), platelets 210 x 10⁹/l (150–400), serum sodium 138 mmol/l (135–146), serum potassium 5.9 mmol/l (3.5–5), creatinine 190 micromol/l (79–118), albumin 24 g/l (35–50), urine protein ++. Which of the following is likely to have provided the most significant contribution to his renal failure?**

    A. Dehydration/pre-renal failure
    B. Acute tubular necrosis
    C. Myeloma kidney
    D. Acute glomerulonephritis.
    E. Membranous nephropathy

52. **A 19-year-old man presents with macroscopic haematuria that has been present for the last three days. He reports having a sore throat for the last week. On further questioning he reveals that a similar episode occurred two years ago but spontaneously resolved. His dipstick is positive for blood and protein. Urine microscopy demonstrates red cell casts. On blood tests his sodium is 136 mmol/l, potassium 4.8 mmol/l, urea 9.2 mmol/l, and creatinine 170 micromol/l. What is the most likely finding on renal biopsy?**

    A. Crescentic glomerulonephritis
    B. Diffuse thickening of the basement membrane
    C. Podocyte process fusion
    D. Mesangial cell proliferation
    E. Focal segmental glomerulosclerosis

53. **A 42-year-old woman returns to the transplant clinic for review some three months after her renal transplant. She is taking a ciclosporin-based regime, and a level pre-clinic is measured at 350, with an upper limit of normal of 300. Her creatinine has deteriorated to 225, from 137 post transplant. Which of the following best describes the mechanism of ciclosporin toxicity?**

    A. MAP kinase inhibition
    B. Increased apoptosis
    C. Renal ischaemia
    D. Calcium channel blockade
    E. Sodium channel blockade

54. **A 50-year-old woman presents to the clinic with lower limb oedema. She has no significant past medical history apart from hypertension which is currently managed with indapamide. On examination BMI is 27, BP is 150/90, she has bilateral pitting odema. Investigations: haemoglobin 12.3 g/dl (11.5–16.5), white cell count 8.1 x 10^9/l (4–11), platelets 232 x 10^9/l (150–400), serum sodium 141 mmol/l (135–146), serum potassium 4.4 mmol/l (3.5–5), creatinine 122 micromol/l (79–118), albumin 24 g/l (35–50), urinary protein 3.5 g/24 h; renal biopsy: consistent with membranous nephropathy. Which of the following is the commonest cause of membranous nephropathy?**

    A. Hepatitis B
    B. Hepatitis C
    C. Occult malignancy
    D. Penicillamine
    E. Idiopathic

55. **A 63-year-old man sustained a myocardial infarct. Echocardiography showed poor left ventricular function and he was started on perindopril, furosemide in addition to aspirin and simvastatin. His serum creatinine on admission to the coronary care unit was 134 micromol/l. He was seen in follow-up two weeks post discharge as he had felt unwell. His pulse was 88 sinus rhythm and blood pressure 142/74 mmHg. Routine blood tests showed a serum creatinine of 451 micromol/l and serum potassium was 5.9 mmol/l.**

    What is the likely cause of his deteriorating renal function?

    A. Drug allergy
    B. Excessive diuretics
    C. Low cardiac output
    D. Poor left ventricular function
    E. Renal artery stenosis

56. A 32-year-woman presents with an erythematous rash and a fever, which has paradoxically worsened after starting a course of amoxycillin for a chest infection. She also has increasing nausea and does not want to eat. On examination her BP is 155/100, her pulse is 79. She has bilateral crackles on auscultation of her chest. Investigations: Hb 10.9, WCC 9.2, eosinophils 0.9 (normal 0.04–0.4), PLT 193, Na 138, K 5.9, Cr 239, urine blood ++, protein +. Which of the following is the most likely diagnosis?

    A. Acute interstitial nephritis
    B. IgA nephropathy
    C. Post streptococcal glomerulonephritis
    D. Membranous nephropathy
    E. Wegener's granulomatosis

57. A 65-year-old woman with known renal impairment is admitted to your ward. Her eGFR according to the Cockroft–Gault equation is 20 ml/min. What stage of chronic kidney disease does she fall in to?

    A. Stage 1
    B. Stage 2
    C. Stage 3
    D. Stage 4
    E. Stage 5

58. A 19-year-old student complains of right loin pain when he goes out drinking a couple of pints of beer with his friends. The pain settles spontaneously but recurs on each occasion. Investigations reveal: haemoglobin 14.3 g/dl, urea 4.3 mmol/l, serum creatinine 93 micromol/l. Liver function tests are normal. What is the most likely cause of his symptoms?

    A. Pelvi-ureteric junction obstruction
    B. Pyelitis
    C. Reflux nephropathy
    D. Retroperitoneal fibrosis
    E. Urolithiasis

59. A 70-year-old man feels increasingly unwell. He tells you that over the past few weeks he has had worsening bony aches and lethargy. He has chronic renal failure related to diabetes. His bloods reveal a mild anaemia, raised creatinine of 195, calcium of 2.06, and 1+ of proteinuria. Which of the following is the most likely diagnosis?

    A. Osteomalacia
    B. Primary hyperparathyroidism
    C. Secondary hyperparathyroidism
    D. Tertiary hyperparathyroidism
    E. Hypoparathyroidism

60. **A 59-year-old man with a history of type 2 diabetes has undergone angioplasty and stenting for a very large anterior myocardial infarction. He initially appears to recover, but the nurses ask you to see him some 48 hours after admission as his legs have deteriorated with livedo reticularis and a blue discoloration to his toes. His BP is 152/81, his pulse is 90, atrial fibrillation. Investigations: haemoglobin 13.4 g/dl (13.5–17.7), white cells 10.7 x 10⁹/l (4–11), eosinophils 0.94 x 10⁹/l (0.04–0.4), platelets 203 x 10⁹/l (150–400), sodium 141 mmol/l (135–146), potassium 6.1 mmol/l (3.5–5), creatinine 285 micromol/l (79–118). Which of the following is the most likely diagnosis?**

A. Renal artery embolus
B. Renal vein thrombosis
C. Saddle embolus
D. Cholesterol embolus
E. Bilateral deep vein thrombosis

61. **A 67-year-old type 2 diabetic is admitted with an acute anterior myocardial infarct and within eight hours undergoes coronary angiography and angioplasty. His serum creatinine on admission was 143 micromol/l. Two days later, on routine screening, it has risen to 231 micromol/l. What is the most likely cause for the deterioration in renal function?**

A. Contrast nephropathy
B. Dehydration
C. Renal artery stenosis
D. Ischaemic nephropathy
E. Acute interstitial nephritis

62. **A 42-year-old woman presents to the emergency room complaining of haemoptysis (fresh red blood) which she finds very distressing indeed. She has been visiting her GP over the last few months to discuss the possibility of plastic surgery because she has had problems with collapse of her nasal bridge. Over the past few days she has also begun to feel increasingly nauseous. On examination her BP is 170/90, her pulse is 88 and regular, she looks short of breath. There are fine crackles on auscultation of the chest. Investigations: Haemoglobin 10.2 g/dl (11.5–16.5), white cell count 11.0 x 10⁹/l (4–11), platelets 178 x 10⁹/l (150–400), serum sodium 139 mmol/l (135–146), serum potassium 5.9 mmol/l (3.5–5), creatinine 320 micromol/l (79–118), cANCA positive; renal biopsy: crescenteric glomerulonephritis. Which of the following is the worst prognostic indicator?**

A. Female sex
B. cANCA positivity
C. High percentage of crescents on renal biopsy
D. Nasal septum symptoms
E. Pulmonary haemorrhage

63. **A 45-year-old man comes to the emergency department with severe tiredness, lethargy, and nausea. He has seen his GP once over the past year to ask for a referral for plastic surgery to his nose as he felt that the shape had changed significantly. Most recently he has become short of breath even walking up the stairs in his house and developed a cough with haemoptysis. His BP is 165/92 and there are bilateral inspiratory crackles. Blood testing reveals mild anaemia, a raised creatinine of 240 micromol/l, raised ESR of 85. Urine is positive to both blood and protein. Which of the following is the most likely diagnosis?**
    A. Churg Strauss syndrome
    B. Wegener's granulomatosis
    C. Membranous nephropathy
    D. Minimal change nephropathy
    E. Alport's syndrome

64. **A 37-year-old man with chronic kidney disease is seen in the A&E department with acute shortness of breath. He has been on chronic ambulatory peritoneal dialysis for two years for the management of end-stage renal failure secondary to Goodpasture's disease. His medication includes perindopril, sevelamer, and alfacaldiol. His chest X-ray shows pulmonary oedema. What is the most appropriate management of this patient?**
    A. Acute haemodialysis
    B. Dopamine
    C. High-dose intravenous diuretics
    D. Isosorbide nitrate infusion
    E. Peritoneal dialysis with icodextrin +/—4.5% glucose dialysate

65. **A 62-year-old man with a history of smoking and hypertension is admitted to the emergency department with central crushing chest pain which is found to be an NSTEMI. His baseline creatinine is 115. Which of the following has been shown to impact on the risk of contrast induced nephropathy in this population?**
    A. Metformin
    B. Rosuvastatin
    C. Fenofibrate
    D. Gelofusin
    E. Ramipril

66. **A 35-year-old man with type 1 diabetes comes to the clinic for review. He is managed with a basal bolus insulin regime and his HbA1c during the past few years has averaged 8.5%. He is currently taking ramipril 10 mg daily and his BP is 110/70. Investigations: haemoglobin 13.8 g/dl (13.5–17.7), white cell count 8.8 x 10⁹/l (4–11), platelets 231 x 10⁹/l (150–400), serum sodium 140 mmol/l (135–146), serum potassium 4.3 mmol/l (3.5–5), creatinine 138 micromol/l (79–118), urinary albumin 310 mg/day (<30).**

    Which of the following is with respect to his renal disease?

    A. Progression to end-stage renal failure is inevitable

    B. He is at increased risk of ischaemic cardiovascular disease

    C. This degree of proteinuria is likely to result in pitting oedema

    D. Diltiazem has no effect on proteinuria

    E. Glitazones are known to accelerate renal disease

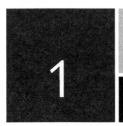

NEPHROLOGY

ANSWERS

1. B. 1 in 5000

Alport's syndrome is an important condition to know for MRCP Part 1. It is the commonest form of hereditary glomerulopathy. Prevalence is 1 in 5000. Type 4 collagen mutation is responsible for this syndrome.

Longmore M et al., *Oxford Handbook of Clinical Medicine*, Eighth Edition, Oxford University Press, 2010, Chapter 7, Renal medicine, Inherited kidney diseases.

2. D. Refer for parathyroidectomy

This patient is not on any calcium-containing phosphate binders (often calcium carbonate is used as first-line therapy for this indication). Newer, non-calcium-containing phosphate binders include sevelamer and lanthanum carbonate. Prevention of severe secondary/tertiary hyperparathyroidism is achieved by adequate (and often early prescription to patients in stage 3–4 chronic kidney disease) alfacacidol therapy. However, in this individual such therapy has been ineffective in trying to reverse his hyperparathyroidism and therefore total parathyroidectomy (in some countries subtotal parathyroidectomy is advocated with removal of 3.5 parathyroid glands) is the treatment of choice if medically fit. Cinacalcet, in the light of its cost, is reserved for those deemed unfit for surgery.

Levy J et al., *Oxford Handbook of Dialysis*, Third Edition, Oxford University Press, 2009, Chapter 10, Complications of ESKD: bone mineral disorders.

3. D. Renal ultrasound

To determine if the deterioration in renal function is due to renal artery stenosis, non-invasive investigations should be undertaken first. An ultrasound (combined, if possible, with Doppler flow studies) may identify disparity in size of the kidneys, hinting about the possibility of shrinkage of the kidney due to renal artery stenosis on one side and therefore possible early stenosis on the opposite side.

Provan D, *Oxford Handbook of Clinical and Laboratory Investigation*, Third Edition, Oxford University Press, 2010, Chapter 10, Renal medicine, Renal imaging.

4. D. IgA nephropathy

IgA nephropathy is the commonest form of glomerulonephritis and is found in approximately 30% of renal biopsies for primary glomerular disorders. It characteristically presents in young adult males with recurrent episodes of macroscopic haematuria which accompany a pharyngitis. IgA nephropathy may occur with systemic manifestations of arthritis, palpable purpura, and gastrointestinal symptoms such as Henoch–Schonlein purpura.

Warrell DA et al., *Oxford Textbook of Medicine*, Fifth Edition, Oxford University Press, 2010, Section 21.8.1, Immunoglobulin A nephropathy and Henoch–Schönlein purpura.

5. C. Papillary necrosis

The presence of anuria makes a urological cause more likely than a renal cause for acute renal failure. Most patients with the other listed conditions will be passing urine. Whilst obstruction from a bladder tumour or a uroepithelial tumour in the ureter may cause anuria, it is unlikely at the age of 38. Long-standing diabetes with microvascular disease may affect those parts of the body without anastamotic arterial supply (e.g. femoral head and renal papilla). The ischaemic papilla may drop off and obstruct the ureter. Diagnosis would be obtained in the first instance by ultrasound showing hydronephrosis. Whilst there is a possibility of acute renal failure secondary to a non-opaque renal stone, the long history of diabetes makes papillary necrosis more likely. Papillary necrosis may also complicate sickle cell disease and phenacetin abuse.

Warrell DA et al., *Oxford Textbook of Medicine*, Fifth Edition, Oxford University Press, 2010, Section 21.17, Urinary tract obstruction.

6. E. Syndrome of inappropriate secretion of antidiuretic hormone

SIADH is most commonly caused by drugs which include chemotherapy (vincristine, vinblastine, and cisplatin), chloropramide, psychiatric drugs, thiazide diuretics, and proton-pump inhibitors. In addition, carbamazepine, one of the most used drugs for trigeminal neuralgia, may also cause SIADH. Whilst the patient might have been taking steroids for his condition, the electrolytes for adrenal insufficiency would have shown an elevated potassium and urea. The low urea is also characteristic due to a dilutional effect. The elevated vasopressin results in inappropriately concentrated urine, dilute plasma, and hyponatraemia with ongoing renal sodium excretion.

Turner H, Wass J, *Oxford Handbook of Endocrinology and Diabetes*, Second Edition, Oxford University Press, 2009, Part 2, Pituitary, Syndrome of inappropriate ADH (SIADH), Definition.

7. D. Systemic lupus erythematosis

This woman's history of joint pains and lethargy is very supportive of an underlying diagnosis of SLE. Whilst we are not given the autoimmune profile, we are given the staining on renal biopsy, and staining for IgG, IgM, and complement is usual in lupus. Disease severity can vary from mild mesangial hypercellularity to focal necrotizing glomerulonephritis. In other systemic vasculitides there is not usually significant immunoglobulin deposition. IgA nephropathy characteristically presents within 24–48 hours of a respiratory tract infection; post-streptococcal glomerulonephritis within two weeks of an episode of streptococcal pharyngitis. Minimal change disease presents with nephrotic syndrome, most commonly in children.

Rahman A, Isenberg MDN, Systemic lupus erythematosus, *England Journal of Medicine* 2008;358:929–939. http://www.nejm.org/doi/pdf/10.1056/NEJMra071297

8. A. Adult polycystic kidney disease

The younger the patient the more likely there may be a secondary cause for hypertension. The presence of renal impairment, together with the family history of a cerebral bleed in the patient's father at the age of 46 (perhaps before significant renal impairment had caused any symptoms), secondary to a subarachnoid haemorrhage, makes adult polycystic kidney (APKD) disease likely. APKD is inherited as an autosomal dominant condition. Of patients with APKD 5–10% may have cerebral aneurysms, a higher percentage in those with a family history of such aneurysms.

Bradley-Smith G et al., *Oxford Handbook of Genetics*, Oxford University Press, 2009, Chapter 5, Common genetic conditions, Autosomal dominant polycystic kidney disease (ADPKD).

9. B. Phenytoin

Acidic drugs undergo significantly reduced protein binding in patients with renal failure. Examples of acidic drugs include digoxin and phenytoin. What this means is that in a patient with renal failure, whilst levels of these drugs may be measured in the normal range, the increase in the unbound fraction can lead to toxicity. Even dose omission can often not prevent toxicity, due to steady state being reached over many days.

Vanholder R et al., Drug protein binding in chronic renal failure: evaluation of nine drugs, *Kidney International* 1988;33(5):996–1004.

10. D. Pre-renal failure

Given that he is under follow-up for his prostatic hypertrophy, post-renal failure is less likely than pre-renal failure. The low urinary sodium and relative hypotension also fit better with pre-renal failure. It is likely that relatively decreased fluid intake and low blood pressure associated with Gram-negative urinary sepsis have precipitated his rise in creatinine. Management is with careful fluid replacement, and omission of the ACE inhibitor and monitoring of his blood pressure. A higher degree of urinary sodium would suggest acute tubular necrosis. Whilst in the toxic range, gentamycin is unlikely to result in a significant creatinine rise after only 24 hours of therapy.

emc+, Gentamicin 40 mg/ml injection, last updated March 2016. http://www.medicines.org.uk/EMC/history/21665/SPC/Gentamicin+40+mg+ml+Injection

11. E. Urine sodium 110 mmol/l

Serum osmolality associated with hyponatraemia is generally low and so would not in itself suggest SIADH. However, in the context of the low plasma osmolality, a high urine osmolality (2* that of the plasma osmolality) with an elevated urine sodium (above 20 mmol/l) is suggestive of this diagnosis.

Longmore M et al., *Oxford Handbook of Clinical Medicine*, Eighth Edition, Oxford University Press, 2010, Chapter 15, Clinical Chemistry, Hyponatraemia

12. C. Haemorrhage into a renal cyst

Hypertension at the age of 22, possible inherited renal impairment, and bilateral renal masses raise the likelihood that this patient has autosomal dominant polycystic kidney disease (ADPKD). ADPKD is associated with the formation of renal cysts, and a common presentation is with loin pain due to haemorrhage into a cyst. Hepatic cysts occur in 50–90% of patients, but pancreatic cysts are much rarer, occuring in 5–10% of patients. There is of course also an association with berry aneurysm formation. Mitral valve prolapse and aortic incompetence are other recognized associations. Ninety percent is due to a mutation on chromosome 16, the other 10% due to a mutation on chromosome 4.

Badani KK et al., Autosomal dominant polycystic kidney disease and pain—a review of the disease from aetiology, evaluation, past surgical treatment options to current practice, *Journal of Postgraduate Medicine* 2004;50:222–226.

13. A. Magnesium

Magnesium deficiency is well recognized to be associated with platinum-based chemotherapeutic regimens. Cisplatin results in both loss from the GI tract due to diarrhoea and vomiting, and loss from renal tubular damage. Oral magnesium glucuronate preparations exist, and chloride or sulphate magnesium salts can be given intravenously. Very rapid infusion for severe palpitations/cardiac compromise should be given under ECG monitoring.

emc+, Cisplatin 1 mg/ml Sterile Concentrate, last updated January 2016. http://www.medicines.org.uk/EMC/medicine/623/SPC/Cisplatin+1+mg+ml+Sterile+Concentrate/

14. D. Sarcoidosis

In this man, the evidence of pulmonary fibrosis and splenomegaly coupled with hypercalcaemia is intended to drive you towards a diagnosis of sarcoidosis. Granulomatous disease of the kidneys is quite rare, but where it occurs it tends to be associated with proteinuria. The relative preservation of renal function, and the fact that we are not told about the presence of haematuria, counts against underlying nephritis. Thankfully, renal sarcoidosis usually responds well to corticosteroid therapy.

Hilderson I et al., Treatment of renal sarcoidosis: is there a guideline? Overview of the different treatment options, *Nephrology Dialysis Transplantation* 2014;10:1841–1847. doi: 10.1093/ndt/gft442.

15. B. Initiation of alpha blockade

Increasingly now, where acute urinary retention is related to benign prostatic hypertrophy as in this case, patients are given a trial without catheter a few days after initiation of alpha-blocker therapy. Control of voiding is restored in 23–40% of cases and surgery can then be planned for a later date if required. An unfavourable outcome can usually be identified by residual volume post voiding, and limited response to initial alpha-blocker therapy. Although the prostate appeared benign on rectal examination, a prostatic specific antigen should be performed to exclude malignancy and, if significantly raised, consideration should be given to transrectal prostatic biopsy under ultrasound control. Whilst his renal impairment might be blamed on his age and hypertension, an ultrasound of his kidneys to exclude some degree of hydronephrosis would also be appropriate.

Callaghan C et al., *Emergencies in Clinical Surgery*, Oxford University Press, 2008, Chapter 15, Urology, Acute urinary retention.

16. A. It often presents with haematuria

Haematuria, due to tumour invasion of the collecting system, remains a common presenting symptom of renal cell carcinoma, occurring in up to 40% of patients. Anaemia is also frequently observed at presentation (50–80% of cases), with symptoms often predating the diagnosis of renal malignancy by many months. Less than 10% of patients present with the 'classic' triad of haematuria, flank pain, and a palpable abdominal mass. With increased use of imaging techniques for other indications, a significant proportion of renal cell carcinomas are identified incidentally (around 30%) and these patients have a markedly better prognosis. Although secondary amyloidosis has been observed in patients with renal cell carcinoma this appears restricted to less than 5% of patients. Von Hippel–Lindau is an autosomal dominant disease due to mutation of the VHL gene on chromosome 3. Around two-thirds of patients develop clear cell renal cancers, usually after the age of 20. Although most renal lesions observed in tuberous sclerosis are benign, these patients are also at greater risk of renal cell carcinomas. There is no evidence that Peutz–Jeghers syndrome is associated with an increased risk of renal cell carcinoma. Males are at increased risk of testicular cancer (hormonally active Sertoli cell tumours), whilst females demonstrate a greater incidence of gynaecological cancers, including breast, ovarian, and cervical. Both sexes are at increased risk of gastrointestinal malignancies.

Verine J et al., Hereditary renal cancer syndromes: an update of a systematic review, *European Urology* 2010;58(5):701–710.

17. D. Membranous GN

Membranous GN is associated with infections such as hepatitis B, as well as some medications and autoimmune diseases. The typical biopsy results are described in the question, and it usually presents with nephrotic syndrome. Minimal change is normal on light microscopy and shows podocyte fusion on electron microscopy. It usually presents with nephrotic syndrome. Mesangiocapillary GN condition often presents with nephrotic syndrome, but can cause nephritic syndrome. On biopsy, there is mesangial proliferation and thickened capillary walls. Immune deposition can be subendothelial or intramembranous. Medullary sponge kidney is a birth defect where cysts are present in the renal medulla. IgA nephropathy usually presents with haematuria. Biopsy shows mesangial proliferation, and IgA deposition is seen on immunofluorescence.

Longmore M et al., *Oxford Handbook of Clinical Medicine*, Eighth Edition, Oxford University Press, 2010, Chapter 7, Renal medicine, Glomerulonephritis.

18. C. Simvastatin

Simvastatin should be used at no more than 10 mg/24 hours in patients with CKD stage 5. With respect to rosuvastatin, it should be avoided in CKD-5. Atorvastatin can be used at normal doses as can pravastatin. Doxasosin is a popular anti-hypertensive in the treatment of hypertension and renal impairment, and can be used across the normal dose range. Some positive data do, however, exist for the combination of simvastatin and ezetimibe, with respect to the combined MACE endpoint used in the SHARP study. Whilst the datasheet for simvastatin does suggest dose reduction to 10 mg, other data suggest that doses up to 20 mg may be safe in CKD-5.

Levy J et al., *Oxford Handbook of Dialysis*, Third Edition, Oxford University Press, 2009, Chapter 17, Drug prescribing in patients on dialysis, Dosing of cardiovascular drugs.

19. A. Sevelamer

This patient has hyperphosphataemia as a result of chronic renal failure. It is unlikely that a low phosphate diet would reduce his phosphate to target. As such, the treatment of choice would be a phosphate binder such as sevelamer. Nausea, diarrhoea, flatulence, and constipation are the commonest side effects.

emc+, Renagel 800 mg film-coated tablets, last updated February 2016. http://www.medicines.org.uk/emc/medicine/18014

20. D. Hypercitraturia

Increased citrate is a protective factor for calcium stones. An increased intake of citrate is recommended for prophylaxis in many patients with calcium stones. Most kidney stones are calcium oxalate stones. Calcium oxalate urinary stones may be associated with any one of several causes of hypercalcaemia, which could also lead to hypercalciuria. Some patients with calcium stones may have associated hyperuricosuria as a cause of their stone. Between 10% and 20% of patients with gout may have kidney stones containing uric acid, calcium oxalate, or phosphate, or a combination. Hypercalciuria is the cause of at least 50% of all kidney stones. Patients with calcium oxalate stones and normal urinary calcium should be investigated for hyperuricaemia.

Micali S et al., Medical therapy of urolithiasis, *Journal of Endourology* 2006;20(11):841–847.

21. A. Pulmonary embolism

The recent onset of shortness of breath and haemoptysis in a patient with nephrotic syndrome should immediately alert the physician to the possibility of pulmonary embolism. This could be preceded by features of renal vein thrombosis such as flank pain, haematuria, and renal impairment. Patients with nephrotic syndrome are at increased risk for thromboembolic events. The loss of antithrombin III and plasminogen in the urine, along with the simultaneous increase in clotting factors, especially factors I, VII, VIII, and X, increases the risk for venous thrombosis. The most common sites of thrombosis in adults are in the deep veins of the lower limb. Thrombosis can also occur in the renal veins and can cause pulmonary embolism. Membranous nephropathy is particularly associated with venous thrombosis and the risk of venous thrombosis is higher when serum albumin is <20–25 g/l. Other items listed in the question are primary pulmonary disorders, and respiratory symptoms are often present at the outset.

Hoyer PF et al., Thromboembolic complications in children with nephrotic syndrome. Risk and incidence, *Acta Paediatrica Scandinavica* 1986;75(5):804–810.

22. A. *Proteus*

Magnesium ammonium phosphate and calcium carbonate apatite are the principal constituents of struvite stones. Struvite stone formation can occur only when ammonia production is increased and the urine pH is elevated. This occurs with upper urinary tract infections with urease-producing organisms such as *Proteus* species. Urease-producing bacteria, including *Ureaplasma urealyticum* and *Proteus* species (most common), *Staphylococcus* species, *Klebsiella* species, *Providencia* species, and *Pseudomonas* species, lead to the hydrolysis of urea into ammonium and hydroxyl ions. *Escherichia coli* does not produce urease and is not associated with struvite stone formation. Other common bacteria that have not been shown to produce urea include *Citrobacter freundii*, *Enterococci*, and *Streptococci*.

Griffith DP, Osborne CA, Infection (urease) stones, *Mineral and Electrolyte Metabolism* 1987;13(4):278–285.

23. E. Alport's syndrome

Anterior lenticonus is a regular conical protrusion on the anterior aspect of the lens due to thinning of the lens capsule. It occurs in 20–30% of males with X-linked Alport syndrome and is pathognomonic of the disease.

Longmore M et al., *Oxford Handbook of Clinical Medicine*, Eighth Edition, Oxford University Press, 2010, Chapter 7, Renal medicine, Inherited kidney diseases.

24. A. Amyloidosis

Amyloidosis formerly complicated chronic infection (chronic osteomyelitis and chronic empyema), but these chronic infections are rarely seen nowadays. The more common causes are chronic inflammation including chronic rheumatoid arthritis, ankylosing spondylitis, Crohn's disease, and psoriatic arthropathy. The hypoalbuminaemia is secondary to renal involvement with nephrotic syndrome (hypoalbuminaemia, 24-hour urinary protein excretion greater than 3 g, dependent oedema, and hyperlipidaemia). There is associated mild renal impairment.

Warrell DA et al., *Oxford Textbook of Medicine*, Fifth Edition, Oxford University Press, 2010, Section 12.12.3, Amyloidosis.

25. D. Type IV

Alport's syndrome is an important condition to know for MRCP Part 1. It is the commonest form of hereditary glomerulopathy. Prevalence is 1 in 5000. Type IV collagen mutation is responsible for this syndrome.

Longmore M et al., *Oxford Handbook of Clinical Medicine*, Eighth Edition, Oxford University Press, 2010, Chapter 7, Renal medicine, Inherited kidney diseases.

26. D. Mitral valve prolapse

This patient has autosomal dominant polycystic kidney disease, ADPKD. ADPKD is associated with hepatic as well as renal cysts; pancreatic cysts occur very much more rarely. There is no association between ADPKD and the development of diabetes or cirrhosis. Only very rarely is the risk of acute pancreatitis increased. Renal stones are increased, with the greatest increase being in urate rather than other stones. With respect to valvular disorders, mitral valve prolapse is the commonest abnormality seen.

Longmore M et al., *Oxford Handbook of Clinical Medicine*, Ninth Edition, Oxford University Press, 2014, Chapter 7, Renal medicine.

27. B. Consider another cause for anaemia if the GFR is >60 ml/min

NICE guidelines recommend considering another cause for anaemia if GFR is >60 ml/min. They also recommend replacing iron first if ferritin is below 100. Once iron is replaced, then Epo preparations can be used, aiming for a target range of haemoglobin of 10–12 g/dl. Concomitant vitamin C or androgens should not be used in an attempt to stimulate haemoglobin, and there is no value in monitoring Epo levels.

NICE Clinical Knowledge Summaries, Anaemia: iron deficiency, February 2013. http://cks.nice.org.uk/anaemia-iron-deficiency

NICE guidelines [CG114], Anaemia management in people with chronic kidney disease, February 2011. https://www.nice.org.uk/guidance/cg114

28. E. Renal vein thrombosis

Amyloidosis formerly complicated chronic infection (chronic osteomyelitis and chronic empyema), but these chronic infections are rarely seen nowadays. The more common causes are chronic inflammation including chronic rheumatoid arthritis, ankylosing spondylitis, Crohn's disease, and psoriatic arthropathy. Renal vein thrombosis may complicate nephritic syndrome, most commonly seen in association with membranous glomerulonephritis.

Warrell DA et al., *Oxford Textbook of Medicine*, Fifth Edition, Oxford University Press, 2010, Section 21.4, Clinical investigation of renal disease.

29. A. Alkaline diuresis

This patient in all likelihood has significant rhabdomyolysis. The positive blood to dipstick on urine testing is consistent with myoglobinuria. Initial treatment of choice is alkaline diuresis, either with 1.26% bicarbonate given peripherally or 8.4% given centrally. Fluid balance is often a problem in the elderly, and as such CVP monitoring is recommended. Patients may well require haemodialysis, although complete recovery of renal function after the acute event is usual.

Ramrakha P et al., *Oxford Handbook of Acute Medicine*, Third Edition, Oxford University Press, 2010, Chapter 4, Renal emergencies.

30. A. Hepatorenal syndrome

Acute renal impairment in the absence of renal pathology in a patient with chronic liver disease is consistent with hepatorenal syndrome. It may develop acutely, or have an insidious onset in patients with refractory ascites. Other causes of renal failure, such as hypovolaemia, GI haemorrhage, and acute sepsis, should be excluded first. A volume challenge with Hartmann's +/− 20% human albumin solution is the initial therapy of choice. Terlipressin is also added; the combination of terlipressin and albumin is thought to lead to resolution of hepatorenal syndrome in about 40% of cases.

Ramrakha P et al., *Oxford Handbook of Acute Medicine*, Third Edition, Oxford University Press, 2010, Chapter 4, Renal emergencies.

31. C. X-linked

X-linked transmission accounts for approximately 80% of affected patients and arises from mutations in the COL4A5 gene on the X chromosome. The autosomal recessive variant accounts for about 15% of patients with Alport syndrome and arises from genetic defects in either the COL4A3 or COL4A4 genes. Autosomal dominant disease accounts for 5% of patients with Alport syndrome and arises from heterozygous mutations in the COL4A3 or COL4A4 genes.

Longmore M et al., *Oxford Handbook of Clinical Medicine*, Eighth Edition, Oxford University Press, 2010, Chapter 7, Renal medicine, Inherited kidney diseases.

32. C. ADAMTS 13

It had long been recognized that inherited forms of TTP appeared to be related to a deficiency of ADAMTS 13, also known as Von Willebrand cleaving factor. Deficiency of ADAMTS 13 is thought to have a key role in the development and continuation of the microangiopathic haemolytic anaemia seen in TTP. Whilst platelet count may be reduced, PT and APTT are only slightly outside the normal range. This patient's role in the nursery is likely to have exposed her to *E. coli* 157, the pathogen recognized as the commonest cause of HUS/TTP. Antibiotics and corticosteroids are thought to have no place in the management of the condition, but plasma exchange or FFP may both remove/dilute antibodies to ADAMTS 13, and replenish active ADAMTS 13.

Michael M et al., Interventions for haemolytic uraemic syndrome and thrombotic thrombocytopenic pupura, *Cochrane Database of Systematic Reviews* 2009;(1):CD003595.

33. C. Locally delivered tPA

Thrombus can also be removed using thrombolytic agents (tissue plasminogen activator (tPA), alteplase, or streptokinase, usually combined with heparin) instilled locally. tPA is used at 0.5–2 mg, and subsequent 0.5 mg aliquots. Standard or pulse spray catheters can be used. Infusion is often continued for several hours. Therapy is usually not successful if patients present more than 48 hours after the onset of thrombosis. Catheters can be used to mechanically disrupt the thrombus as an alternative. The construct should, however, be investigated for any areas of stenosis which may have precipitated the formation of thrombus. An alternative approach to locally delivered tPA is surgical thrombectomy, where available, as this may allow correction of any anatomical abnormality at the same time.

Levy J et al., *Oxford Handbook of Dialysis*, Third Edition, Oxford University Press, Chapter 2, Haemodialysis, Thrombosis of fistulae and grafts.

34. A. IV calcium gluconate

This patient is at imminent risk of cardiac arrest and therefore the first priority is IV calcium gluconate. The reason for giving calcium gluconate initially and immediately is that it stabilizes the cardiac cell membranes, reducing the risk of arrhythmia. This can be followed by insulin and dextrose IV, which essentially 'buys time' whilst the cause of renal failure/hyperkalaemia determined and definitive therapy is instituted. Repeated salbutamol nebulizers may also be useful in driving K+ into the intracellular space. Calcium resonium is less useful in the acute situation as it will not significantly reduce potassium until at least 2–3 doses have been given.

Ramrakha P et al., *Oxford Handbook of Acute Medicine*, Third Edition, Oxford University Press, 2010, Chapter 4, Renal emergencies.

35. B. *S. epidermidis*

S. epidermidis is one of the commonest causes of line infection in dialysis patients. Given the fact his urine is normal and his chest is clear, this is the most likely cause of the patient's fevers. Vancomycin, rifampicin, gentamicin, and linezolid are all potential anti-bacterial agents. The line should be removed as colonization is virtually impossible to eradicate, and therapy is needed for at least six weeks.

Levy J et al., *Oxford Handbook of Dialysis*, Third Edition, Oxford University Press, 2009, Chapter 2, Haemodialysis, Management of access (catheter) infections.

36. C. Weekly 1-alpha calcidol supplementation

This patient has mild hyperphosphataemia, low calcium, and raised PTH. As such he fits the criteria for vitamin D supplementation. Standard supplementation is with weekly vitamin D. As the measured phosphate is also above the upper limit of normal, he should be encouraged to follow a low phosphate diet if possible, reducing his intake of dairy products and eggs. Treatment of renal bone disease is only initiated after PTH has breached twice the upper limit of normal, because of the risk of inducing adynamic bone disease. If addition of vitamin D leads to a rise in serum phosphate, the addition of phosphate binders to his medication list may be required.

Longmore M et al., *Oxford Handbook of Clinical Medicine*, Ninth Edition, Oxford University Press, 2014, Chapter 7, Renal medicine.

37. E. Observe

This woman in all probability has hyperparathyroidism. Indications for parathyroidectomy include calcium levels above 3 mmol/l, renal stone formation, reduced bone mineral density and fracture, acute episodes of hypercalcaemia, or impaired renal function. This patient should be observed with six-monthly calcium, renal function, and physical examination including blood pressure. She should have a repeat BMD every 2–3 years. If she progresses to surgery, it is crucial that parathyroidectomy is performed by an experienced surgeon who does more than 20 parathyroidectomies per year.

Guidelines on management of hyperparathyroidism, *Journal of Clinical Endocrinology & Metabolism* 2009;94(2):335–339. http://www.ncbi.nlm.nih.gov/pubmed/19193908?dopt=Abstract

38. E. Familial hypocalciuric hypercalcaemia (FHH)

The man is asymptomatic and well. His PTH is at the lower end of the normal range and serum ACE is well within the normal limits indicating that he does not have primary hyperparathyroidism or sarcoidosis. In hyperparathyroidism the PTH is either elevated or at the upper end of the normal range. There is reduced excretion of calcium as shown by the reduced urinary calcium to creatinine ratio. This is a feature of benign FHH. In this condition, there is a defect in the calcium-sensing receptor (a G-protein embedded in the plasma membrane). No treatment is required for the hypercalcaemia. Rarely patients are seen who suffer from recurrent pancreatitis.

Longmore M et al., *Oxford Handbook of Clinical Medicine*, Eighth Edition, Oxford University Press, 2010, Chapter 15, Clinical Chemistry, Hypercalcaemia

39. C. 10 mmol/l

A rise in sodium greater than 10 mmol/l over the first 24 hours runs the risk of central pontine myelolysis. If the patient is unconscious with seizures, as here, then sodium replacement with hypertonic (3%) saline may be considered. The increase in serum sodium in response to 1 litre of 3% saline can be calculated using the following equation: 513—[serum Na?]/(total body water + 1). Total body water is calculated as weight x 0.6 for males and weight x 0.5 for females. Three precent saline is usually delivered at 50–60 ml/h for the first few hours; then the rate of delivery is slowed significantly, to a maximum of around 30 ml/h.

Ramrakha P et al., *Oxford Handbook of Acute Medicine*, Third Edition, Oxford University Press, 2010, Chapter 4, Renal emergencies.

40. D. X-linked dominant

X-linked Alport's (the diagnosis here) presents with hearing loss and haematuria in females, but with more severe symptoms in males due to the fact they only carry one X chromosome. This leads to the need for renal replacement therapy in many cases. Ocular lens abnormalities also occur, with retinopathy characterized by a dot and fleck appearance.

Collier J et al., *Oxford Handbook of Clinical Specialties*, Eighth Edition, Oxford University Press, 2009, Chapter 10, Unusual eponymous syndromes.

41. C. Keep his BP medication the same

It is a common misconception that, as creatinine rises in diabetic nephropathy, ACE inhibition should be discontinued. On the contrary, it is still effective with respect to renoprotection at this stage, and in the presence of controlled BP, it should be continued. Of course, it is a rapid rise in creatinine associated with ACE inhibitor initiation which is of most concern as it may signify renovascular disease.

Turner H, Wass J, *Oxford Handbook of Endocrinology and Diabetes*, Third Edition, Oxford University Press, 2014, Chapter 13, Diabetes.

42. A. *S. epidermidis*

S. epidermidis is the commonest cause of CAPD-related peritonitis, and as such the majority of treatment protocols involve instillation of vancomycin into the CAPD fluid. A quinolone or cephalosporin is usually added to the regime. Treatment is continued for a period of 10–14 days. Up to 10–20% of patients may unfortunately require catheter removal, and repeated peritonitis may result in peritoneal adhesions and a decrease in the efficiency of peritoneal dialysis over the longer term.

McLatchie G et al., *Oxford Handbook of Clinical Surgery*, Third Edition, Oxford University Press, 2007, Chapter 7, Upper gastrointestinal surgery, Acute peritonitis.

43. A. Oral trimethoprim

This patient has an uncomplicated urinary tract infection. As such guidelines recommend oral trimethoprim as first-line therapy. There is significant *E. coli* resistance to amoxycillin; this is therefore no longer recommended as treatment. In patients who are penicillin allergic, nitrofurantoin, or cephalexin are appropriate options. Where fluoroquinolone resistance is low, oral quinolones may remain an option for uncomplicated pyelonephritis.

SIGN guidelines on the management of UTI, A national clinical guideline. Updated July 2012. http://www.sign.ac.uk/pdf/sign88.pdf

44. B. Calcium oxalate

Short bowel syndrome is a recognized consequence of extensive small bowel resection for inflammatory bowel disease or ischaemic bowel. In short bowel syndrome, there is increased delivery of free oxalate to the colon, where it is readily absorbed. This increases the risk of calcium oxalate stone formation because of raised urinary oxalate excretion. In total, calcium containing renal stones represent approximately 80% of the total, 10–15% are ammonium magnesium phosphate, and 5–10% are uric acid stones. Limitation of oxalate consumption, such as by reducing consumption of chocolate, tea, nuts, rhubarb, and strawberries may reduce the risk of stone formation.

Reynard J et al., *The Oxford Specialist Handbook of Urological Surgery*, Oxford University Press, 2008, Chapter 6, Stone disease.

45. B. Polycystic kidney disease

There are clues from the history, examination, and investigation findings which support a diagnosis of polycystic kidney disease. Hypertension and a history of sudden death due to stroke in the family are pointers, as is the right-sided renal mass. It is likely that the patient has undergone haemorrhage into a cyst, which has led to the pain and haematuria. The renal impairment also supports the diagnosis. The normal ESR counts against either cancer or an inflammatory disorder. An ultrasound of the abdomen would be adequate to confirm the diagnosis, with control of hypertension, primarily via ACE inhibition, the most important aim of therapy.

Longmore M et al., *Oxford Handbook of Clinical Medicine*, Ninth Edition, Oxford University Press, 2014, Chapter 7, Renal medicine.

46. D. Dextrose

Standard dialysis fluid contains dextrose, the most commonly used concentrations being 1.36% and 2.27% dextrose. The fluid works as a method of dialysis because an osmotic gradient is set up between the blood and the fluid in the bag. The major adverse metabolic effect of concern is the extra calorie load afforded by the dextrose, a particular problem in patients with diabetes mellitus. Out of the other options both icodextrin and bicarbonate have advantages versus dextrose dialysis solution, but this comes at significantly greater cost.

Levy J et al., *Oxford Handbook of Dialysis*, Fourth Edition, Oxford University Press, 2016.

47. A. Vancomycin and gentamicin in combination delivered intraperitoneally

Intraperitoneal vancomycin and gentamicin are generally recommended as initial therapy of choice in dialysis-related bacterial peritonitis. The regime can then be tailored once the causative organism has been identified. Causative organisms and typical regimens for treatment are outlined as follows:

Staphlycoccus epidermidis: Stop gentamicin, continue vancomycin for 14 days according to levels.

Staphlycoccus aureus: Stop gentamicin. Continue vancomycin according to levels, consider adding rifampicin 300mg bd orally (discuss with microbiologists). Aim for 21 days therapy in total.

Enterococcus spp: Continue gentamicin 0.6mg/kg IP daily (according to levels), add amoxicillin 125mg/l to each exchange. Patient needs to inject these themselves just before use. If patient unable to inject own bags, further treatment should be vancomycin alone. Total duration of therapy 14 days.

Culture negative: Continue vancomycin according to levels, stop gentamicin. Start ciprofloxacin 500mg bd orally. Total duration of therapy 14 days.

Gram-negative rod: Continue gentamicin 0.6mg/kg IP daily (according to levels). Total duration of therapy 14 days.

Pseudomonas spp: Continue gentamicin (according to levels) AND discuss with microbiologists to choose appropriate second agent. Consider catheter removal. Total duration of therapy 21 days.

Fungal: ADMIT TO HOSPITAL. Flucytosine loading dose 50mg/kg orally in four divided doses and then 500mg bd (monitor blood levels) AND fluconazole, 200mg orally or IP daily. If no improvement by day 3, remove catheter. If improving continue antifungal treatment (with low threshold for catheter removal). Total duration of therapy 4–6 weeks or seven days after catheter removal.

Levy J et al., *Oxford Handbook of Dialysis*, Fourth Edition, Oxford University Press, 2016, Chapter 4, Peritoneal dialysis.

48. E. Ammonium magnesium phosphate

Proteus infection drives formation of ammonium magnesium phosphate (struvite) crystals and calcium phosphate. These do not permit complete clearance of *Proteus* infection, and lead to a vicious cycle of repeated infection and further crystal formation. Oxalate crystals are found in patients with short bowel syndrome and in those who consume large amounts of dietary oxalate (e.g. rhubarb). Urate stones are associated with gout. Cystinuria is autsomal recessive, it drives increased urinary cystine excretion and hence stone formation.

Reynard J et al., *Oxford Handbook of Urology*, Third Edition, Oxford University Press, 2013, Chapter 9, Stone disease.

49. C. Phenytoin

Nephrotic syndrome impacts most significantly on drugs which are protein bound. Out of those listed, phenytoin is highly protein bound, hence a decrease in plasma proteins leads to an increase in free phenytoin and potentially increases the risk of toxicity. Acute renal failure and a fall in pH also increase the percentage of free phenytoin and can lead to symptoms of toxicity at 'therapeutic' phenytoin levels. For all of the other options listed, protein binding does not significantly impact on their metabolism.

Steddon S et al., *Oxford Handbook of Nephrology and Hypertension*, Oxford University Press, Second Edition, 2014, Chapter 12, Drugs and the kidney.

50. E. Amanita phalloides

Amanita phalloides or death cap is a source of severe poisoning in response to mushroom ingestion. It cause severe vomiting and diarrhoea which recovers during the initial period, but is followed around three days later by further nausea, lethargy, and acute renal failure. Cortinarius is also associated with acute renal failure, but initial symptoms are much milder. Liberty cap is a type of mushroom commonly used in magic mushroom preparations.

West PL, *Amanita smithiana* mushroom ingestion: a case of delayed renal failure and literature review *Toxicology Reviews, Journal of Medical Toxicology* 2009:5:32–38. http://www.springerlink.com/content/v67835h11116w913/

51. C. Myeloma kidney

The clues here include the chronic back pain, low serum albumin, and proteinuria. The combination of the three is highly suggestive of an underlying diagnosis of myeloma. Myeloma can lead to light chain deposition within the kidney/amyloidosis. Of course, a portion of the creatinine of 190, given the patient's postural drop, may be related to hypovolaemia because of his acute gastrointestinal illness. Chronic renal failure due to myeloma is usually not reversible to any great extent, but treatment of the underlying myeloma may slow further elevation in the creatinine.

Dimopoulos MA et al., Pathogenesis and treatment of renal failure in multiple myeloma, *Leukemia* 2008;22:1485–1493; doi:10.1038/leu.2008.131; published online 5 June 2008. http://www.nature.com/leu/journal/v22/n8/full/leu2008131a.html

52. D. Mesangial cell proliferation

The case described is a classical presentation of IgA nephropathy, also known as IgA nephritis or Berger's disease. The term synpharyngitic nephritis is sometimes used to refer to the onset of haematuria and sore throat virtually simultaneously, as in this case. In post-streptococcal glomerulonephritis the onset of renal disease is usually some time (weeks) after the upper respiratory illness. Mesangial widening, inflammation, and mesangial cell proliferation are common features on renal biopsy in IgA nephropathy. Granular IgA deposits on immunofluorescence are the hallmark of the disease and give it its name. IgA nephropathy may occasionally present as a crescentic glomerulonephritis. In such cases renal function is unlikely to be even relatively preserved as in this case. Crescentic changes are more often associated with ANCA-positive vasculitides or anti-GBM disease. Diffuse membrane thickening is found in membranous glomerulonephritis, podocyte fusion in minimal change disease, and focal segmental glomerulosclerosis is found in the disease of the same name.

Longmore M et al., *Oxford Handbook of Clinical Medicine*, Eighth Edition, Oxford University Press, 2010, Chapter 7, Renal medicine, Glomerulonephritis.

53. C. Renal ischaemia

Ciclosporin leads to renal artery vasospasm when administered at toxic levels, and the subsequent renal ischaemia leads to elevated creatinine. Monitoring of ciclosporin levels is very important, particularly during the first six months after transplant when increased levels of immunosuppression are required, to differentiate between rejection and ciclosporin toxicity. A reduction in ciclosporin dose leads to a rapid resolution of renal ischaemia and an improvement in creatinine. Co-administration with other substrates of CYP 450 3A4 may lead to toxicity, and care should be taken to avoid drugs such as statins or antibiotics metabolized through this pathway where possible.

emc+, Neoral Soft Gelatin Capsules, last updated March 2016. http://www.medicines.org.uk/EMC/medicine/1307/SPC/Neoral+Soft+Gelatin+Capsules%2c+Neoral+Oral+Solution/

54. E. Idiopathic

Occult malignancy, gold or penicillamine therapy, infections including hepatitis B and C, and SLE are all causes of membranous nephropathy. Seventy percent of cases are said to be idiopathic, but often a detailed medical history may reveal an inflammatory disorder related to development of the condition. Unfortunately, membranous nephropathy is poorly responsive to therapy with corticosteroids. Limited results suggest a benefit from corticosteroids and chlorambucil in combination, especially in patients with a creatinine of less than 170 micromol/l at the time of diagnosis. Limited evidence suggests a possible benefit from the anti-CD20 agent rituximab, but further studies are awaited.

Mansur A, Membranous glomerulonephritis, *Medscape*, January 2014. http://emedicine.medscape.com/article/239799-overview

55. E. Renal artery stenosis

A patient with ischaemic heart disease has, by definition, generalized arteriosclerosis, and therefore a high index of suspicion regarding the possibility of renal artery stenosis needs to be borne in mind. Indeed a significant number of patients undergoing coronary angiography are found to have some degree of renal artery disease: in one series (Leandri et al., J Radiol 2004;85:627–638) 9% of patients with normal kidney function and 32.5% of patients with mild renal insufficiency had renal artery stenosis. As a result of ACE inhibitors, both afferent and efferent arterioles are dilated (unlike other antihypertensive drugs when only the afferent arterioles are dilated) with a consequent drop in glomerular pressure which, when combined with the drop in arterial pressure distal to the stenosis of the renal artery, results in further reduction in glomerular pressure and consequent acute renal failure.

Warrell DA et al., *Oxford Textbook of Medicine*, Fifth Edition, Oxford University Press, 2010, Section 21.4, Clinical investigation of renal disease.

56. A. Acute interstitial nephritis

The clue here is the proximity to a recent course of antibiotic therapy and the presence of a marked eosinophilia. Taken together with the acute renal impairment and blood and proteinuria, acute interstitial nephritis is the most likely cause. Management involves cessation of antibiotic therapy, and recovery usually occurs over subsequent days. Unfortunately up to 30% of patients may require short-term renal replacement therapy.

Longmore M et al., *Oxford Handbook of Clinical Medicine*, Eighth Edition, Oxford University Press, 2010, Chapter 7, Renal medicine, Inherited kidney diseases.

57. D. Stage 4

The eGFR is used to estimate kidney function. It takes into account the serum creatinine as well as some patient characteristics such as age and gender. As renal function declines, the GFR decreases. The eGFR is therefore often used to classify chronic kidney disease as follows: eGFR greater than 90 ml/min, with some sign of kidney damage on other tests = CKD stage 1 (if all kidney tests are normal, there is no CKD). eGFT 60–90 ml/min with some sign of kidney damage = CKD stage 2 (if all the kidney tests are normal, there is no CKD). eGFR 30–59 ml/min = CKD stage 3, a moderate reduction in kidney function. eGFR 15–29 ml/min = CKD stage 4, a severe reduction in kidney function. eGFR less than 15 ml/min = CKD stage 5, established kidney failure. At this stage, renal replacement therapy (dialysis or transplantion) may be considered. With an eGFR of 20, this woman falls into the category of CKD stage 4. It is important to know this classification system as it is often used to define a patient's renal function. It is also useful to think about how severe the impairment is and whether it may be necessary to consider renal replacement therapy.

UK National Kidney Federation website. http://www.kidney.org.uk

58. A. Pelvi-ureteric junction obstruction

This is a typical scenario in which an increased load on the kidneys as manifested by a few pints of beer results in an inability to achieve a diuresis in the presence of a functional disturbance of the pelvi-ureteric junction peristalsis. Diagnosis is confirmed by furosemide renography. An Anderson–Hynes pyeloplasty, first described in 1949, will relieve the obstruction. If the diagnosis is delayed, renal function may deteriorate and subsequent hydronephrosis may occur and then a nephrectomy may be required.

Warrell DA et al., *Oxford Textbook of Medicine*, Fifth Edition, Oxford University Press, 2010, Section 21.17, Urinary tract obstruction.

59. C. Secondary hyperparathyroidism

The picture of mild hypocalcaemia, coupled with chronic renal failure and bone pain is typical of secondary hyperparathyroidism which occurs due to a decrease in levels of 1,25-OH vitamin D. In an effort to preserve calcium levels, parathyroid hormone production is then elevated. The threshold for treatment, however, is taken to be PTH levels of twice normal; this is to avoid the risk of adynamic bone disease which is significantly elevated in this population.

Longmore M et al., *Oxford Handbook of Clinical Medicine*, Eighth Edition, Oxford University Press, 2010, Chapter 7, Renal medicine, Inherited kidney diseases.

60. D. Cholesterol embolus

Cholesterol emboli are associated with arterial instrumentation, and are recognized to occur after coronary artery instrumentation when access occurs via the femoral artery. Fragments from cholesterol plaques are dislodged and then travel distally. The blue discoloration of the toes and livedo reticularis fit well with the diagnosis. Management is supportive, but unfortunately no therapies are known to definitively impact on renal function.

Kronzon I, Saric M, Cholesterol embolization syndrome, *Circulation* 2010;122:631–641.

61. A. Contrast nephropthy

The risk of contrast nephropathy is increasingly being recognized as a cause for acute renal impairment. Debate continues about the best way to prevent it. Patients undergoing such procedures, deemed at risk because of pre-existing renal impairment, are advised to be well hydrated. However, the use of intravenous fluids, especially bicarbonate, as well as acetyl cysteine, remains controversial.

Ramrakha PS et al., *Oxford Handbook of Acute Medicine*, Third Edition, Oxford University Press, 2010, Chapter 4, Renal emergencies, Contrast nephropathy.

62. E. Pulmonary haemorrhage

The symptoms given here, with renal failure and c-ANCA positivity, raise the possibility of Wegener's granulomatosis. Out of those factors given, pulmonary haemorrhage is the one which most closely indicates a poor prognosis. c-ANCA itself is not related to poor prognosis. With respect to renal function, early presentation is crucial; the percentage of crescents seen on biopsy does not necessarily impact negatively on prognosis if treatment with steroids and cyclophosphamide are instigated early enough. The response to therapy after two weeks does, however, link closely to long-term prognosis.

Schilder AM, Wegener's granulomatosis vasculitis and granuloma, *Autoimmunity Reviews* 2010;9:483–487.

63. B. Wegener's granulomatosis

The central mucosal involvement leading to collapse of the nasal bridge is typical of Wegener's granulomatosis. The diagnosis is supported by the evidence of pulmonary haemorrhage and renal vasculitis (blood and protein in the urine). Wegener's is associated with cANCA positivity, and renal biopsy is usually employed to obtain a tissue diagnosis. Steroids and cyclophosphamide are the mainstay of therapy, with early presentation crucial with respect to achieving a good prognosis.

Chapman S et al., *Oxford Handbook of Respiratory Medicine*, Third Edition, Oxford University Press, 2014.

64. E. Peritoneal dialysis with icodextrin +/–4.5% glucose dialysate

The patient is 'fluid overloaded' due to inadequate removal of fluid by dialysis. Intravenous diuretics, even furosemide 250 mg, are ineffective in established end-stage renal disease in patients on dialysis, although often wrongly prescribed. Fluid needs to be removed and rather than inflict central line catheterization and haemodialysis on this individual, fluid can be removed with high-glucose-containing fluid or icodextrin with frequent exhanges on peritoneal dialysis, resulting in ultrafiltration and consequent removal of the excess fluids and relief of the symptoms.

Harrison J et al., *Oxford Handbook of Key Clinical Evidence*, Oxford University Press, 2009, Chapter 16, Renal medicine.

65. B. Rosuvastatin

The PRATO-ACS examined the effect of high-dose rosuvastatin versus placebo on risk of contrast induced nephropathy in patients presenting with NSTEMI. Results revealed a significantly lower incidence of contrast-induced nephropathy in the rosuvastatin group compared with the placebo group (6.7% versus 15.1%; adjusted OR = 0.38; 95% CI, 0.2–0.71). This finding persisted after application of different criteria for acute kidney injury and in higher-risk patients, such as those with baseline estimated creatinine clearance <60 mL per minute (adjusted OR = 0.36; 95% CI, 0.15–0.87); in those who had a high-risk clinical profile (adjusted OR = 0.44; 95% CI, 0.23–0.86); and in those who underwent PCI (adjusted OR = 0.41; 95% CI, 0.19–0.89). The researchers also noted a significantly lower 30-day incidence of major adverse clinical events in the rosuvastatin group, as compared with the control group (3.6% versus 7.9%; P = 0.036). Metformin is actually thought to increase the risk of contrast nephropathy, and there is no positive evidence to support the use of gelofusin, fenofibrate or ramipril in this situation.

Tropeano F et al., Impact of rosuvastatin in contrast-induced acute kidney injury in the elderly: post hoc analysis of the PRATO-ACS tTrial, *Journal of Cardiovascular Pharmacology and Therapeutics* 2016;21(2):159–166.

66. B. He is at increased risk of ischaemic cardiovascular disease

This man has albuminuria, but not at the level which is likely to result in significant peripheral pitting oedema. Apart from ACE inhibitors and ARBS, one small trial of non-dihydropyridine calcium antagonists did suggest an impact on the degree of proteinuria. Apart from increased risk of progression of renal disease, the endothelial damage suggested by albuminuria is also associated with increased risk of ischaemic cardiovascular disease. For this reason patients with albuminuria are managed to a tight HbA1c target, a BP target of 120 mmHg systolic, and with other cardiovascular risk reduction agents such as statins.

NICE Guidance [CG15], Type 1 diabetes: diagnosis and management of type 1 diabetes in children, young people and adults, July 2004. https://www.nice.org.uk/guidance/cg15

1. **A 27-year-old healthy woman presents with headache, neck stiffness, photophobia, and vomiting. Cerebrospinal fluid analysis shows white cells at 600 (99% lymphocytes), protein 1.5 g/l, and glucose 4.8 mmol/l; Herpes simplex virus-2 (HSV-2) antibodies were detected. This type of meningitis:**
   A. Is a complication of primary genital herpes
   B. Has a mortality rate of 50%
   C. Recurrence after complete recovery is extremely rare
   D. Convulsions are distinctive features
   E. Vaccination would offer protection in 85% of cases

2. **A 68-year-old woman with a history of type 2 diabetes comes to the emergency department after returning home from a holiday in Spain. She has a history of type 2 diabetes for which she takes metformin and sulphonylurea, her glucose is relatively well controlled with an HbA1c of 7.2%, and she smokes 20 cigarettes per day. She tells you she was admitted to hospital in Spain with a TIA. Current other medication includes aspirin 75 mg which pre-dated the TIA, ramipril, and atorvastatin. Her BP in the clinic is 144/81. Which of the following is the most appropriate additional therapy to reduce her stroke risk?**
   A. Amlodipine
   B. Clopidogrel
   C. Warfarin
   D. Ezetimibe
   E. Dipyridamole MR

3. A 45-year-old man comes to the neurology clinic complaining of muscle weakness. He has been finding it increasingly difficult with respect to walking over the past few months and finds that he has been tripping over his feet. In particular he tells you that he has problems with washing his hair, getting out of a chair, and climbing the stairs. On examination his BP is 112/75, his pulse is 70 and regular. His BMI is 22. There is bilateral lower limb spasticity and foot drop. You also notice proximal shoulder weakness and fasciculation on examination of his tongue. There is no sensory loss. Which of the following is the most likely diagnosis?

    A. Motor neuron disease
    B. Hereditary spastic paraplegia
    C. Charcot–Marie–Tooth
    D. Hereditary mixed motor and sensory neuropathy
    E. Metabolic myopathy

4. A 62-year-old man is referred to the clinic with possible Parkinson's disease. His wife has noticed that he has become increasingly slow to mobilize over the past few months and has developed a tremor. He has also given up handwriting and asks her to write letters to friends on his behalf now. On examination his BP is 130/70, pulse 70, and there are no significant postural changes. There is obvious cogwheel rigidity and a pill-rolling tremor worse on the left than the right. Investigations: Hb 13.1, WCC 8.1, PLT 203, Na 138, K 4.3, Cr 102, CT head—normal. Which of the following is the most appropriate initial therapy?

    A. Entacepone
    B. Selegiline
    C. Benzhexol
    D. Apomorphine
    E. Ropinirole

5. A 33-year-old woman is referred because of recent onset headache and double vision. Neurological examination shows abducted right eye looking down and absent light reflex in the right pupil. What is the most likely diagnosis?

    A. Right third nerve palsy due to diabetes mellitus
    B. Posterior communicating artery aneurysm
    C. Myasthenia gravis
    D. Multiple sclerosis
    E. Progressive external ophthalmoplegia

6. A 22-year-old woman is brought to the emergency department by her
    boyfriend. She has suffered the worst headache of her life, vomiting,
    and blurred vision for the past 48 hours. Past history of note includes
    a left leg DVT after a flight from Australia, and her only medication is
    the combined oral contraceptive pill. On examination she is drowsy, her
    BP is elevated at 155/80, and she has bilateral papilloedema and severe
    photophobia. Investigations: Hb 12.3, WCC 9.1, PLT 187, Na 137, K 4.3,
    Cr 100; CT head unremarkable; lumbar puncture—raised opening
    pressure (22 cm H$_2$O). Which of the following is the most likely diagnosis?

    A. Inferior petrosal sinus thrombosis
    B. Cavernous sinus thrombosis
    C. Transverse sinus thrombosis
    D. Sigmoid sinus thrombosis
    E. Sagittal sinus thrombosis

7. A 32-year-old woman presents with diplopia, ptosis, and numbness over
    the left half of her forehead, which came on gradually over three days.
    She is in good health generally, but recently had a dental abscess treated
    by her dentist. Examination of eye movements reveals ophthalmoplegia
    suggestive of a palsy of the left third and fourth cranial nerves. There is
    miosis and complete ptosis of the left eye. The most likely diagnosis is:

    A. Cavernous sinus thrombosis
    B. Tolosa–Hunt syndrome
    C. Pontine tumour
    D. Neurosarcoidosis
    E. Carotid artery aneurysm

8. A 32-year-old man presents with a severe holocranial headache,
    associated with photophobia, vomiting, neck stiffness, iritis, and fever,
    which came on over the course of yesterday afternoon. There are no
    focal neurological deficits on examination. There are no petechiae or
    purpura, although there are acneiform papules over his chest and back,
    and two herpetiform oral lesions. This is his fourth episode in the past
    six months, each time with very similar symptoms. On his last admission
    three weeks ago he had a normal MRI head and routine bloods, except
    for a CRP of 48. An HIV test and ANA were negative. A lumbar
    puncture showed: CSF wcc 5 (all lymphocytes), rcc 10, protein 0.66 g/dl,
    glucose 3.4 mmol/l (serum 5.7), xanthochromia negative, bacterial
    cultures negative, viral PCR negative. His past medical history includes
    diabetes type I and childhood meningitis. The most likely diagnosis is:

    A. Behçet's disease
    B. Syphilis meningitis
    C. Migraine
    D. Systemic lupus erythematosis
    E. TB meningitis

9. **An 82-year-old right-handed man with a past medical history of hypertension and hypercholesterolaemia presents to hospital with a right-sided weakness after being found slumped in bed by his carers. Upon arrival to hospital he was unable to answer any questions but could follow commands. He is noted to have a dense right-sided hemiparaesis (MRC grade 2/5) alongside a right-sided visual defect although direct visual confrontational assessment is difficult. What would be the classification of this man's stroke?**
   A. Partial anterior circulation stroke
   B. Total anterior circulation stroke
   C. Lacunar stroke
   D. Posterior circulation stroke
   E. Lateral medullary syndrome

10. **A 73-year-old man comes to the clinic with his wife. He has suffered three grand mal seizures with incontinence of urine over the past four months, but each time refused to go to hospital. He has a history of vascular disease with two previous myocardial infarctions and a stroke three years ago that has left him with spastic weakness of his left arm. In the clinic he looks well, his BP is 141/83, his pulse is 74 and regular. Investigations reveal a raised creatinine of 153 micromol/l, but his other bloods are unremarkable, as is his ECG. Which of the following is the optimal next step?**
   A. CT head
   B. Start sodium valproate
   C. Carotid ultrasound
   D. Echocardiogram
   E. EEG

11. **A 17-year-old boy comes to the neurology clinic. He complains of persistent fatigue and numbness in his feet. He tells you that his mother told him not to worry about it as she too has tired legs but is just able to 'get on with it'. On examination there is bilateral weakness of ankle dorsi and plantar flexion. There is also bilateral forearm weakness. Reflexes are depressed bilaterally, there is bilateral pes cavus, and sensory loss over a glove and stocking distribution. Which of the following is the most likely diagnosis?**
   A. HMSN-1
   B. HMSN-2
   C. HMSN-X
   D. Distal spinal muscular atrophy
   E. Friedrich's ataxia

12. **A 64-year-old woman with a past medical history of hypertension and angina presents to hospital with an acute-onset headache whilst she was driving which was maximal within seconds of onset. She often gets headaches but this was more severe than her usual headaches. She did not lose consciousness at the onset of the headache and had suffered from no focal weakness. She managed to get home and found that the lights at home made her headache worse, following which she suffered from several vomiting episodes. She has also noted that her neck has become stiff and she is no longer able to touch her chin on her chest. She is on several antihypertensive medications and smokes 25 cigarettes per day and consumes 21 units of alcohol per week. She has been otherwise well prior to her presentation. What is her most likely diagnosis?**
    A. Alcohol withdrawal
    B. Subarachnoid haemorrhage
    C. Infective meningitis
    D. Intracerebral haemorrhage
    E. Tension headache

13. **An 80-year-old woman, who is otherwise well, is found to have asymptomatic atrial fibrillation. You are asked to advise her regarding warfarin treatment. Roughly what is her annual risk of stroke if she is untreated?**
    A. 0.1%
    B. 0.3%
    C. 3%
    D. 10%
    E. 30%

14. **An 80-year-old woman with known cerebrovascular disease was admitted to the emergency department having been found by her carers unresponsive in her bed in the morning. Glasgow Coma Score (GCS) was 5/15 with flaccid weakness of her left arm. Baseline blood tests and ECG recording were unremarkable. An acute stroke was suspected and she had an urgent CT head scan which showed an old right parietal infarct with no evidence of haemorrhage. An acute ischaemic stroke was diagnosed and the family was warned that the outlook was poor. She was treated symptomatically and by the following morning her GCS had improved to 14 and she had weakness 4/5 in her left upper limb. Over the ensuing 24 hours, she returned to her baseline function with no discernible motor weakness and independent mobility. What was the most likely cause of her coma and limb paralysis?**
    A. Dementia with Lewy bodies
    B. Stokes–Adams attack
    C. Transient global amnesia
    D. Transient ischaemic attack
    E. Todd's paresis after a convulsion

15. **You see a patient in clinic who says that her mother has von Recklinghousen's disease (Neurofibromatosis type 1, NF1). You know that she is at risk of having inherited this autosomal dominant condition, and examine her for features. Which of these features are not part of the diagnostic criteria?**
    A. First-degree relative with NF1 (who does fulfil the diagnostic criteria)
    B. Six or more cafe-au-lait spo
    C. Inguinal freckling
    D. Two or more neurofibromas
    E. Carcinoid syndrome

16. **Which of the following is regarding malignant spinal cord compression?**
    A. Lung cancer, prostate cancer, and thyroid cancer account for the majority of cases
    B. Painless weakness is characteristic
    C. Only one in four patients with paraplegia due to malignant cord compression will regain the ability to walk following appropriate treatment
    D. It is a medical emergency and treatment should begin within hours of diagnosis
    E. Surgery for spinal cord compression has no role in patients with metastatic cancer

17. **An 82-year-old right-handed man with a past medical history of hypertension and hypercholesterolaemia presented to hospital with a right-sided numbness and immobility after being found by his carers. Upon closer history and examination it became apparent that the patient is also suffering from reduced sensation on the left side of his face alongside a ptosis of his left eye, vertical diplopia, and nystagmus on left lateral gaze. He also has right-sided sensory loss to light touch and pain. There is also some left-sided finger-nose dysmetria. The diagnosis is:**
    A. Basilar artery aneurysm
    B. Multiple sclerosis
    C. Lateral medullary syndrome
    D. Posterior circulation stroke
    E. Miller–Fisher syndrome

18. **A 56-year-old male presents with slurred speech, bilateral facial weakness, difficulty swallowing, and ptosis following a holiday to India when he had bad diarrhoea. The symptoms have been getting worse over a couple of weeks, and now he feels weak all over and needs to rest his chin on his hand in order to lift his head up. Having confirmed a diagnosis of myasthenia with a raised anti-ACh receptor antibody titre, what further investigation should you perform?**
    A. CT chest
    B. MRI head
    C. Barium swallow
    D. Prostate-specific antigen level
    E. CT chest/abdo/pelvis

19. **A 26-year-old right-handed builder was bending over to tie his shoelaces when he collapsed. His wife found him on the floor two hours later with his phone broken in pieces. His speech was slow and effortful with numerous word-finding difficulties. His past medical history includes: fractured tibia and fibula a couple of years ago and appendicitis last year. No family history of note. Non-smoker. His BP was 120/70, ECG showed normal sinus rhythm. Neurological examination revealed right-sided hemiparesis with an expressive dysphasia. What is the most likely diagnosis?**

A. Stroke affecting the right side of his brain
B. Subarachnoid haemorrhage affecting the right side of his brain
C. Subarachnoid haemorrhage affecting the left side of his brain
D. Subdural haematoma affecting the left side of his brain
E. Cryptogenic stroke due to paradoxical embolism

20. **An 83-year-old man presents to the neurology outpatient clinic complaining of pain and imbalance. Upon further questioning it becomes apparent that the pain is like 'lightning', occurs in both legs, and causes his legs to 'spasm'. This had occurred over a long period of time. More recently he has found that he would lose balance easily, particularly at night and with no preceding symptoms. To counter this he has taken to 'stomping' his feet so he can feel where they are going. He also reluctantly admits that he has developed urge incontinence as well. His past medical history includes insulin-controlled type II diabetes mellitus. Upon neurological examination his power is entirely normal but he is noted to have proprioceptive loss to the ankle and lack of vibration sense to the knee. He is Romberg's sign positive. His reflexes are diminished in the lower limbs but normal elsewhere. He is noted to have one pupil larger than the other, which did not react to light. His gait was normal but he was noted to concentrate on his foot placement. The most likely diagnosis is:**

A. Tabes dorsalis
B. Diabetic peripheral neuropathy
C. Chronic inflammatory demyelinating polyneuropathy
D. Hypovitaminosis E
E. Spinocerebellar ataxia

21. **Which onconeural antibody is associated with the following neurological presentation? Mood and sleep disturbance associated with memory loss, frontotemporal deficit in cognition, hallucinations, and seizures. MR imaging reveals high signal in the limbic structures, especially on T2 sequences. Electroencephalogram shows foci of epileptic activity in the temporal lobes and occasionally focal or generalized slowing.**

    A. Anti-Yo antibodies
    B. Anti-voltage-gated potassium antibodies
    C. Anti-voltage-gated calcium channel antibodies
    D. Anti-Hu antibodies
    E. Anti-NMDA receptor antibodies

22. **A 45-year-old man presents with a five-day history of back pain, and progressive parasthesiae and numbness in his legs. The parasthesiae started in his calves and spread up the whole of both legs. It now extends up to the level of his umbilicus. In the past 48 hours he reports weakness in his legs too. He is able to pass urine and open his bowels normally. He had a diarrhoeal illness two weeks ago. On examination he has a sensory level at T6, weakness at his ankles and knees in both legs, absent leg reflexes, flexor plantars, and normal anal tone. The most important investigation to do immediately is:**

    A. Forced vital capacity
    B. MRI of the cervical and thoracic spine
    C. MRI of the head
    D. Lumbar puncture
    E. Nerve conduction studies

23. **Which onconeural antibody is associated with the following neurological presentation? Subacute limb ataxia followed by truncal ataxia associated with dysarthria and dysphagia. Downbeat nystagmus is present on clinical examination. Patients may become hyporeflexic and develop a mild sensory deficit. Emotional lability and memory deficits may also occur.**

    A. Anti-voltage-gated potassium antibodies
    B. Anti-Yo antibodies
    C. Anti-voltage-gated calcium channel antibodies
    D. Anti-Hu antibodies
    E. Anti-NMDA receptor antibodies

24. **A 48-year-old chronic alcohol abuser is admitted with a five-day history of painful and tender lower limb muscles. On getting up in the morning after a heavy night-time alcohol binge and 12 hours' sleep, he found that he could not walk on his own because of marked pain in the muscles of the lower limbs and weakness. There is no history of trauma, convulsions, or coma. Two days later, his urine output decreased and he was brought to the hospital. He admits to passing cola-coloured urine. Neurological examination confirms 3/5 weakness in lower limbs with no sensory or reflex abnormalities. CT scan of the brain was reported as normal. The most likely diagnosis is:**

    A. Guillain–Barré syndrome
    B. Cauda equina lesion
    C. Subdural haematoma
    D. Osteomalacia
    E. Rhabdomyolysis

25. **A 19-year-old woman presents to A&E with a severe headache and meningism that she woke with two days earlier. She admits to a mild headache that has been present intermittently for a month, ever since a bad cold. GCS is 15/15 and there are no focal neurological signs. During your examination she gets focal clonic movements in the right arm and face that develop into a secondary generalized tonic-clonic seizure. An urgent CT head shows a small high signal area surrounded by low signal in the right frontal lobe, and a second low density area in the left temporal lobe. The most likely diagnosis is:**

    A. Dural sinus thrombosis
    B. Subarachnoid haemorrhage
    C. Herpes simplex encephalitis
    D. Subdural haemorrhage
    E. Neurocysticercosis

26. **A 24-year-old woman presents with a two-month history of headaches that are worse in the morning. She denies visual symptoms. She is on the oral contraceptive pill only. She has a BMI of 35 and bilateral mild papilloedema, but the systemic and neurological examination is otherwise normal. CT head is normal. The opening pressure when a lumbar puncture is performed is 40 mm CSF. The most important next management step is:**

    A. MR venography
    B. Goldmann field perimetry
    C. MRI head with contrast to look for a brain tumour
    D. MRI head to look for obstructive hydrocephalus
    E. Repeat lumbar puncture in one month's time to see if the opening pressure is still high

27. **A patient presents to you with foot drop and ulnar nerve palsy. Which of these is the least likely cause?**
    A. Diabetes
    B. Lyme disease
    C. Sarcoidosis
    D. Vasculitis
    E. Alcohol excess

28. **You see a 67-year-old man in outpatients with a six-month history of a rest tremor in the right arm. On examination there is cog-wheel rigidity and bradykinesia of the right arm, and reduced armswing on the right when walking. You suspect he has idiopathic Parkinson's disease. All of the following features of the history or examination might make you concerned that this was not idiopathic Parkinson's disease except:**
    A. Postural drop in blood pressure
    B. Brisk knee jerks
    C. Failure of downgaze that corrects with the doll's head manoeuvre
    D. Postural instability
    E. Anosmia

29. **Regarding late side effects following whole brain radiotherapy which of the following is true?**
    A. Pituitary dysfunction occurs in one in five patients
    B. Infertility is most commonly caused via effects on the frontal lobe
    C. Radiation necrosis typically occurs within 3–6 months following treatment
    D. Cranial irradiation in childhood is usually associated with a significant reduction in verbal I
    E. There is an increased risk of stroke in children.

30. **A 72-year-old presents to a neurology outpatient clinic with a several-month history of reduced mobility, falls, and stiffness. He complains about an inability to roll over in bed and has found it hard to initiate walking. His wife states that once he does start to walk he staggers from side to side much like someone who is drunk. Most worryingly he has started to have falls which would happen without warning and are always backwards. He notices this happens especially when walking up stairs. His wife also notes that his personality has changed slightly, but she had put this down to frustration with his symptoms. She has also noted that he will stare often and barely blink. The patient is not aware of this. Examination is notable for a limitation of downgaze, reduced blinking, and an overactivation of frontalis. The most likely diagnosis is:**
    A. Parkinson's disease
    B. Multiple systems atrophy
    C. Corticobasal degeneration
    D. Progressive supranuclear palsy
    E. Whipple's disease

31. **A 42-year-old man presents with an 18-month history of progressive weakness and wasting of the muscles of the arms and neck. There is no dysphagia, and his legs are not affected. On examination, he is unable to extend his neck, and there is global wasting and weakness of the sternocleidomastoids and trapezii, and throughout both arms. Tendon reflexes are present, plantar responses are flexor, and sensation to light touch appears intact. He is a type I diabetic, and in his childhood had radiotherapy for a Hodgkin's lymphoma. The most likely cause of his weakness is:**

A. Myasthenia

B. Motor neuron disease

C. Brachial neuritis

D. Radiation-induced neuropathy

E. Diabetic amyotrophy

32. **A 74-year-old man is admitted from a residential home with an eight-month history of progressive cognitive decline and falls. He has particular difficulty with his memory and attention. He has a past medical history of well-controlled hypertension, for which he takes bisoprolol 5 mg OD and ramipril 2.5 mg OD, and he was diagnosed recently by his GP with benign prostatic hypertrophy, with symptoms of urinary frequency and urgency. He has a family history of strokes. Examination reveals normal tone and power, but brisk reflexes globally and extensor plantars. His gait is shuffling, with the feet appearing almost glued to the ground as he walks. Romberg's test is negative. His MMSE is 22/30. What would you expect to see on brain imaging?**

A. Enlarged ventricles with cortical atrophy

B. Enlarged ventricles without cortical atrophy

C. Normal ventricles and no atrophy

D. Cortical atrophy with an anterior gradient

E. Cortical atrophy with a posterior gradient

33. **A 27-year-old man is brought to the emergency department having been thrown off his motorbike at approximately 60 miles per hour. He arrives boarded and collared; he is grunting but opens his eyes to painful stimulus. When you attempt to put in the intravenous cannula he pulls his arm away. You try to tell him to keep still but he is unable to comply with your request and you seek assistance from the nursing staff. You next assess his Glasgow coma score (GCS). What score would he get?**

A. 6

B. 7

C. 8

D. 9

E. 10

34. **A 55-year-old woman presents with a six-month history of difficulty walking, and more recently with swallowing. Her husband notes that she has been forgetful, irritable, and prone to unprovoked tearfulness over the past few months. She has also been eating more sweet foods than she would normally. On examination, she has mild weakness of shoulder abduction, grip and hip/knee flexion bilaterally but worse on the left. There are no fasciculations or wasting. Reflexes are brisk throughout, and tone in both arms and legs is increased. Plantar responses are extensor bilaterally. The most likely diagnosis is:**

    A. Amyotrophic lateral sclerosis
    B. Stiff man syndrome
    C. Frontotemporal dementia
    D. Multiple system atrophy
    E. Vascular dementia

35. **A 55-year-old woman presents with a six-month history of difficulty walking, and more recently with swallowing. Her husband notes that she has been forgetful, irritable and prone to unprovoked tearfulness over the past few months. She has also been eating more sweet foods than she would normally. On examination, she has mild weakness of shoulder abduction, grip and hip/knee flexion bilaterally but worse on the left. There are no fasciculations or wasting. Reflexes are brisk throughout, and tone in both arms and legs is increased. Plantar responses are extensor bilaterally. The most helpful diagnostic investigation is likely to be:**

    A. MRI head
    B. MRI spine
    C. Electromyography
    D. CSF analysis
    E. Neuropsychometric evaluation

36. **A 74-year-old man is admitted from a residential home with an eight-month history of progressive cognitive decline and falls. He has particular difficulty with his memory and attention. He has a past medical history of well-controlled hypertension, for which he takes bisoprolol 5 mg OD and ramipril 2.5 mg OD, and he was diagnosed recently by his GP with benign prostatic hypertrophy, with symptoms of urinary frequency and urgency. He has a family history of strokes. Examination reveals normal tone and power, but brisk reflexes globally and extensor plantars. His gait is shuffling, with the feet appearing almost glued to the ground as he walks. Romberg's test is negative. His MMSE is 22/30. What is the most likely diagnosis?**

    A. Normal pressure hydrocephalus
    B. Vascular dementia
    C. Multiple system atrophy
    D. Alzheimer's disease
    E. Prostatic carcinoma with brain metastases

37. **A 74-year-old man is admitted from a residential home with an eight-month history of progressive cognitive decline and falls. He has particular difficulty with his memory and attention. He has a past medical history of well-controlled hypertension, for which he takes bisoprolol 5 mg OD and ramipril 2.5 mg OD, and he was diagnosed recently by his GP with benign prostatic hypertrophy, with symptoms of urinary frequency and urgency. He has a family history of strokes. Examination reveals normal tone and power, but brisk reflexes globally and extensor plantars. His gait is shuffling, with the feet appearing almost glued to the ground as he walks. Romberg's test is negative. His MMSE is 22/30. Which test is most likely to be the most helpful for prognosis?**

    A. Lumbar puncture tap test
    B. MRI head
    C. DAT scan
    D. Postural BPs
    E. PSA

38. **A 22-year-old woman complains of severe headaches. She has had them since her late teens, but over the past year they have become more frequent and now occur most weeks. The headaches are unilateral and throbbing, and associated with nausea, photophobia, and phonophobia. They last up to two days at a time. There is no postural exacerbation. She is on the oral contraceptive pill, and inhalers for her asthma, but is otherwise well. Neurological examination is normal. Routine bloods and MRI head are normal. Which of the following is not a recognized prophylactic for this woman's headache?**

    A. Propranolol
    B. Topiramate
    C. Sumatriptan
    D. Amitriptyline
    E. Pizotifen

39. **A 22-year-old asthmatic woman complains of severe headaches. She has had them since her late teens, but over the past year they have become more frequent and now occur most weeks. The headaches are unilateral and throbbing, and associated with nausea, photophobia, and phonophobia. They last up to two days at a time. There is no postural exacerbation. She is on the oral contraceptive pill, and inhalers for her asthma, but is otherwise well. Neurological examination is normal. Routine bloods and MRI head are normal. Which of the following is the most appropriate treatment for this woman's headache?**

    A. Propranolol
    B. Indomethacin
    C. Topiramate
    D. Pizotifen
    E. Verapamil

40. A 25-year-old woman presents following a second episode of loss of consciousness. She describes a brief rising sensation in her abdomen prior to the loss of consciousness. It is clear from the witness account that she went on to have a generalized tonic-clonic seizure. There is nothing in the history to suggest that this was a provoked seizure. Which anti-convulsant drug should you start her on?

A. Carbamazepine

B. Lamotrigine

C. Sodium valproate

D. Levetiracetam

E. Nothing—she does not need one

41. A 47-year-old woman presents with vertigo, difficulty with her speech and balance, and headache. The headache is sharp and throbbing, over her right occiput, with no associated features. It came on suddenly last night as she was walking home after an evening out. She has a past history of migraine with visual auras, and she has a sister who had breast cancer at the age of 45. Neurological examination reveals dysarthric speech, gaze-evoked nystagmus, and ataxic finger–nose pointing on the right. Her gait is broad-based and ataxic. Tone, power, and reflexes are normal in all four limbs, as is the remainder of the cranial nerve examination. The most likely clinical diagnosis is:

A. Basilar migraine

B. Vertebral artery dissection

C. Breast cancer with cerebellar metastases

D. Atherosclerotic cerebellar stroke

E. Multiple sclerosis

42. A 24-year-old man complains of a constant worsening headache. It is holocranial, dull, and has no associated features. He has suffered with migraines since childhood, which have generally responded well to co-codamol, but now the headache has become constant and does not improve with the co-codamol, despite taking it regularly. He has no other past medical history, and no other medications. Neurological examination is entirely normal. The most likely clinical diagnosis is:

A. Medication overuse headache

B. Obstructive sleep apnoea

C. Intracranial tumour

D. Idiopathic intracranial hypertension

E. Venous sinus thrombosis

43. **A 50-year-old obese man attends outpatients complaining of morning headaches. The headaches are bilateral and frontal. They are not associated with nausea or sensory hypersensitivity. He also thinks that his memory and concentration have deteriorated recently. Neurological examination is normal. His past medical history includes hypertension and type II diabetes, and he smokes a pack of cigarettes each day. The most likely diagnosis is:**

    A. Obstructive sleep apnoea
    B. Venous sinus thrombosis
    C. Intracranial tumour
    D. Idiopathic intracranial hypertension
    E. Migraine

44. **A 32-year-old man presents with a severe holocranial headache, associated with photophobia, vomiting, neck stiffness, iritis, and fever, which came on over the course of yesterday afternoon. There are no focal neurological deficits on examination. There are no petechiae or purpura, although there are acneiform papules over his chest and back, and two herpetiform oral lesions. This is his fourth episode in the past six months, each time with very similar symptoms. On his last admission three weeks ago he had a normal MRI head and routine bloods, except for a CRP of 48. A lumbar puncture showed: CSF wcc 5 (all lymphocytes), rcc 10, protein 0.66 g/dl, glucose 3.4 mmol/l (serum 5.7), xanthochromia negative, bacterial cultures negative, viral PCR negative. His past medical history includes diabetes type I and childhood meningitis. The most likely test to return a positive result is:**

    A. ANA
    B. HIV serology
    C. Pathergy testing
    D. dsDNA
    E. TB culture with CSF

45. **An 86-year-old female is referred to the emergency department after falling out of bed whilst leaning out to switch her bedside light off. She was unable to get herself up and lay on the floor overnight until her carer arrived the next morning. She suffered no loss of consciousness and did not sustain any bone injury. She lives alone with a four-times-a-day care package. Her past medical history includes: lumpectomy for carcinoma left breast (11 years earlier), hypertension (diagnosed five years earlier), and gastro-oesophageal reflux disease (GORD—diagnosed one year earlier). Her medication is letrozole 2.5 mg, atenolol 100 mg, amlodipine 5 mg, simvastatin 40 mg all taken once daily, and gaviscon 10 ml four times a day. Physical examination is normal. Her MMSE is 15/30. Blood pressure is 130/72 mmHg. Heart rate 76 bpm. Investigations: Hb 13.6 g/dl, WBC 8.0 (4–11), PLT 15 (150–400), urea 7.0 mmol/l (2.5–7.0), Na 135 mmol/l (137–144), K 4.5 mmol/l (3.5–4.9), Cr 160 micromol/l (60–110), bilirubin 18 micromol/l (1–22), ALT 25 U/l (5–35), ALP 186 U/l (45–105). Blood glucose 5.6 mmol/l (4–7), ECG normal, CXR normal, CT head scan: diffuse periventricular white matter lucencies, cortical atrophy in keeping with diffuse small vessel ischaemia. Established left frontal infarct. No intra-cranial haemorrhage or space-occupying lesion. What would be the best option in respect of minimizing her risk of future stroke?**

    A. Change amlodipine to perindopril 4 mg OD
    B. Leave her medication unchanged.
    C. Start aspirin 75 mg daily
    D. Start aspirin 75 mg daily and clopidogrel 75 mg daily
    E. Start dipyridamole MR 200 mg twice daily

46. **A 77-year-old woman is referred to the hospital with confusion that has worsened significantly over the past few weeks. This is accompanied by incontinence of urine and a change in her gait to a slow, broad-based shuffling appearance. Clinical examination reveals a BP of 155/82, a regular pulse of 72. There are no heart murmurs and her chest is clear. There is no papilloedema but there is heel–shin ataxia and finger–nose dysmetria on neurological examination. Investigations: Hb 12.9, WCC 6.7, PLT 200, Na 137, K 4.2, Cr 110. CT head: ventricular enlargement. CSF: normal opening pressure and normal constituents. Which of the following is the best predictor of positive outcome in this condition?**

    A. Response to large-volume lumbar puncture
    B. Ventricular size on CT scan
    C. Opening pressure on lumbar puncture
    D. CSF protein
    E. CSF glucose

47. **A right-handed 47-year-old man, with a background of atrial fibrillation (AF), hypertension, and type 1 diabetes, presents with a one-hour history of sudden onset right-sided weakness. On further questioning he volunteers that his only other past medical history was 'a hole in the heart as a child'. Clinical examination confirms a flaccid paralysis of the right arm and leg, right-sided facial weakness, and dysarthria. The most appropriate initial investigation is:**

A. Erythrocyte sedimentation rate (ESR)

B. Transoesphageal echocardiogram (TOE)

C. Finger prick glucose ('BM')

D. Computed tomography (CT) of head

E. International normalized ration (INR)

48. **A 62-year-old man presents with a one-year history of progressive weakness in both hands and difficulty walking. On examination, there is wasting of the intrinsic muscles of the hands on both sides, and commensurate weakness. There is also weakness of shoulder abduction, knee extension, hip flexion, and, to a lesser degree, extension. Plantar responses are flexor. He has a waddling gait. The most likely diagnosis is:**

A. Inclusion body myositis

B. Syringomyelia

C. Motor neurone disease

D. Polymyositis

E. Multifocal motor neuropathy with conduction block

49. **A 63-year-old lady presents with a one-month history of rapidly worsening nausea, imbalance, slurred speech, and difficulty with fine manual dexterity. She has lost 2 stone in weight over the past six months. On examination she has a gaze-evoked nystagmus bilaterally, absent vestibulo-ocular reflex, dysarthria, and gross ataxia of all four limbs and gait. There are no palpable lymph nodes or abdominal masses. You suspect she may have a paraneoplastic syndrome. Which tumour is most commonly associated with a progressive symmetrical paraneoplastic cerebellar syndrome?**

A. Ovary

B. Thymoma

C. Pancreas

D. Small cell lung

E. Melanoma

50. **Which of the following finding is characteristic of an Argyll Robertson pupil?**
    A. Normal light reflex
    B. Dilated pupils
    C. Intact accommodation reflex
    D. Ptosis
    E. Central scotoma

51. **A 37-year-old woman was referred to the neurology unit for further assessment. When asked to look to the left she was noticed to have impaired adduction in the right eye and nystagmus of the left abducting eye. Lesion of which of the following structures is responsible for this presentation?**
    A. Medial longitudinal fasciculus
    B. Cerebellum
    C. Labyrinth
    D. Vestibular nuclei
    E. Temporal lobe

52. **A 25-year-old man presents following his second episode of loss of consciousness. The witness account is highly suggestive that these are epileptic seizures, and a routine EEG shows intermittent epileptiform discharges. You make a diagnosis of epilepsy and start carbamazepine. You should discuss all of the following issues except:**
    A. The need to stop driving and inform the DVLA of the diagnosis
    B. Safety advice including avoidance of heights and bathing
    C. Public transport freedom pass
    D. Exemption from prescription charges
    E. Advice regarding the teratogenic risk of anti-convulsants to an unborn child

53. **A 29-year-old woman presents with her second episode of blurred vision in her right eye. The last episode occurred eight months ago. Two years ago she had a three-week episode of weakness in her left arm. On examination she has disc pallor on the right, brisk reflexes in her left arm and leg, and an extensor plantar on the left. Which of the following is not associated with MS?**
    A. Pulfrich's effect
    B. Uhthoff's phenomenon
    C. Lhermitte's sign
    D. Gelineau syndrome
    E. Marcus Gunn sign

54. **A 69-year-old man presents with a six-month history of a rest tremor and a shuffling gait. On examination there is a rest tremor affecting the right arm and leg, and mild cogwheel rigidity and bradykinesia of both arms. He has brisk tendon reflexes in his legs, and his right plantar response is extensor. His gait is stiff and shuffling, as if his feet are stuck to the floor. As far as he can recall, his past medical history includes gout, type 2 diabetes, and hypertension. The most likely diagnosis is:**
   A. Lewy body dementia
   B. Cortico-basal degeneration
   C. Progressive supra-nuclear palsy
   D. Cerebrovascular disease
   E. Multiple system atrophy

55. **A 25-year-old woman presents following her third witnessed episode of loss of consciousness. She is fearful that she will be told she is not allowed to drive and had not presented sooner because she had hoped they would stop. All of the following features in the history of loss of consciousness could occur with psychogenic seizures except:**
   A. Cyanosis
   B. Tongue-biting
   C. Urinary incontinence
   D. Opisthotonus
   E. Only ever happens when witnessed

56. **A 24-year-old woman who is four weeks postpartum presents to hospital having had three seizures at home. She has no other neurological history and has never had seizures before. She is teetotal currently but has never consumed alcohol to excess. Once stabilized she gives a history of an increasingly worsening headache over the last two weeks. The headache is global in location and is worse in the mornings and when she coughs or sneezes and would be 10/10 in severity on occasion. There were no other neurological problems at that time. Her examination was notable for papilloedema and no other neurological deficits. She had felt otherwise well other than her headache. What is the most likely diagnosis?**
   A. Subarachnoid history
   B. Subdural abscess
   C. Central venous sinus thrombosis
   D. Generalized epilepsy
   E. Eclampsia

57. A 63-year-old lady presents with a one-month history of rapidly worsening nausea, imbalance, slurred speech, and difficulty with fine manual dexterity. She has lost 2 stone in weight over the past six months. On examination she has a gaze-evoked nystagmus bilaterally, absent vestibulo-ocular reflex, dysarthria, and gross ataxia of all four limbs and gait. There are no palpable lymph nodes or abdominal masses. You suspect she may have a paraneoplastic syndrome. Which antibody is most commonly associated with a progressive symmetrical cerebellar syndrome?

   A. Anti-Yo
   B. Anti-amphiphysin
   C. Anti-Ri
   D. Anti-Ma1
   E. Anti-Ma2

58. You see a 73-year-old man in outpatients with an eight-year history of progressive Parkinsonism. On examination there is cog-wheel rigidity and bradykinesia of both arms, worse on the right arm, and reduced armswing on the right when walking. He is hypomimic and hypophonic. A sample of his writing exhibits micrographia. You suspect he has idiopathic Parkinson's disease. Which of the following non-motor features would not be expected with a diagnosis of idiopathic Parkinson's disease?

   A. Anosmia
   B. Non-REM sleep disorder
   C. Constipation
   D. Depression
   E. Abdominal pain

59. A 25-year-old man presents with a five-day history of double vision and balance problems when walking. He has had a prolonged upper respiratory tract infection for the past couple of weeks, and is a type 1 diabetic, but is otherwise well. Examination reveals a complex ophthalmoplegia, global areflexia, and an ataxic gait. Power and sensation in the face and limbs are preserved, although Romberg's test is positive. Finger–nose pointing is mildly ataxic. The most likely diagnosis is:

   A. Myasthenia
   B. Miller Fisher syndrome
   C. Tolosa-Hunt syndrome
   D. Multiple sclerosis
   E. Vitamin E deficiency

60. **A 73-year-old woman presents with a one-year history of increasing difficulty using her left arm. It is not specifically weak, but rather she tells you she is not sure how to make it work. On direct questioning, she tells you that occasionally it will interfere with the action of her dominant right arm, for example when picking something up. On examination, her left arm shows significant lead-pipe rigidity and mild cogwheeling. Her MMSE is 22/30. The other physical sign you would expect to find is:**

   A. Failure of downgaze that corrects with the doll's head manoeuvre
   B. Left arm apraxia
   C. Palmo-mental response on the left
   D. Brisk knee jerks bilaterally
   E. Extensor plantar responses bilaterally

61. **A 69-year-old man presents with a six-month history of falls. He finds that he is increasingly unsteady on his feet. On examination there is pronounced truncal rigidity, symmetrical cogwheel rigidity, and bradykinesia of both arms, but no tremor. There is postural instability when you challenge his balance. His MMSE is 30/30. The other physical sign you would expect to find in this man is:**

   A. Failure of downgaze that corrects with the doll's head manoeuvre
   B. Limb apraxia
   C. Palmo-mental response
   D. Brisk knee jerks
   E. Extensor plantar responses

62. **A 69-year-old man presents with a six-month history of a shuffling gait and the feeling of being about to faint when he stands up. He has also been incontinent of urine a few times over the past few months, which he has found most unusual and embarrassing. His wife says he has been becoming increasingly forgetful. On examination there is pronounced symmetrical cogwheel rigidity and bradykinesia of both arms, but no rest tremor. He has brisk tendon reflexes in his legs, and flexor plantar responses. His gait is shuffling with reduced arm swing. Blood pressure measurements reveal a postural drop of 26 mmHg between lying and standing. The most likely diagnosis is:**

   A. Lewy body dementia
   B. Cortico-basal degeneration
   C. Progressive supra-nuclear palsy
   D. Cerebrovascular disease
   E. Multiple system atrophy

63. **A 69-year-old man presents with a six-month history of a shuffling gait and the feeling of being about to faint when he stands up. He has also been incontinent of urine a few times over the past few months, which he has found most unusual and embarrassing. His wife says he has been becoming increasingly forgetful. On examination there is pronounced symmetrical cogwheel rigidity and bradykinesia of both arms, but no rest tremor. He has brisk tendon reflexes in his legs, and flexor plantar responses. His gait is shuffling with reduced arm swing bilaterally. Blood pressure measurements reveal a postural drop of 26 mmHg between lying and standing. The other physical sign you would expect to find in this man is:**

A. Failure of downgaze that corrects with the doll's head manoeuvre
B. Limb apraxia
C. Finger–nose ataxia
D. Positive Romberg's test
E. Postural instability

64. **A 56-year-old male presents with slurred speech, bilateral facial weakness, difficulty swallowing, and ptosis following a holiday to India when he had bad diarrhoea. The symptoms have been getting worse over a couple of weeks, and now he feels weak all over and needs to rest his chin on his hand in order to lift up his head. You suspect he may have myasthenia. What is the most reliable test to confirm your suspicion?**

A. Anti-ACh receptor antibody titres
B. Repetitive stimulation EMG
C. Single-fibre EMG
D. Edrophonium test
E. Trial of treatment

65. **What disease is associated with widespread central nervous demyelination, immunodeficient states, and the JC virus?**

A. Multiple sclerosis
B. Tumefactive multiple sclerosis
C. Limbic encephalitis
D. Acute disseminated encephalomeningitis
E. Progressive multifocal leukoencephalopathy

66. **A 30-year-old man presents to A&E having had a witnessed convulsive episode lasting three minutes. There was no warning before he lost consciousness, and he was confused afterwards, and is still confused now. He has bitten his tongue but is not incontinent of urine or faeces. He has no other medical problems and has been completely well recently. He had malaria eight years ago. He is not febrile, and the neurological examination is normal. His CT shows a hypodense area within the white matter of the anterior portion of the left temporal lobe. There is no mass effect. The most important investigation to do next is:**

    A. CSF analysis
    B. MRI head
    C. Acute viral serology
    D. Serum for anti-voltage-gated K+ channel antibodies
    E. MRV

67. **A 45-year-old woman with no significant past medical history presents with progressive weakness over a two-week period associated with diminished sensation. Her weakness was graded as 4/5 and she had a symmetrical sensory loss to all modalities. Her ankle jerks were absent but her knee jerks were present. Two weeks previously she had a short-lived cough and fever. The most likely cerebrospinal fluid findings for this condition are:**

    A. Protein >4 g/dl, 2×10^6/l white blood cells, glucose consistent with serum glucose
    B. Protein >4 g/dl, 15×10^6/l white blood cells, 90% polymorphs, glucose consistent with serum glucose
    C. Protein >4 g/dl, 15×10^6/l white blood cells, 90% lymphocytes, glucose consistent with serum glucose
    D. Protein <4 g/dl, 2×10^6/l white blood cells, glucose less than half of serum glucose
    E. Protein <4 g/dl, 2×10^6/l white blood cells, glucose consistent with serum glucose

68. **A 45-year-old man presents with a five-day history of back pain, and progressive parasthesiae, and numbness in his legs. The parasthesiae started in his calves and spread up the whole of both legs. It now extends up to the level of his umbilicus. In the past 48 hours he reports weakness in his legs too. This man needs investigating for all of the following differential diagnoses except:**

    A. Guillain–Barré syndrome
    B. Spinal cord infarct
    C. Multiple sclerosis
    D. HIV
    E. Thoracic disc prolapse

69. **A 94-year-old woman was admitted from a residential home after having a tonic-clonic seizure lasting for more than five minutes. Her first seizure was four months earlier and it was unclear how many she had had in the intervening period. She had lost about 4 kg weight in the last four months. Her past medical history included angina, diet controlled type 2 diabetes, glaucoma, atrial fibrillation, and polymyalgia rheumatica. She was taking the following drugs: once daily aspirin 75 mg, digoxin 125 mcg, isosorbide mono-nitrate MR 60 mg, omeprazole 20 mg, senna 15 mg, and amitriptyline 25 mg at night. On examination, she was in atrial fibrillation at 80 bpm with a blood pressure of 110/75 mmHg. Her GCS was 12/15 (E3, M6, V3). She had a left lower motor neurone VII nerve palsy and minimal scalp tenderness on that side. There were no other abnormalities. Investigations: Hb 9.3 g/dl (11.5–16.5), WBC 8.7 x 10^9/l (4–11), neutrophils 7.2 x 10^9/l (1.5–7.0), platelets 624 x 10^9/l (150–400), CRP 147 (< 10), ESR 105 mm/1st h (<30), urea 5.5 mmol/l (2.5–7.0), creatinine 65 micromol/l (60–110), Na 133 mmol/l (137–144), K 4.7 mmol/l (3.5–4.9), CSF opening pressure 9 cm, cells/organisms nil, protein 0.4, glucose 3.9 (serum glucose 5.5); virology HSV, VZV not detected on PCR; CXR: unfolded aorta, lung fields clear; CT head: cerebral atrophy, no intra cranial space-occupying lesion, infarct or haemorrhage; vasculitic screen: ANA –ve, antihistone antibodies +ve, antiglial antibodies –ve, complement C3 and C4 normal. What is the most likely cause of her seizures?**

    A. Cerebrovascular disease
    B. Encephalitis
    C. Giant cell arteritis
    D. Malignancy
    E. Meningitis

70. **A 73-year-old man is brought to outpatient clinic by his wife. They had returned early from the holiday apartment that they owned in Benidorm, as his wife did not feel confident in managing his altered behaviour. He was found bewildered near the swimming pool of the apartment complex, after his morning swim. He was repeatedly asking the other residents where he was and what was happening. When his wife arrived at the poolside he knew who she was but had no recollection of where they were or why they were there. He could not understand why he was in swimwear and could not recall his way to their apartment. He also complained of a generalized headache. He had been taken to the local hospital where the doctors could not find any abnormality on clinical examination except disorientation in time, place, and person. His wife had a letter from the hospital stating that his full blood count, U&Es, liver function, thyroid function, ECG, and CT head scan had all been normal. He was not kept in hospital. His wife had arranged their return home the next day, on the first available flight. He has no recollection of the event but remembers the journey back very clearly. He has a past medical history of migraine, hypertension, and impaired glucose tolerance. His current medication is aspirin 75 mg, simvastatin 40 mg and lisinopril 5 mg daily. No abnormality is detected on general physical or systemic examination. Urine dipstick is positive for leucocytes but not for nitrites. What is the most likely diagnosis?**

    A. Acute delirium
    B. Migraine with aura
    C. Subdural haematoma
    D. Transient global amnesia
    E. Transient ischaemic attack

71. **An 82-year-old woman is admitted with a two-week history of progressive deterioration in mobility to the point that she has become immobile. Over the same time period she complains of worsened bilateral hand tremor. Tremor was first noticed by the patient and her daughter four months ago and started in the right hand, moving to the left hand two months later. She has lived with her daughter for 30 years since her husband died and has only needed assistance with personal care in the last two months. She had a permanent cardiac pacemaker inserted four years ago for complete heart block and is taking aspirin 75 mg, simvastatin 40 mg, and amlodipine 10 mg once daily. Examination reveals resting tremor of both hands and right leg, and generalized increase in tone in all limbs. There is a right facial droop. She is in atrial fibrillation at a rate of 80 bpm and blood pressure is 116/78 resting. What is the most likely cause of her tremor?**

    A. Amlodipine
    B. Essential tremor.
    C. Idiopathic Parkinson's disease
    D. Thyrotoxicosis
    E. Vascular Parkinsonism

72. **A 33-year-old man known to suffer with AIDS presents with an altered level of consciousness, general weakness, and slurred speech. MRI of the brain reveals multiple, bilateral, hypodense, ring-enhancing lesions with associated brain oedema. The most likely cause of this clinical presentation is:**

A. Primary CNS lymphoma
B. Toxoplasmosis
C. Kaposi's sarcoma
D. Cryptosporum meningitis
E. Pneumococcal meningitis

73. **A 27-year-old woman with a background of type 1 diabetes mellitus presents with uncontrolled blood sugars. She admits that she has not been concordant with her insulin regimen. Further questioning reveals that she is currently ten weeks pregnant and has been experiencing severe nausea and recurrent vomiting for the last two weeks. A full neurological examination at this time is entirely normal. Admission urinalysis confirms the presence of ketones. Arterial blood gas analysis reveals a severe metabolic acidosis with a pH of 7.13. She is treated overnight with an intravenous insulin infusion and intravenous fluids (dextrose and saline) on a high dependency unit. Her blood sugars return slowly to normal range overnight; her arterial pH also normalizes. Her morning bloods reveal entirely normal electrolytes, unchanged from admission. On the morning ward round, however, the patient is now confused. She scores an abbreviated mental test score of 5/10. Examination of eye movements reveals evidence of horizontal gaze nystagmus and bilateral lateral rectus palsies. Assessment of gait reveals marked unsteadiness on standing and is therefore abandoned. Assessment of upper limb coordination (via the finger–nose test) reveals ataxia. An urgent CT scan of the head is arranged and is normal. Lumbar puncture is performed and is unremarkable. What is the most likely cause of the neurological symptoms in this lady?**

A. Cerebral oedema
B. Posterior fossa neoplasm
C. Multiple sclerosis
D. Wernicke's encephalopathy
E. Freidrich's ataxia

74. An 80-year-old woman is brought to the hospital by the police after being found wandering in the streets at 2 am in her nightdress. She is bewildered, agitated, and aggressive towards staff when approached but settles with reassurance and allows them to examine her. She claims that she was going to the dairy to help milk the cows. The police have identified that she lives alone in an isolated cottage 6 miles from where she was found. There is no known next of kin but a local farmer's wife visits her once a week to check that she is alright. Her blood pressure is 140/78 and she is in sinus rhythm at 80 bpm. Examination of chest and abdomen is unremarkable as is neurological examination. Her abbreviated mental test score (AMTS) is 2/10. She is unconcerned about being incontinent of urine whilst being examined. Blood results showed CRP 35, WBC 11.3, with neutrophils 7.8. Urinalysis is trace positive for protein and blood. Urine culture does not grow any bacteria. Chest X-ray and electrocardiogram are normal. A search of the hospital computer system reveals that she has been admitted to the hospital twice in the last year under similar circumstances and on each occasion had been treated for a urinary tract infection. Further cognitive assessment was as follows: MMSE (Mini-Mental State Examination) 15/30, CLOX 1 (clock drawing test) 8/15, CAM (Confusion Assessment Method) positive, and IQCODE (Informant Questionnaire on Cognitive Decline in the Elderly) 4.5. What is the most likely diagnosis?

A. Acute on chronic confusion
B. Agitated depression
C. Delirium
D. Dementia
E. Psychotic depression

75. A 70-year-old man with small cell lung cancer develops muscle weakness, and you suspect Lambert–Eaton myasthenic syndrome. Which of these autoantibodies would you expect to be positive?

A. Voltage-gated calcium channel (VGCC) antibodies
B. Voltage-gated potassium channel (VGKC) antibodies
C. Voltage-gated sodium channel (VGNC) antibodies
D. Voltage-gated hydrogen channel (VGHC) antibodies
E. Acetyl choline receptor (AChR) antibodies

76. **A 27-year-old woman is admitted to the emergency department after an unprovoked seizure. She has no past medical history of note, takes no regular medication, and only drinks 3 units of alcohol per week. Neurological examination is entirely normal, and investigations including MRI brain are unremarkable. Which of the following correctly represents her risk of a recurrent seizure during the next two years?**
    A. 5%.
    B. 10%.
    C. 20%.
    D. 40%.
    E. 80%.

77. **An isolated sixth nerve palsy, or eye movements simulating a sixth nerve palsy, are least likely to be seen with:**
    A. Guillain–Barré syndrome
    B. Myasthenia gravis
    C. Duane syndrome
    D. As a side effect of retinoic acid medication
    E. Multiple sclerosis

78. **A 42-year-old woman who is just completing a course of steroids for an exacerbation of asthma is brought to the clinic by her husband. He is very concerned as she has become very confused, believing that there is dog barking at the bottom of the garden, and she walked home from the supermarket having forgotten that she left her car there. On examination she has a temperature of 37.8°C. She is clearly confused but there is no focal limb weakness. She has bilateral decreased coordination. Investigations reveal: Hb 12.8, WCC 11.2, PLT 184, Na 137, K 4.3, Cr 102. MRI brain: frontal and temporal oedema. Lumbar puncture: mildly elevated protein, low glucose, lymphocytic pleocytosis. Which of the following is the most likely diagnosis?**
    A. Enterovirus meningitis
    B. Herpes simplex encephalitis
    C. Middle cerebral artery stroke
    D. CMV meningitis
    E. Bacterial meningitis

79. **A 45-year-old man presents to the emergency department following three days of an unrelenting right-sided headache. The pain is centred around his right orbit and he suffers from brief episodes of stabbing pain which last for about a minute and then disappear as quickly as they occur. The pain is severe and occurs up to three times an hour. During attacks he has noticed his right eye becomes red and tears. The attacks sometimes start if he touches the right side of his face. What is the diagnosis?**

A. Migraine

B. Paroxsymal hemicrania

C. Cluster headache

D. Tension headache

E. Short-lasting unilateral neuralgiform headache attacks with conjunctival injection and tearing (SUNCT)

80. **A 30-year-old woman is referred by her GP to a neurologist. She describes a two-year history of intermittent neurological symptoms that include sensory loss, leg weakness, and blurred vision. Which of the following is the single best investigation to confirm the likely diagnosis?**

A. Non-contrast CT brain

B. Non-contrast MRI brain

C. Contrast-enhanced CT brain

D. Contrast-enhanced MRI brain

E. Contrast-enhanced MRI spine

81. **A 24-year-old woman who is four weeks postpartum presents to hospital having had three seizures at home. She has no other neurological history and has never had seizures before. She is teetotal currently but has never consumed alcohol to excess. Once stabilized she gives a history of an increasingly worsening headache over the last two weeks. The headache is global in location and is worse in the mornings and when she coughs or sneezes and would be 10/10 in severity on occasion. There are no other neurological problems at this time. Her examination is notable for papilloedema and no other neurological deficits. She has felt well other than her headache. What is the most appropriate initial investigation?**

A. CT head

B. CT head with contrast

C. MR venography

D. Lumbar puncture

E. Formal perimetry

82. **A 60-year-old man with a history of previous TIAs presents to A&E with acute onset left hemiplegia, of 12 hours' duration. He has an urgent non-contrast CT of the brain. Which of the following CT findings are least compatible with the history?**

A. Loss of grey–white matter differentiation in the right MCA territory

B. High attenuation within the right middle cerebral artery

C. Dilatation of the third and lateral ventricles

D. A normal CT

E. Acute haemorrhage within the right cerebral hemisphere parenchyma

83. **A 34-year-old woman is referred for investigation of visual symptoms, irregular menses, and galactorrhoea. Initial investigation reveals an elevated serum prolactin. The definitive investigation of choice is:**

A. Lateral skull X-ray to assess size of the pituitary fossa

B. Contrast-enhanced CT brain

C. MRI spectroscopy of the brain

D. Contrast-enhanced MRI of the brain

E. Non-contrast CT brain with sagittal reformat views

84. **An 80-year-old man is brought to A&E due to concerns from his family regarding confusion. His family also report that he has been increasingly drowsy over the past 24 hours. Initial biochemistry reveals the following: sodium 150 mmol/l, bicarbonate 30 mmol/l, potassium 5 mmol/l, chloride 110 mmol/l, urea 10 mmol/l, glucose 40 mmol/l. Which of the following is the most likely diagnosis?**

A. Diabetic ketoacidosis

B. Meningitis

C. Subdural haematoma

D. Post-ictal

E. Hyperosmolar non-ketotic coma

85. **A 23-year-old woman is admitted to the emergency department after suffering her second tonic clonic seizure in a month; her third overall. She is five months pregnant. Past medical history is unremarkable. Physical examination, including full neurological examination is normal. Bloods including a full blood count and metabolic screen are unremarkable. Assuming the diagnosis of epilepsy is confirmed, which of the following would be the most appropriate option for her?**

A. No treatment

B. Sodium valproate

C. Carbamazepine

D. Vigabatrin

E. Lamotrigine

86. **A 72-year-old man is reviewed in the clinic some six weeks after a stroke which has left him with left arm weakness. He has a history of ischaemic heart disease and type 2 diabetes and was taking aspirin before the most recent event. On examination his BP is 145/72, pulse is 70 and regular. The results of an ECHO reveal a normal sized left atrium and left ventricle. Which of the following is the most appropriate prophylaxis against a further stroke?**
   A. Continue aspirin 75 mg
   B. Increase aspirin to 300 mg
   C. Add dipyridamole 200 mg MR
   D. Change to clopidogrel 75 mg
   E. Change to warfarin

87. **A 62-year-old man who is known to drink 2–3 bottles of wine per day is brought into the emergency department by ambulance. Concern had been raised for his health after his son had to break into his property because the patient had not been seen for some time. His son found him confused and unable to stand. On examination he is confused and agitated, has bilateral gaze-evoked nystagmus and a conjugate gaze palsy. When you ask him how he got to hospital, he says that his friend Jim drove him in his car. Which of the following is the most likely cause of his confusion?**
   A. B12 deficiency
   B. Thiamine deficiency
   C. Subdural haematoma
   D. Delerium tremens
   E. Hypoglycaemia

88. **A 65-year-old man is brought by ambulance to the emergency department. He has suffered an acute stroke with left hemiparesis. He has a history of atrial fibrillation (for which he takes aspirin 300 mg), hypertension, and type 2 diabetes mellitus. On examination his BP is 170/90 and his pulse is in atrial fibrillation at a rate of 80. There is evidence of left hemiparesis and expressive dysphasia. A CT scan shows no evidence of haemorrhage and you elect to discuss the risk benefit of thrombolysis. Which of the following is true?**
   A. Risk of haemorrhage is increased two-fold by thrombolysis
   B. Tissue plasminogen activator (TPA) should be given within three hours if possible
   C. Abdominal surgery approximately six months earlier is a contraindication
   D. Approximately 20 people need to be thrombolysed within three hours to save one person from death or dependency
   E. Tissue plasminogen activator (TPA) should be delivered locally via a catheter placed under radiological control

89. **A 62-year-old woman comes to the clinic for review. She complains of blurring of in her left eye and that she is increasingly uncomfortable in bright lights. This has been a problem for the past few days. There is a history of hypertension for which she takes a combination of ramipril and amlodipine. Her left pupil is fixed and dilated, and she has lost accomodation. There is no ptosis on the left or right. There is some loss of adduction for the left eye when movements are examined. Her BP is 142/82, her fasting glucose is 6.9 mmol/l. Which of the following is the most likely cause of her presentation?**

   A. Giant cell arteritis
   B. Diabetes mellitus
   C. Posterior communicating artery aneurysm
   D. Anterior communicating artery aneurysm
   E. Idiopathic

90. **A 71-year-old man presents with neck stiffness, fever, and photophobia. He has recently returned from a trip to France where he ate a number of unpasteurized soft cheeses. The A&E FY2 doctor decided to give IV ceftriaxone 2 g. Given the history, which of the following organisms would you be concerned about not being adequately covered?**

   A. *Escherichia coli*
   B. *Haemophilus influenzae type b*
   C. *Streptococcus pneumoniae*
   D. *Neisseria meningitidis*
   E. *Listeria monocytogenes*

91. **A 45-year-old man presents with a ten-week history of progressive weakness and parasthesiae in his legs. The parasthesiae started in his toes and has spread up both legs to just above the knees. He has begun to notice that the tips of his fingers are also beginning to feel numb. The weakness is mild, and affects only the ankles. He is able to pass urine and open his bowels normally. You note absent knee and ankle jerks on examination. He is generally well, but has been a type 2 diabetic for ten years and had a bad 'cold' in the spring, a few weeks before the start of his symptoms. The most likely diagnosis is:**

   A. Guillain–Barré syndrome
   B. Multiple sclerosis
   C. Diabetic neuropathy
   D. Chronic inflammatory demyelinating radiculoneuropathy (CIDP)
   E. Lumbar disc prolapse

92. **An 82-year-old man in hospital recovering from pneumonia is reviewed by the ward physiotherapist. They report that his mobility is limited owing to previously undiagnosed bilateral foot drop. This is not associated with any pain and the patient reports it has been present for several years. He usually eats a normal diet and has never consumed significant amounts of alcohol. Neurological examination shows normal tone, impaired dorsiflexion, reduced vibration and light touch sensation distally, and attenuated ankle jerks in both lower limbs. Investigations show a mild degree of renal impairment and a normal full blood count, B12, folate, ESR, and vasculitis screen. A fasting venous glucose is 4.6 mmol/l (3.9–5.5 mmol/l). Which of the following is the next most appropriate investigation?**

    A. Glucose tolerance test
    B. HbA1c
    C. MRI lumbar spine
    D. Nerve conduction studies
    E. Syphilis serology

93. **Which onconeural antibody is associated with the following neurological presentation? A proximal muscle weakness with mild autonomic dysfunction (particularly a dry mouth) and depressed tendon reflexes. Approximately half of the patients have a mild ptosis. MR is usually normal. Electromyography shows an increase in compound muscle action potential following maximum voluntary contraction.**

    A. Anti-Yo antibodies
    B. Anti-voltage-gated potassium antibodies
    C. Anti-voltage-gated calcium antibodies.
    D. Anti-Hu antibodies
    E. Anti-NMDA receptor antibodies

94. **A 45-year-old woman with no significant past medical history presents with progressive weakness over a two-week period associated with diminished sensation. Her weakness is graded as 4/5 and she has a symmetrical sensory loss to all modalities. Her ankle jerks are absent but her knee jerks are present. Two weeks ago she had a short-lived cough and fever. The most likely diagnosis is:**

    A. Multiple sclerosis
    B. Guillain–Barré syndrome
    C. Transverse myelitis
    D. Myasthenia gravis
    E. Subacute chronic demyelinating inflammatory polyneuropathy

95. A 63-year-old retired surveyor with no past medical history presents to hospital alongside his wife with increasing confusion over two months which did not appear to fluctuate and becoming increasingly poor on his feet. There are no infective symptoms alongside the confusion. His wife has noted a general deterioration in his mood as well and that his sleep has become erratic. She has also noted some jerky movements of his limbs especially when startled. Routine blood tests and a **CT** head scan are all normal. His **MMSE** is **19/30** with a global reduction in scores. The most likely diagnosis is:

    A. Alzheimer's disease
    B. Sporadic Creutzfeldt–Jakob disease
    C. Huntington's chorea
    D. Depression
    E. Huntington's chorea

96. A 24-year-old man presents with a several-month history of ankle weakness and wasting. He has no other past medical history and was a keen football player. He found that he would trip over easily, especially if trying to turn on his ankle. Occasionally he finds that he stubs his toes whilst walking. Alongside this he has found that his feet have become 'numb' and that he often cannot feel his feet unless he stamps them. Examination is notable for pes cavus, 4/5 weakness particularly of the ankle extensors, absent ankle jerks, and a global sensory loss to the ankles. His arms are not affected. There is no family history of neurological disease but the patient reports that his father also has high-arched feet. The most likely diagnosis is:

    A. Diabetic neuropathy
    B. Friedreich's ataxia
    C. Entrapment neuropathy
    D. Multiple sclerosis
    E. Charcot–Marie–Tooth disease

97. A 82-year-old right-handed man with a past medical history of hypertension and hypercholesterolaemia presents to hospital with a right-sided weakness after being found slumped in bed by his carers. Upon arrival at hospital he is able to answer questions and can follow commands. He is noted to have a dense right-sided hemiparaesis (MRC grade 2/5) but with no evidence of inattention or a hemianopia. What would be the classification of this man's stroke?

    A. Partial anterior circulation stroke
    B. Total anterior circulation stroke
    C. Lacunar stroke
    D. Posterior circulation stroke
    E. Lateral medullary syndrome

98. **A 74-year-old man presents to his GP with progressive difficulties swallowing, worse for liquids than solids, and finds that he would often get a sore jaw when chewing, especially meat. His wife has noticed that his speech had become quite nasal over a few months. He is not otherwise weak but gets quite tired after gardening all day. Upon examination he had a nasal speech but with no evidence of ophthalmoplegia. What autoimmune antibody is associated with this condition?**

    A. Anti-acetylcholine receptor antibodies
    B. Anti-voltage-gated calcium channel antibodies
    C. Anti-voltage-gated potassium channel antibodies
    D. Anti-Hu antibodies
    E. Anti-NMDA receptor antibodies

99. **A 45-year-old presents to the emergency department with a three-day history of intense right-sided headaches. The headache always starts about an hour after he goes to bed and is located around his right orbit. The pain is very intense although the patient is clear that it is not throbbing in nature. The pain lasts for 30 minutes before disappearing. Simple analgesia has no effect on the pain. He otherwise notes that his nose 'runs' from the right nostril and that he becomes very restless. His wife notes that his eye looks red and that his eyelid becomes droopy. The headaches have started at the same time for the last three nights. His neurological examination is entirely normal and he has no past medical history other than cigarette smoking. The diagnosis is:**

    A. Migraine
    B. Paroxysmal hemicrania
    C. Cluster headache
    D. Tension headache
    E. Short-lasting unilateral neuralgifom headache attacks with conjunctival injection and tearing (SUNCT)

100. **Which of the following suggests an alternative diagnosis to Duchenne muscular dystrophy?**

    A. Inability to rise from the floor
    B. Absence of a family history
    C. Respiratory failure in adolescence
    D. Normal serum creatine kinase
    E. Calf muscle hypertrophy

101. **A 32-year-old gymnastics teacher suffers a spinal cord injury and hemisection at the level of T1. You review her a few weeks later in the neurology clinic. Which of the following neurological features is likely to be found?**

A. Ipsilateral loss of pain sensation
B. Contralateral loss of temperature sensation
C. Babinski sign contralateral to the lesion
D. Contralateral loss of fine touch
E. Contralateral loss of vibration sense

102. **The presenilin-1 (PSEN1) gene associated with early-onset Alzheimer's disease is found on which chromosome?**

A. 14
B. 1
C. 21
D. 20
E. 5

103. **A 64-year-old woman with a past medical history of hypertension and angina presents to hospital with an acute-onset headache whilst she was driving which was maximal within seconds of onset. She often gets headaches but this was more severe than her usual headaches. She did not lose consciousness at the onset of the headache and had suffered from no focal weakness. She managed to get home and found that the lights at home made her headache worse, following which she suffered from several vomiting episodes. She also noted that her neck had become stiff and she was no longer able to touch her chin on her chest. She is on several antihypertensive medications, smokes 25 cigarettes per day, and consumes 21 units of alcohol per week. She has been otherwise well prior to her presentation. What is the most appropriate initial course of action?**

A. Routine CT head
B. Urgent CT head
C. Immediate lumbar puncture
D. 12-hour lumbar puncture
E. Intravenous cephalosporin and acyclovir

104. **A 22-year-old car mechanic presents to an outpatient clinic with a long history of clumsiness, particularly with his hands, and frequent falls. Upon further questioning he notes that he has always had problems letting go of things held with his hands. This is particularly noticeable when he is at work and cannot release his tools straight away. His girlfriend has noted that his eyelids have become increasingly droopy, but the patient is adamant that they have always been like this. His past medical history is notable for being a 'borderline diabetic' and that he has noticed he is becoming bald. Examination is notable for an inability to release his hands, distal weakness, bilateral ptosis, and marked facial atrophy. The patient reports his father has similar problems but not as severe as his. The diagnosis is:**

A. Charcot–Marie–Tooth disease.

B. Lambert–Eaton myasthenic syndrome

C. Myasthenia gravis

D. Myotonic dystrophy

E. Inclusion body myositis

105. **Which onconeural antibody is associated with the following neurological presentation? Patients may present with psychiatric disturbance which may include anxiety, agitation, bizarre behaviour, delusions, paranoia, hallucinations, or memory loss. Alongside this there is a demonstration of autonomic instability and a high chance of progression to a reduction in conscious state and catatonia. More than half will have some form of movement disorder such as an orofacial dyskinesia or choreoathetosis. In 90% of cases the disease is seen in female patients. Death can ensue rapidly due to central hypoventilation.**

A. Anti-Yo antibodies

B. Anti-voltage-gated potassium antibodies

C. Anti-voltage-gated calcium channel antibodies

D. Anti-Hu antibodies

E. Anti-NMDA receptor antibodies

106. **A 16-year-old girl presents to clinic with a deteriorating gait and noticeably slurred speech. Whilst she has always been a 'clumsy' child, she and her parents have noticed that she has been becoming increasingly unstable on her feet and that over the last few months she developed a slurring of her speech. Her examination is notable for a wide-based gait, reduced vibration and proprioception to her ankles, absent lower limb reflexes, upgoing plantars, dysarthria, and pes cavus. Her past medical history and family history are unremarkable. What is the most likely diagnosis?**
    A. Friedreich's ataxia
    B. Hypovitaminosis A
    C. Congenital syphilis
    D. Refsum's disease
    E. Myelopathy secondary to prolapsed lumber disc

107. **Which of the following diagnoses is not associated with dysphonia?**
    A. Myasthenia gravis
    B. Supranuclear palsy
    C. Parkinson's disease
    D. Cerebellar disease
    E. Dominant-hemispheric partial or total anterior circulation stroke

108. **A 69-year-old man presents with an 18-month history of recurrent falls and progressive decline in mobility. His family has noticed recent personality change. On examination the patient has low monotonous speech, hypokinesia, and cogwheel rigidity, but no tremor or fasciculations. There is no muscle weakness or sensory loss. The cranial nerves examination is intact apart from limitation of upward movement of both eyes. The most likely diagnosis is:**
    A. Parkinson's disease
    B. Alzheimer's disease
    C. Multiple sclerosis
    D. Progressive supranuclear palsy
    E. Motor neuron disease

109. **You are keen to start a 50-year-old man with Parkinson's disease on the dopamine agonist ropinirole. Which of these side effects, strongly associated with this class of drug, is it vital to warn him about?**
    A. Reduced fertility
    B. Impulse control disorders such as hypersexuality
    C. Malignancy
    D. Depression
    E. Hypertension

110. **A 20-year-old woman, who was previously well, has three tonic-clonic seizures over the course of three months. After investigations, she is diagnosed with epilepsy and started on medication. She is keen to start driving again. If she has no further seizures, then how long since the last seizure must she wait before she drives again?**

A. 4 months

B. 6 months

C. 1 year

D. 2 years

E. She is never allowed to drive again

111. **An otherwise well 67-year-old man hass noticed a tremor in his left hand. This does not disturb him when performing intricate tasks and is more evident at rest. He denies any other symptoms. His wife reports that his handwriting has deteriorated slightly over the past 12 months and she also wonders if he is becoming depressed. He is not on any medication. On examination he has a 5 Hz resting tremor of his left hand. There is minimal increased rigidity of his left upper limb with slight cogwheeling. He is able to mobilize unaided with a normal gait with a walking speed of 1.1 metres/second. Finger snap frequency was reduced in his left hand compared to his right. Folstein Mini-Mental State Examination (MMSE) was 30/30, clock drawing test was normal, and Geriatric Depression Score (GDS) was 3/15. Which of the following would be the most appropriate next step?**

A. A diagnostic trial of levodopa

B. Arrange a CT brain scan

C. Arrange a DaT (dopamine transporter) scan to confirm the diagnosis

D. Initiate treatment with a dopamine agonist

E. No further diagnostics or treatments and review in six months

112. **You are an SHO in the general neurology clinic where you see a patient with epilepsy who wants to know more about his condition. What is nearest estimate of the prevalence of this condition in the UK?**

A. 1 in 1,000,000

B. 1 in 100,000

C. 1 in 10,000

D. 1 in 1000

E. 1 in 100

113. **A 41-year-old woman presents with a rapid painless loss of vision associated with a rapid onset weakness of both her arms and legs. She has been otherwise well prior to this. Upon examination she is found to have a symmetrical spastic paraparesis of her arms and legs and a sensory level to all modalities up to C5. The patient also suffers from profound urinary incontinence. She undergoes MR imaging which finds two central white matter lesions with evidence of optic neuritis and an extensive cervical cord lesion. Her CSF demonstrates a pleocytosis with oligoclonal bands. She is positive for aquaporin 4 antibodies. Her diagnosis is:**

    A. Multiple sclerosis
    B. Anterior ischaemic optic neuropathy
    C. Neuromyelitis optica
    D. Sjogren's syndrome
    E. Acute disseminated encephalomyelitis

114. **You are called to see a 34-year-old man who suffered bilateral femoral and pelvic fractures in a road traffic accident on his motorbike 18 hours ago. Twelve hours previously he had the femurs pinned. He drank some tea that evening, but the nurse has called you as he is now shouting, pulling out his intravenous line, and attempting to pull out his urinary catheter. What is the most likely aetiology of his condition?**

    A. Alcohol withdrawal
    B. Anaphylaxis
    C. Fat embolism
    D. Inhalation
    E. Pulmonary embolism

115. **A 72-year-old woman complains of a severe aching/stabbing pain over her left cheek. She says this pain can come on without warning and is made worse by movement or exposure to cold air, or even sometimes when she is stressed. She says it is driving her mad. There are no associated headaches, and neurological examination is entirely unremarkable. Which of the following is the most appropriate treatment for her?**

    A. Amitryptilline
    B. Carbamazepine
    C. Sodium valproate
    D. Prednisolone
    E. Acyclovir

116. **A 28-year-old woman comes to the clinic for review. She wishes to get pregnant but has a previous history of generalized epilepsy. She takes sodium valproate 500 mg BD and has had no fits for the past 3.5 years. She does not drive as she can walk to work and her partner has a car. Which of the following is the best advice with respect to her anti-epileptic medication?**

A. Start folic acid in addition to her valproate
B. Consider stopping her valproate
C. Switch to lamotrigine
D. Switch to topiramate
E. Try reducing the valproate to 500 mg

117. **A 29-year-old woman presents with a second episode of blurred vision in her right eye. The last episode occurred 8 months ago. Two years ago she had a three-week episode of weakness in her left arm. On examination she has disc pallor on the right, brisk reflexes in her left arm and leg, and an extensor plantar response on the left. Which is not associated with optic neuritis?**

A. Pulfrich's effect
B. Uhthoff's phenomenon
C. Lhermitte's sign
D. Relative afferent pupillary defect
E. Marcu Gunn sign

1. A. Is a complication of primary genital herpes

Whereas herpes simplex virus encephalitis is a life-threatening medical emergency warranting empiric antiviral treatment, herpes simplex virus meningitis is a self-limiting condition in patients with normal immunity. Herpes simplex virus meningitis is a complication of primary genital herpes, especially with HSV-2. Meningitis due to HSV-2 can recur, especially in women with primary genital infection. Clinical recurrences have been described in 20–50% of cases, both with and without genital symptoms. Convulsions are features of viral encephalitis. There is no effective vaccination.

Wald A et al., Reactivation of genital herpes simplex type infection in asymptomatic seropositive persons, *New England Journal of Medicine* 2000;342:844–850.

2. E. Dipyridamole MR

Whilst the addition of clopidogrel to aspirin showed a reduction in the risk of stroke events in patients with unstable coronary syndromes, the data in secondary stroke prevention is much stronger from the ESPS-2 study, which used aspirin and dipyridamole in combination. This demonstrated a reduction of 23% in further strokes versus aspirin alone. There is no obvious indication for warfarinization here, and the aspirin would need to be stopped prior to warfarin initiation.

Diener H et al., European stroke prevention study, 2: dipyridamole and acetylsalicylic acid in the secondary prevention of stroke, *Journal of the Neurological Sciences* 1996;143:1–13.

3. A. Motor neuron disease

This picture of mixed upper and lower motor neuron signs, coupled with a lack of sensory deficit, raises the possibility of motor neuron disease. Diagnosis is via a combination of brain and spinal cord MRI to rule out structural disorders, lumbar puncture to exclude inflammatory disease, and neurophysiology to rule out mimicking motor neuropathies. Unfortunately, only riluzole is thought to extend life, and this is by an average of three months only.

Longmore M et al., *Oxford Handbook of Clinical Medicine*, Eighth Edition, Oxford University Press, 2010, Chapter 10, Neurology, Motor neuron disease (MND)

4. E. Ropinirole

Ropinirole is a non-ergot dopamine agonist used in the initial management of Parkinson's disease in an attempt to delay use of L-dopa. Benzhexol is an anti-cholinergic which may reduce tremor but with increasing risk of confusion in the elderly. Selegiline is a MAO-B inhibitor; side effects include postural hypotension and increased risk of atrial fibrillation. Apomorphine is given by subcutaneous infusion and is normally used late in the disease.

Longmore M et al., *Oxford Handbook of Clinical Medicine*, Eighth Edition, Oxford University Press, 2010, Chapter 10, Neurology, Parkinson's disease (PD).

5. B. Posterior communicating artery aneurysm

Diplopia and sluggish or absent reaction to light is most likely due to compression injury to the oculomotor nerve (cranial nerve III). Pupillary dilatation and sluggish or absent reaction to light result from involvement of parasympathetic fibres that originate in the Edinger–Westphal subnucleus of the third cranial nerve complex and are situated very superficially within the nerve trunk, and hence are damaged by compression injury most often seen with posterior communicating artery aneurysm. A third nerve palsy with pupillary sparing is often termed a medical third palsy and frequently has an ischaemic or diabetic aetiology. The ischaemic injury will damage the inner tissues of the nerve trunk and spare the superficial parasympathetic fibres which have an alternative blood supply. The pupil is never involved in myasthenia gravis or other ocular myopathy although these patients typically present with diplopia. Internuclear ophthalmoplegia (INO) is the most common ocular motility dysfunction in MS. The patient will manifest an adduction deficit on the involved side and a nystagmus of the fellow eye in extreme abduction. It is caused by lesions through the medial longitudinal fasciculus (MLF) in the pons. The pupil is not involved.

Dimopoulos VG et al., Literature review regarding the methodology of assessing third nerve paresis associated with non-ruptured posterior communicating artery aneurysms, *Neurosurgical Review* 2005;28(4):256–260.

6. E. Sagittal sinus thrombosis

These symptoms are consistent with a cerebral sinus thrombosis, of which a sagittal sinus thrombosis is the most likely (47% of events) versus 35% for transverse sinus thrombosis. The history of a previous deep vein thrombosis raises the possiblity of an inherited thrombophilic disorder. CT may be normal in the early stages and the raised intracranial pressure supports the diagnosis. Heparin may be of value in improving outcome.

Longmore M et al., *Oxford Handbook of Clinical Medicine*, Eighth Edition, Oxford University Press, 2010, Chapter 10, Neurology, Intracranial venous thrombosis (IVT).

7. A. Cavernous sinus thrombosis

Cavernous sinus syndrome typically presents with a progressive ophthalmoplegia involving any or all of the ipsilateral third, fourth, and sixth cranial nerves, with associated ptosis and miosis, and numbness in the ophthalmic and sometimes the maxillary divisions of the fifth cranial nerve. There may also be headache and/or proptosis. The differential diagnosis of a cavernous sinus syndrome is wide, being broadly classified into: tumours (e.g. meningioma, nasopharyngeal tumour, pituitary, metastatic); thrombosis (often following a local sinus or dental infection); infection (e.g. Herpes zoster, fungal); inflammation (e.g. Tolosa–Hunt, neurosarcoidosis, Wegener's); vascular (e.g. carotid artery aneurysm, A-V fistula); trauma. MRI and gadolinium of the orbits may show a mass or inflammatory changes. MR angiography may reveal a carotid artery aneurysm or A-V fistula. MR venography may suggest thrombosis, although a normal MRV does not exclude the diagnosis.

Kattah JC, Cavernous sinus syndrome, *Medscape*, February 2014. http://emedicine.medscape.com/article/1161710-overview

8. A. Behçet's disease

This man presents with a recurrent meningitis. The CSF is essentially normal, with the white cell count (all lymphocytes) and protein at the upper end of the normal range. Bacterial cultures are negative. This would therefore be described as an aseptic meningitis. Drug reactions, Lyme disease, and viruses such as Coxsackie, echovirus, and HIV can all cause an aseptic meningitis, but they would not be recurrent as in this case. Recurrent aseptic meningitis is typically caused by a systemic inflammatory or granulomatous process, such as Behçet's disease, SLE, Wegener's granulomatosis, sarcoidosis, or TB. The question stem includes a number of symptoms of Behçet's disease—uveitis, oral herpetiform ulcers, and an acneiform papulopustular rash over the trunk—pointing to this as the likely diagnosis. Other features include oral aphthous ulcers, genital ulcers, a non-deforming arthropathy, and erythema nodosum.

Alnaimat FA, Behçet's disease, *Medscape*, April 2016. http://emedicine.medscape.com/article/329099-overview

9. B. Total anterior circulation stroke

This man has suffered from a total anterior circulation stroke (TACS). The Bamford stroke classification is as follows: (1) Total anterior circulation stroke (TACS). All three of: unilateral motor or sensory deficit (two or three of face, arm, and leg), higher function dysfunction (receptive or expressive dysphasia, inattention/neglect), and homonymous hemianopia. (2) Partial anterior circulation stroke (PACS). Two out of three of the features for a TACS. (3) Lacunar infarct. Five lacunar syndromes exist: pure motor weakness (presenting with unilateral motor weakness with the thrombus within the corona radiate as it passes through the basal ganglia), pure sensory loss (lesion to the contralateral thalamus), mixed sensorimotor (lesion to the thalamus and adjacent internal capsule), ataxic hemiparesis (lesion within the internal capsule and pons), and dysarthria or clumsy hand (pons lesion). (4) Posterior circulation stroke (POCS). This may be associated with any of the following: cranial nerve palsy and contralateral motor/sensory defect, bilateral motor or sensory defect, eye movement problems (e.g. nystagmus), cerebellar dysfunction, and isolated homonymous hemianopia. The MRC power grades are as follows: (0) No movement. (1) A flicker of movement or fasciculations are present. (2) Movement with the force of gravity. (3) Anti-gravity power is present. (4) Reduced muscle strength but the muscle is able to move against resistance. (5) Muscle contracts normally against resistance.

Manji H et al., *Oxford Handbook of Neurology*, Oxford University Press, 2006, Chapter 4, Neurological disorders, Cerebrovascular disease: stroke.

10. C. Carotid ultrasound

The major concern would be to rule out the possibility of carotid disease leading to vascular insufficiency and seizures, as intervention may be possible. An MRI may be useful in defining the cause of epilepsy as it will reveal possible structural abnormalities. EEG is difficult to interpret in the elderly population because of pre-existing cerebrovascular disease. Starting sodium valproate without defining the cause of the seizures is not advisable.

Ramrakha PS et al., *Oxford Handbook of Acute Medicine*, Third Edition, Oxford University Press, 2010.

11. C. HMSN-X

The picture of distal motor and sensory loss coupled with pes cavus and diminished reflexes fits best with hereditary motor and sensory neuropathy (HSMN). The comparison with the more mild symptoms in the patient's mother suggests that he has the X-linked semi-dominant form, linked to a mutation in connexin-32. HMSN-2 tends to be associated with milder symptomatology.

Bradley-Smith G et al., *Oxford Handbook of Genetics*, Oxford University Press, 2009, Chapter 5, Common genetic conditions, Hereditary motor sensory neuropathy (HMSN/CMT).

12. B. Subarachnoid haemorrhage

The most likely diagnosis here is a subarachnoid haemorrhage (SAH), which would certainly need to be excluded. The incidence is approximately 8 per 100,000 and would normally account for 3% of the patients presenting to emergency departments with headache. The prognosis is poor with up to half of patients dying and a third of survivors remaining dependent. Early diagnosis and treatment is key. The headache of SAH typically peaks within seconds to minutes and lasts for more than one hour. It may be associated with meningitic features such as nuchal rigidity, nausea and vomiting, and light intolerance/photophobia. SAH should also be considered in the differential diagnosis of someone presenting with an acute deterioration in GCS. SAH is more common in those who have pre-exisiting cardiovascular disease and who smoke, are hypertensive, and drink more than recommended quantities of alcohol. Subarachnoid haemorrhage is graded in various ways but the most common is the WFNS classification which utilizes the GCS. The grades are: grade I: GCS 15 with no focal neurological deficits; grade II: GCS 13–14 with no focal neurological deficits; grade III: GCS 13–14 with focal neurological deficit; grade IV: GCS 7–12 with or without focal neurological deficit; grade V: GCS < 7 with or without focal neurological deficit. Management requires an urgent CT scan. If negative, a 12-hour lumbar puncture should be performed for haemoglobin breakdown products in the CSF (xanthochromia). SAH patients should be transferred to a neurosurgical unit for ongoing treatment but initial treatments should include oral nimodipine 60 mg every four hours and intravenous fluids (both to prevent cerebral vasospasm). Endovascular aneurysmal coiling is preferred to clipping in most circumstances.

Al-Shahi R et al., Subarachnoid haemorrhage, *British Medical Journal* 2006;333:235–240.

13. C. 3%

Untreated, the risk of stroke is often estimated using the CHADS2 score. This scoring system helps to predict annual risk of stroke so that informed decisions can be made about treatment. The risk of stroke increases as the number of points increases. Individual circumstances are considered when deciding treatment. However, in the absence of other factors, patients with a score of 0 are usually treated with aspirin. Those with a score of 1 may be given aspirin or warfarin, and those with 2 or more are advised to take warfarin. In this case, the patient has a score of 1 for her age, and so according to this data her risk is about 2.8%. The best answer here is therefore 3%.

Gage BF et al., Validation of clinical classification schemes for predicting stroke, Results from the National Registry of Atrial Fibrillation, *Journal of the American Medical Association* 2001;285:2864–2870.

14. E. Todd's paresis after a convulsion

It is highly likely this woman had a focal seizure with secondary generalization related to her previous stroke prior to admission and that her limb weakness is due to Todd's paresis. Of patients with stroke 11.5% are at risk of developing post-stroke seizures by five years. Dementia with Lewy bodies may present with profound variations in either cognitive or physical function and even syncopal attacks; however, focal neurological deficits would be unusual. Although cardiac syncope could result in cerebral hypoxia, thereby inducing a transient ischaemic attack or seizure, there is no evidence of a history of cardiac disease and the ECG is reassuring.

A Stokes–Adams attack is therefore unlikely. Transient global amnesia and transient ischaemic attacks are not associated with loss of or an altered state of consciousness, with the rare exception of brainstem ischaemia.

Myint PK et al., Post-stroke seizure and post-stroke epilepsy, *Postgraduate Medical Journal* 2006;82:568–572, doi:10.1136/pgmj.2005.041426. http://pmj.bmj.com/content/82/971/568

15. E. Carcinoid syndrome

NF1 is an autosomal dominant condition caused by a mutation on chromosome 17. It affects neural crest cells, which proliferate. The tumours caused are usually benign but can undergo malignant transformation. There are a variety of dermatological and other manifestations. There are some criteria used for diagnosis, and the diagnosis can be made if two or more of these are found (see Box 2.1). All the options are part of this criteria except carcinoid syndrome. Carcinoid syndrome is a rare complication of this condition, but is not part of the criteria. Phaeochromocytoma has a slightly greater association with NF1, and must be considered if the patient presents with symptoms or signs which may be suggestive (e.g. hypertension).

Longmore M et al., *Oxford Handbook of Clinical Medicine*, Ninth Edition, Oxford University Press, 2010, Chapter 10, Neurology, Neurofibromatosis.

16. D. It is a medical emergency and treatment should begin within hours of diagnosis

Lung, prostate, and breast cancer are the malignancies most frequently associated with spinal cord compression, accounting for around 60% of cases in total. Multiple myeloma, non-Hodgkins lymphoma, and renal cell carcinoma account for most of the remaining cases. Metastatic thyroid cancer can cause spinal cord compression but it is much less common. Although up to 80% of patients will demonstrate motor weakness at the time of diagnosis, worsening back pain, often in a radicular distribution, is the most common initial symptom and typically precedes weakness by 1–2 months. By the time the diagnosis of malignant spinal cord compression is confirmed most patients are no longer ambulatory. Once a patient has become paraplegic <5% will recover the ability to walk, despite treatment. Patients who are ambulatory at diagnosis have a median survival of around six months, compared to only 1–3 months for those who were non-ambulatory at diagnosis. For this reason, worsening back pain in a patient with known malignancy must never be overlooked. Investigations should be carried out urgently. Almost all patients benefit from urgent treatment within hours (usually radiotherapy), in order that quality of life is maximized. In carefully selected patients, surgery followed by radiotherapy offers the optimum chance of regaining useful function, hence the need to discuss all patients with neurosurgical or oncology teams as soon as possible.

Cassidy J et al., *Oxford Handbook of Oncology*, Third Edition, Oxford University Press, 2010, Chapter 31, Spinal cord compression and bone marrow suppression.

17. C. Lateral medullary syndrome

The diagnosis here is lateral medullary syndrome. This diagnosis comes as a consequence of occlusion of any of the five arteries: vertebral, posterior inferior cerebellar, or superior, middle, or inferior lateral medullary arteries. Lesions in the lateral medulla cause primarily sensory and cerebellar problems with relative motor sparing (the pyramids being located in the medial medulla). Lesions here involve the vestibular nuclei (causing vertigo, nystagmus, oscilloscopia, vomiting); spinothalamic tract (causing contralateral sensory loss—this site is prior to the spinothalamic decussation); descending sympathetic tract (causing an ipsilateral Horner's syndrome); otolithic

---

Box 2.1 Diagnostic criteria for neurofibromatosis

NFL (von Recklinghausen's disease)

Diagnosis is made if 2 of the following are found:

≥6 café-au-lait macules >5 mm (prepubertal) or >15 mm (post-pubertal)

≥2 neurofibromas of any type or 1 plexiform

Freckling in the axillary or inguinal regions

Optic glioma

≥2 Lisch nodules

Distinctive osseous lesion typical of NF1, e.g. sphenoid dysplasia

First-degree relative with NF1 according to the above criteria

Differential:

McCune—Albright syndrome (OHCS p649), multiple lentigenes, urticaria pigmentosa

NF2

Diagnosis is made if either of the following are found:

Bilateral vestibular Schwannomas seen on MRI or CT

First-degree relative with NF2, and either:

(a) Unilateral vestibular Schwannoma; or

(b) One of the following:

• Neurofibroma

• Meningioma

• Glioma

• Schwannoma

• Juvenile cataract (NF2 type)

Differential:

NF1, Schwannomatosis

Adapted from Longmore M et al., *Oxford Handbook of Clinical Medicine*, Ninth Edition, 2014 with permission from Oxford University Press.

---

nuclei (causing vertical diplopia); spinocerebellar tracts (causing ipsilateral ataxia), and the descending fibres and nucleus of the trigeminal nerve (causing impaired sensation of the ipsilateral face). Fragmentary syndromes also exist with variations on the lesions seen. Treatment is via secondary prevention as with most cerebrovascular syndromes, and physiotherapy, and patients often recover good function afterwards.

Manji H et al., *Oxford Handbook of Neurology*, Oxford University Press, 2006, Chapter 4, Neurological disorders.

18. A. CT chest

Approximately 15% of myasthenics have a thymoma evident on CT chest, and the majority achieve better control of their myasthenia after thymectomy. Thymomas are benign tumours of the thymus gland. PSA and CT chest/abdomen/pelvis would be indicated if a diagnosis of Lambert–Eaton myasthenic syndrome was suspected, as prostatic carcinoma is one of the more common causes, but there is no association with myasthenia.

Skeie GO et al., European Federation Guidelines on treatment for myasthenia, *European Journal of Neurology* 2010, doi:10.1111/j.1468-1331.2010.03019.x. http://www.efns.org/fileadmin/user_upload/guidline_papers/EFNS_guideline_2010_autoimmune_neuromuscular_transmission_disorders.pdf

19. E. Cryptogenic stroke due to paradoxical embolism

This man has a patent foramen ovale (PFO) causing cerebral artery occlusion. The action of bending forward to tie his shoelaces is a Valsalva manoeuvre. An embolus would have traversed from the right atrium to the left to then enter the left middle cerebral artery resulting in an ischaemia/infarct to that territory. A bubble-contrast echocardiogram would demonstrate the patency of the PFO.

Longmore M et al., *Oxford Handbook of Clinical Medicine*, Eighth Edition, Oxford University Press, 2010, Chapter 10, Neurology, Stroke

20. A. Tabes dorsalis

This patient is most likely to suffer from tabes dorsalis or tabetic neurosyphilis. Characteristically, tabes dorsalis presents initially with neuropathic pain usually in the legs, although the upper limbs and body may be involved as well. Patients then go on to develop urge incontinence and eventually a sensory ataxia as the dorsal columns become more involved. This may present with falls, especially at night when visual information is limited. The areflexia is thought to be due to the dorsal column loss resulting in less proprioceptive information arriving to the spinal reflex arc. CSF examination may show a pleocytosis. Continued, untreated tabes dorsalis may eventually lead to a neuropathic joint or Charcot joints in which there is a painless destruction of the joints (especially ankles and knees). Treatment is of the infection although the neurological impairment is unlikely to recover.

Manji H et al., *Oxford Handbook of Neurology*, Oxford University Press, 2006, Chapter 4, Neurological disorders, Chronic inflammatory demyelinating polyneuropathy (CIDP).

21. B. Anti-voltage-gated potassium antibodies

This is limbic encephalitis associated with anti-voltage-gated potassium antibodies. Of these patients 71% present with cognitive impairment, with a further 10% presenting with hallucinations. Patients may present with more subtle neuropsychiatric changes such as a change in personality and memory difficulties (representing the frontotemporal component) or with depression or agitation. A minority of patients may present with parkinsonism, tremor, or chorea. MR imaging demonstrates high signal in the limbic structures especially on T2 sequences. Other sites may be involved as well (i.e. brainstem). Electroencephalogram shows foci of epileptic activity in the temporal lobes and occasionally focal or generalized slowing. Cerebrospinal fluid analysis may show a raised protein, pleocytosis with a predominance of lymphocytes, and unpaired oligoclonal bands. The principal tumour types associated with limbic encephalitis are: lung, testicle, Hodgkin's lymphoma, teratoma, and thymoma.

Gozzard P, Maddison P, Which antibody and which cancer in which paraneoplastic syndromes? *Practical Neurology* 2010;10:260–270.

22. A. Forced vital capacity

This man presents with a typical history for Guillain–Barré syndrome, with an ascending numbness and weakness over several days. It is commonly associated with back pain. Triggers include diarrhoeal illness (especially *Campylobacter jejuni*) and upper respiratory tract infections. Appropriate investigations include imaging the spine to look for a cord compression or tranverse myelitis, and analysis of the CSF looking for a raised protein typical of Guillain-Barré syndrome. However, the most immediate threat to his safety is neuromuscular respiratory failure due to weakness of the respiratory muscles, which needs immediate assessment then monitoring, with measurements of forced vital capacity (FVC) every four hours. If the FVC is falling, ITU will need to be made aware that he may need ventilatory support soon. Cardiac monitoring is also necessary in severe cases of Guillain–Barré syndrome due to the risk of arrhythmias (from vagal nerve involvement). Nerve conduction studies are not generally performed for Guillain–Barré syndrome unless there is some doubt about the diagnosis, but if performed they would be expected to show a demyelinating neuropathy. Guillain–Barré syndrome is one of the acute inflammatory demyelinating polyradiculoneuropathies (AIDP—others include the Miller Fisher variant). It is monophasic, and therefore treatment with IVIg is needed only once. In contrast, chronic inflammatory demyelinating polyradiculoneuropathy (CIDP) is, as the name suggests, a chronic and relapsing disease, and so regular treatment with IVIg every 2–3 months is usually necessary for symptom control.

Guillain-Barre Syndrome et al., Guillain-Barre syndrome, *Medscape*. http://emedicine.medscape.com/article/315632-overview

23. B. Anti-Yo antibodies

This is paraneoplastic cerebellar degeneration associated with anti-Yo antibodies. The antibodies are directed against the Purkinje cells of the cerebellum. A hundred percent of patients present with a subacute (i.e. three months) cerebellar syndrome comprising of limb ataxia followed by truncal ataxia. Eventually dysarthria and dysphagia also occur. Downbeat nystagmus is often seen on examination. Alongside this 47% of patients develop hyporeflexia, or a mild sensory disturbance as a peripheral neuropathy can also occur. Emotional lability and memory deficits may occur in 18% of patients. MR imaging is usually normal; occasionally cerebellar swelling and contrast enhancement may be seen in the acute phase. Cerebellar atrophy is seen in the chronic phase only. Cerebrospinal fluid analysis may show a raised protein, pleocytosis with a predominance of lymphocytes, and unpaired oligoclonal bands. The principal underlying tumour types are (in descending order): lung, gynaecological, Hodgkin's lymphoma, breast, thymoma, and testicle cancer.

Gozzard P, Maddison P, Which antibody and which cancer in which paraneoplastic syndromes? *Practical Neurology* 2010;10:260–270.

24. E. Rhabdomyolysis

The possibility of rhabdomyolysis should be considered in any intoxicated patient with acute muscle weakness. Ethanol is not a well-recognized cause of acute non-traumatic rhabdomyolysis. However, it is a well-known cause of chronic myopathy. In alcohol-related acute muscle injury cases, other mechanisms may also be playing a role (i.e. the patient may be comatose and lying in one position for a prolonged period causing continuous pressure on certain parts of the body). This would result in muscle compression and capillary occlusion, leading to ischaemia and subsequent rhabdomyolysis. The usual complication of acute rhabdomyolysis is acute renal failure. When more groups of muscles are injured, myoglobin is deposited in renal tubules causing acute renal failure and myoglobinuria (dark red-coloured urine). In cauda equina lesions and Guillain-Barré syndrome there is often associated sensory and reflex loss. Subdural haematoma needs to be seriously considered as there is a higher incidence in this group of patients and the initial presentation could be generalized weakness and inability to walk. The CT scan of the brain is very sensitive during the acute stage. Osteomalacia can be encountered in patients with chronic alcoholism and liver disease. The proximal muscle weakness is often gradual and of insidious onset.

Sauret JM et al., Rhabdomyolysis, *American Family Physician* 2002;65(5):907–912.

25. A. Dural sinus thrombosis

Dural venous sinus thrombosis typically presents with a progressive headache (though thunderclap headache is also possible), culminating in venous infarcts that are often haemorrhagic. They are commonly associated with seizures. There may be focal neurological signs due to cerebral infarction, or they may be silent, as in this case. There may be a history of a prothrombotic state, dehydration, or local ENT infection or inflammation (e.g. in the sphenoid or maxillary sinus) prior to the onset of the headache. The CT findings in this case suggest haemorrhage with surrounding oedema, which is consistent with either a haemorrhagic infarct or a subarachnoid haemorrhage. The prolonged history and two areas of signal abnormality argue against subarachnoid haemorrhage. Neurocysticercosis may present with headaches and seizures (it is the most common acquired cause of seizures in the developing world), but there are typically multiple high signal ring lesions (cysts with a calcified rim). In dural sinus thrombosis CT may, but does not always, show a delta sign, caused by thrombus in the sagittal sinus. MR venography may show the absence of a sinus, although the absence of a transverse sinus may also occur as a normal variant. MRI with T2* gradient echo helps to visualize the thrombus and infarction directly. The key feature that distinguishes a venous infarct from an arterial one is when it crosses multiple arterial territories. Dural sinus thrombosis with venous infarcts is a medical emergency requiring immediate treatment with an IV heparin infusion, even if haemorrhage is present. The thrombosis causes venous stasis, and therefore reduced oxygen delivery to the area of cortex drained by that vein. Infarction leads to cytotoxic oedema and ultimately death due to brainstem herniation. The increased pressure in the capillary beds makes haemorrhage into the infarct much more likely than in arterial infarcts. If there is extensive oedema, referral to a neurosurgical unit may be necessary for decompressive craniotomy. A loading dose of phenytoin may be given for symptomatic treatment of seizures, followed by regular dosing (e.g. 100 mg TDS IV).

Patel MR et al., Brain imaging in venous sinus thrombosis, *Medscape*, 2011. http://emedicine.medscape.com/article/338750-overview

26. B. Goldmann field perimetry

Idiopathic intracranial hypertension (IIH, also called pseudotumor cerebri) presents with signs and symptoms suggestive of an intracranial mass when in fact none is present: headache that is worse when lying, bending over, straining, or coughing; blurred vision; reduced peripheral vision; papilloedema; tinnitus; diplopia (sixth cranial nerve palsy); nausea/vomiting. Risk factors include obesity, the oral contraceptive pill, tetracycline antibiotics, atypical cerebral venous drainage, and several systemic disorders including anaemia, obstructive sleep apnoea, Behçet's, and SLE. Management consists of excluding an intracranial mass with CT or MRI, and confirming the diagnosis of raised intracranial pressure by lumbar puncture (opening pressure >25 mmCSF). Plain CT or MRI should be sufficient to exclude a tumour—if a tumour were exerting sufficient mass effect to present with papilloedema it should be readily apparent and contrast imaging should not be necessary. If there are atypical features (such as focal neurological signs), MR venography is important to look for dural sinus thrombosis. Untreated, IIH can lead to permanent visual loss, so the decision on whether to treat medically is based on the risk to the patient's vision. Weight loss is the single most effective way of reducing the morbidity associated with IIH and preventing recurrence—as little as 5–10% weight loss may be sufficient. However, if there is evidence of reduced peripheral vision on formal (Goldmann or Humphrey) perimetry then treatment with acetazolamide should be started immediately. Progress should be followed with serial perimetry rather than lumbar puncture for the same reason. Medically resistant IIH can be treated surgically either with a ventriculo-peritoneal shunt (preferably), or with optic nerve sheath fenestration.

Longmore M et al., *Oxford Handbook of Clinical Medicine*, Eighth Edition, Oxford University Press, 2010, Chapter 10, Neurology, Idiopathic intracranial hypertension.

27. E. Alcohol excess

This presentation is strongly suggestive of a mononeuritis multiplex. Causes of this include diabetes mellitus, sarcoid, cancer, PAN, amyloid, leprosy, and Lyme disease. Alcohol causes peripheral neuropathy but not mononeuritis multiplex.

Simon C et al., *Oxford Handbook of General Practice*, Third Edition, Oxford University Press, 2009, Chapter 16, Neurology, Neuropathy.

28. E. Anosmia

Parkinson's Plus syndromes present with a variable degree of parkinsonism, and a variety of other features that are not found in the early stages of idiopathic Parkinson's disease. Lewy body dementia: visual hallucinations, marked fluctuation in cognition from day to day. Vascular parkinsonism: legs more affected than arms, marche à petit pas, pyramidal signs. Multiple system atrophy: autonomic features (postural hypotension, bladder dysfunction), pyramidal signs, rigidity more prominent than tremor, cerebellar signs. Progressive supranuclear palsy: supranuclear gaze palsy, no tremor, truncal rigidity, symmetrical onset, postural instability, dysphagia. Cortico-basal degeneration: asymmetrical akinetic rigidity, apraxia, alien limb phenomenon, cortical sensory loss (e.g. astereognosis). Anosmia is one of the more common non-motor features of idiopathic Parkinson's disease, and often precedes the onset of motor symptoms by a few years.

Longmore M et al., *Oxford Handbook of Clinical Medicine*, Eighth Edition, Oxford University Press, 2010, Chapter 10, Neurology: Parkinson's disease.

29. E. There is an increased risk of stroke in children

Whole brain radiotherapy for malignancy is associated with late side effects in the majority of surviving patients. Pituitary dysfunction is particularly prevalent and patients benefit from surveillance because serum hormone levels typically fall well before patients report symptoms. Over 90% will become growth hormone deficient. Thyroid dysfunction (via an effect on TSH) and gonadal failure (via LH/FSH), with potential infertility, are also common. Cranial irradiation in children is associated with a reduction in attention span, short-term memory, and IQ. Initially, this may be difficult to identify as verbal IQ is frequently preserved and hence the child can appear to be functioning well. In addition survivors of childhood leukaemias and brain tumours, treated with radiotherapy, have a significantly increased risk of CVA. This effect appears limited to protocols in which higher doses of radiation are used (>30 Gy) and may be exacerbated by other anti-cancer treatments received, such as certain chemotherapies. Radiation necrosis, due to fibrinoid necrosis of small arteries within the radiation field, most commonly occurs 1–3 years following radiation. Presentation may be with focal abnormalities, or more diffuse neurological symptoms such as seizures.

Bowers DC et al., Late occurring stroke among long-term survivors of childhood leukaemias and brain tumors: a report from the Childhood Cancer Survivor Study, *Journal of Clinical Oncology* 2006;24(33):5277–5282.

30. D. Progressive supranuclear palsy

The most likely diagnosis is progressive supranuclear palsy (PSP). The hallmarks of 'classic' PSP are a lurching gait (like that of a 'drunken sailor') and unexplained falls backwards. Usually most patients with PSP will develop personality changes, cognitive slowing, and executive dysfunction (associated with the developing frontal lobe dementia). Patients often get non-specific ocular symptoms such as: dry, red, and sore eyes, photophobia, blurred vision, and difficulty in focusing. The classic supranuclear palsy may not be present on initial presentation but may develop years into the disease. Limitation of downgaze is the most sensitive oculomotor change but eventually there is a limitation of upgaze as well. Patients may develop an apraxia of eyelid closure and reduced blink rate giving them a staring expression. This is heightened by the overactivation of frontalis, procerus, and corrugator muscles, which cause further eyelid retraction. PSP patients are said to have a 'worried' expression on their face due to these changes. Initial investigations might include an MRI of the brain which could show midbrain atrophy with enlargement of the third ventricle and interpenduncular fossa. There is often a hyperintense signal on T2-weighted images in the periaqueductal grey matter and globus pallidus. In keeping with the frontal lobe dementia there may be fronto-temporal lobe dementia. There are no good medications for PSP although amantidine could be tried. Eventually bulbar weakness develops leading to dysphagia. Aspiration pneumonia is the most common cause of death.

Williams DR, Lees AJ, Progressive supranuclear palsy: clinicopathological concepts and diagnostic challenges, *Lancet Neurology* 2009;8:270–279.

31. D. Radiation-induced neuropathy

This question may appear difficult, but if approached by excluding each of the more familiar options in turn, it becomes clear that only one answer fits the rather unusual clinical picture. Brachial neuritis is usually unilateral, but if bilateral, might cause the localized arm symptoms through inflammation of the brachial plexuses. Typically, it would not affect the neck (because the neck is supplied by the spinal accessory nerve rather than the brachial plexus), but rare variants may involve the lower cranial nerves too. However, onset of brachial neuritis is very acute and it is usually very painful. The history will often reveal a prodromal viral illness. Myasthenia and MND would be expected to present with more global symptoms, given the severity of the symptoms locally. Diabetic amyotrophy is a diabetic neuropathy affecting the lumbosacral plexus, and therefore presents with wasting and weakness of the legs, rather than the arms. It is often painful, and onset is proximal, affecting the thighs first. The remaining option is radiation damage to the brachial plexuses (arm weakness) and the spinal accessory nerves (neck weakness). The clinical symptoms of radiation neuropathy may occur many years after the original exposure, and may be progressive once it has started. It is caused by progressive fibrosis of the nerve fascicles and perineurium. Neuropathic pain is uncommon, occurring only in about 10% of cases. Radiation doses used for radiotherapy a few decades ago were far in excess of what is now considered necessary, so the occurrence of such side effects is more common in this age group. Radiation-induced brachial plexopathy is most commonly seen after radiotherapy for breast or apical lung cancer, and lymphoma in the cervical chain.

Stephenson RO et al., Radiation-induced brachial plexopathy, *Medscape*, 2015. http://emedicine.medscape.com/article/316497-overview

32. B. Enlarged ventricles without cortical atrophy

This man presents with the classic triad of gait disturbance, cognitive impairment, and urinary urgency/frequency, which points to a diagnosis of normal pressure hydrocephalus (NPH). The description of a gait in which the feet appeared almost glued to the floor is very characteristic. Brisk reflexes and extensor plantars without spastic tone are a common finding in NPH. The cognitive impairment is typically fronto-subcortical, with memory loss, poor concentration, inattention, executive dysfunction and difficulty processing complex information. Imaging with CT or MRI typically shows enlarged ventricles with no evidence of cortical atrophy (i.e. normal gyral volume and no prominent sulci). If cortical atrophy is seen then the ventricular enlargement is probably secondary to the atrophy (e.g. small vessel ischaemia) and not NPH. Where cortical atrophy is present, the bias towards atrophy of anterior or posterior structures creates an apparent gradient of atrophy that can be diagnostically helpful. Fronto-temporal dementia, for example, typically affect anterior structures first, while Alzheimer's typically involves parietal and hippocampal structures first.

Schneck MJ et al., Normal pressure hydrocephalus, *Medscape*, 2015. http://emedicine.medscape.com/article/1150924-overview

33. C. 8

The Glasgow Coma Scale (GCS) was developed to give a reliable, reproducible, and objective way of measuring a patient's neurological state after a head injury. The scale is made up of three components: eye, verbal, and motor responses. Best eye response (E) comprises four grades: (1) No eye opening. (2) Eye opening in response to pain. (3) Eye opening to speech. (4) Eyes opening spontaneously. Best verbal response (V) comprises five grades: (1) No verbal response. (2) Incomprehensible sounds (grunting/moaning). (3). Inappropriate words. (4) Confused. (5) Oriented. Best motor response (M) comprises six grades: (1) No motor response. (2) Extension to pain (decerebrate response). (3) Abnormal flexion to pain (decorticate response). (4) Flexion/Withdrawal to pain. (5) Localizes to pain (purposeful movements towards painful stimuli). (6) Obeys commands. The individual categories as well as the sum of the score are important. The patient in the example given would have a calculated GCS of 8/15, E2M4V2. The score is not only used to look at neurological function over time but it is also useful to classify brain injury into severity: severe, with GCS? 8; moderate, GCS 9–12; minor, GCS? 13.

Ramrakha PS et al., *Oxford Handbook of Acute Medicine*, Third Edition, Oxford University Press, 2010, Chapter 6, Neurological emergencies, Glasgow Coma Scale (GCS).

34. A. Amyotrophic lateral sclerosis

Amyotrophic lateral sclerosis is the most common disease within the family of disorders known as motor neurone disease (MND). There is typically a mixture of upper and lower motor neurone signs, affecting bulbar muscles and upper and lower limbs, but the presentation is very variable, especially in the early stages of the disease. This patient has typical UMN signs and symptoms of arms and legs, and probably of bulbar muscles given the dysphagia. Fasciculations and wasting may not be apparent until later on in the disease. About 20% of patients have symptoms of fronto-temporal dementia at the time of presentation, typified by emotional lability, impulsive, disinhibited, or irritable behaviour, and a preference for sweet foods. Other MND variants are progressive bulbar palsy (bulbar only; poor prognosis), primary lateral sclerosis (UMN only), and progressive muscular atrophy (LMN only; better prognosis). The most important principle when making the diagnosis of MND is to be certain that it is not an atypical variant of another, treatable disease. Common mimics include chronic inflammatory demyelinating polyneuropathy (CIDP), polymyositis, inclusion body myositis, and cervical spondylosis. There is no simple diagnostic test for MND. The revised El Escorial diagnostic criteria do, however, include EMG as supportive evidence.

Sathasivam S, Motor neurone disease: clinical features, diagnosis, diagnostic pitfalls and prognostic markers, *Singapore Medical Journal* 2010;51(5):367–372. http://smj.sma.org.sg/5105/5105ra1.pdf

35. C. Electromyography

Amyotrophic lateral sclerosis is the most common disease within the family of disorders known as motor neurone disease (MND). There is typically a mixture of upper and lower motor neurone signs, affecting bulbar muscles and upper and lower limbs, but the presentation is very variable, especially in the early stages of the disease. This patient has typical UMN signs and symptoms of arms and legs, and probably of bulbar muscles given the dysphagia. Fasciculations and wasting may not be apparent until later on in the disease. About 20% of patients have symptoms of frontotemporal dementia at the time of presentation, typified by emotional lability, impulsive, disinhibited, or irritable behaviour, and a preference for sweet foods. Other MND variants are progressive bulbar palsy (bulbar only; poor prognosis), primary lateral sclerosis (UMN only), and progressive muscular atrophy (LMN only; better prognosis). The most important principle when making the diagnosis of MND is to be certain that it is not an atypical variant of another, treatable disease. Common mimics include chronic inflammatory demyelinating polyneuropathy (CIDP), polymyositis, inclusion body myositis, and cervical spondylosis. There is no simple diagnostic test for MND. The revised El Escorial diagnostic criteria do, however, include EMG as supportive evidence.

Longmore M et al., *Oxford Handbook of Clinical Medicine*, Eighth Edition, Oxford University Press, 2010, Chapter 10, Neurology: Motor neuron disease.

36. A. Normal pressure hydrocephalus

This man presents with the classic triad of gait disturbance, cognitive impairment, and urinary urgency/frequency, which points to a diagnosis of normal pressure hydrocephalus (NPH). The description of a gait in which the feet appeared almost glued to the floor is very characteristic. Brisk reflexes and extensor plantars without spastic tone are a common finding in NPH. The cognitive impairment is typically fronto-subcortical, with memory loss, poor concentration, inattention, executive dysfunction, and difficulty processing complex information. Vascular dementia can look similar, and he has one risk factor for it—hypertension—but it would not account for the urinary symptoms, and the gait disturbance is classical. Similarly, Alzheimer's would not cause a gait disturbance or urinary symptoms. MSA could cause the combination of urinary symptoms, cognitive impairment, and gait disturbance, but you would expect extrapyramidal signs such as cogwheel rigidity, and a rather more Parkinsonian gait. Imaging with CT or MRI typically shows enlarged ventricles with no evidence of cortical atrophy (i.e. normal gyral volume and no prominent sulci). If cortical atrophy is seen then the ventricular enlargement is probably secondary to the atrophy (e.g. small vessel ischaemia) and not NPH. The aim of a tap test is to demonstrate improvement in gait and cognitive function after the removal of a significant quantity of CSF. The patient should have an MMSE and be timed and videoed walking 10 metres, before, one hour after, and 24 hours after a lumbar puncture in which up to 50 ml CSF should be removed. The reason for performing the test is to demonstrate that benefit would be gained from insertion of a ventriculo-peritoneal shunt, and so should not be performed (just to prove the diagnosis) if the patient would not be a suitable candidate for a neurosurgical procedure.

Schneck MJ et al., Normal pressure hydrocephalus, *Medscape*, 2015. http://emedicine.medscape.com/article/1150924-overview

37. A. Lumbar puncture tap test

This man presents with the classic triad of gait disturbance, cognitive impairment, and urinary urgency/frequency, which points to a diagnosis of normal pressure hydrocephalus (NPH). The description of a gait in which the feet appeared almost glued to the floor is very characteristic. Brisk reflexes and extensor plantars without spastic tone are a common finding in NPH. The cognitive impairment is typically fronto-subcortical, with memory loss, poor concentration, inattention, executive dysfunction, and difficulty processing complex information. Vascular dementia can look similar, and he has one risk factor for it—hypertension—but it would not account for the urinary symptoms, and the gait disturbance is distinct. Similarly, Alzheimer's would not cause a gait disturbance or urinary symptoms. MSA could cause the combination of urinary symptoms, cognitive impairment, and gait disturbance, but you would expect extrapyramidal signs such as cogwheel rigidity, and a rather more Parkinsonian gait. The aim of a tap test is to demonstrate improvement in gait and cognitive function after the removal of a significant quantity of CSF. The patient should have an MMSE and be timed and videoed walking 10 metres, before, one hour after, and 24 hours after a lumbar puncture in which up to 50 ml CSF should be removed. The reason for performing the test is to demonstrate that benefit would be gained from insertion of a ventriculo-peritoneal shunt, and so should not generally be performed just to prove the diagnosis if the patient would not be a suitable candidate for a neurosurgical procedure. Imaging with CT or MRI typically shows enlarged ventricles with no evidence of cortical atrophy (i.e. normal gyral volume and no prominent sulci). If cortical atrophy is seen then the ventricular enlargement is probably secondary to the atrophy (e.g. small vessel ischaemia) and not NPH.

Schneck MJ et al., Normal pressure hydrocephalus, *Medscape*, 2015. http://emedicine.medscape.com/article/1150924-overview

38. C. Sumatriptan

This woman presents with a typical history for common migraine (migraine without aura). It is severe enough to warrant treatment with a prophylactic agent. Sumatriptan is of course an acute treatment for migraine rather than a prophylactic. First-line prophylactic agents for migraine are propranolol, amitriptyline, and topiramate. Other second-line options include pizotifen, anti-convulsants such as sodium valproate, lamotrigine, and gabapentin, and calcium-channel blockers such as verapamil and flunarizine. Pizotifen is as effective as the first-line prophylactics, but often causes weight gain that would be unwelcome in a young woman.

Fenstermacher N et al., Pharmacological prevention of migraine, *British Medical Journal* 2011;342, doi: http://dx.doi.org/10.1136/bmj.d583. http://www.bmj.com/content/342/bmj.d583.long

39. C. Topiramate

This woman presents with a typical history for common migraine (migraine without aura). It is severe enough to warrant treatment with a prophylactic agent. First-line prophylactic agents for migraine are propranolol, amitriptyline, and topiramate. Other second-line options include pizotifen, anti-convulsants such as sodium valproate, lamotrigine, and gabapentin, and calcium-channel blockers such as verapamil and flunarizine. Of the options offered here, only propranolol and topiramate would be first-line prophylactics for migraine, of which the propranolol is contraindicated due to the asthma. Pizotifen is as effective as the first-line prophylactics, but often causes weight gain that would be unwelcome in a young woman. Verapamil is more commonly used for cluster headache. Indomethacin is used for the treatment of hemicrania continua.

Fenstermacher N et al., Pharmacological prevention of migraine, *British Medical Journal* 2011;342, doi: http://dx.doi.org/10.1136/bmj.d583. http://www.bmj.com/content/342/bmj.d583.long

40. B. Lamotrigine

The history is suggestive of complex partial seizures. The SANAD trial suggests that the efficacy of lamotrigine is as good as carbamazepine for partial seizures, and better tolerated. Levetiracetam is increasingly being used as a first-line treatment for both primary generalized and partial seizures, but there is currently less evidence to support its use.

Marson AG et al., The SANAD study of effectiveness of carbamazepine, gabapentin, lamotrigine, oxcarbazepine, or topiramate for treatment of partial epilepsy: an unblinded randomised controlled trial, *Lancet* 2007;369(9566):1000–1015. http://www.ncbi.nlm.nih.gov/pmc/articles/PMC2080688/pdf/nihms-686.pdf

41. B. Vertebral artery dissection

This patient has signs and symptoms suggestive of a cerebellar insult. The sudden onset of symptoms is highly suggestive of a vascular event, in this case a cerebellar stroke. Vertebral artery dissection is most common in people in their 40s and 50s, and often follows awkward neck movements or minor neck trauma, such as star-gazing, RTAs, and sudden neck manoeuvres in chiropractice. The arterial dissection can cause either complete luminal occlusion, or a thrombogenic partial occlusion that throws off emboli. Atherosclerosis is certainly a possibility, but less likely in this age group without significant risk factors.

Lang ES et al., Vertebral artery dissection, *Medscape*, 2015. http://emedicine.medscape.com/article/761451-overview

42. A. Medication overuse headache

This is a common situation for migraineurs who take increasing amounts of simple analgesics when their migraines become more severe. The migrainous features of the headache become less apparent (i.e. the nausea, photophobia, auras, etc.) and the headache becomes constant and featureless. Paracetamol and codeine are the worst culprits for this, but non-steroidals and tramadol are nearly as bad. An MRI is of course indicated to exclude a space-occupying tumour, but it is an unlikely differential diagnosis. Management is by withdrawal of the offending medications before starting migraine prophylaxis—this is important because continuing use of the simple analgesia will continue to propagate the medication overuse headache and the patient will perceive that the migraine prophylaxis is not working. The patient must be educated as to the cause of the chronic headache and that use of simple analgesics should be limited to no more than six days per month.

Longmore M et al., *Oxford Handbook of Clinical Medicine*, Eighth Edition, Oxford University Press, 2010, Chapter 10, Neurology: Headache.

43. A. Obstructive sleep apnoea

Morning headaches are often associated with high intracranial pressure, due to the postural effect of lying down or bending over increasing intracranial pressure. However, obstructive sleep apnoea (OSA) also causes morning headaches (but not headaches later in the day that are worse when bending over). Other features of OSA include daytime somnolence and reduced libido. A partner may comment on loud snoring ± apnoeic episodes at night. Management is through weight loss, avoidance of tobacco and alcohol, and CPAP to support the airway at night.

Longmore M et al., *Oxford Handbook of Clinical Medicine*, Eighth Edition, Oxford University Press, 2010, Chapter 4, Chest Medicine: Obstructive sleep apnoea syndrome.

44. C. Pathergy testing

This man presents with a recurrent meningitis. The CSF is essentially normal, with the white cell count (all lymphocytes) and protein at the upper end of the normal range. Bacterial cultures are negative. This would therefore be described as an aseptic meningitis. Drug reactions, Lyme disease, and viruses such as Coxsackie, echovirus, and HIV can all cause an aseptic meningitis but they would not be recurrent as in this case. Recurrent aseptic meningitis is typically caused by a systemic inflammatory or granulomatous process, such as Behçet's disease, SLE, Wegener's granulomatosis, sarcoidosis, or TB. The question stem includes a number of symptoms of Behçet's disease—uveitis, oral herpetiform ulcers, and an acneiform papulopustular rash over the trunk—pointing to this as the likely diagnosis. Other features include oral aphthous ulcers, genital ulcers, a non-deforming arthropathy, and erythema nodosum. Pathergy testing leads to papule formation within 48 hours.

Alnaimat FA, Behçet's disease, *Medscape*, April 2016. http://emedicine.medscape.com/article/329099-overview

45. B. Leave her medication unchanged

Her cognitive impairment does not preclude adjusting her medication regime as she has a substantial care package to include medication supervision. However, the thrombocytopaenia precludes the use of any anti-platelet agent and her blood pressure is well controlled (optimal target < 130/80) so there is no need to adjust her antihypertensives. The PROGRESS trial compared the benefit of blood pressure lowering with perindopril (+/- inadpamide) with placebo. The group receiving combination therapy showed a significant reduction in risk for both ischaemic and haemorrhagic stroke. The group receiving perindopril monotherapy did not show this benefit. It seems likely that this reduction in risk resulted from the absolute reduction in blood pressure, rather than the actual agents used, although head-to-head trials would be needed to substantiate this. The evidence is not strong enough to warrant alterations in blood pressure treatments, providing satisfactory control is achieved. This patient's medication regime should therefore be left unchanged and investigations into the cause of her thrombocytopaenia undertaken. Unchecked, this may predispose to haemorrhagic stroke.

Nice Guidance [CG127], Hypertension in adults: diagnosis and management,

NICE guidelines [CG127] Published date: August 2011. https://www.nice.org.uk/guidance/CG127

46. A. Response to large volume lumbar puncture

The clinical picture is highly suspicious of normal pressure hydrocephalus. The response in terms of relief of symptoms to large volume lumbar puncture is highly predictive of long-term response to therapy. If symptoms are significantly improved then both repeated lumbar puncture and acetazolamide are potential options; otherwise, surgical shunt insertion is a possible longer-term solution.

Bowker LK et al., *Oxford Handbook of Geriatric Medicine*, Oxford University Press, 2006, Chapter 9, Psychiatry, Normal pressure hydrocephalus.

47. C. Finger prick glucose ('BM')

This gentleman's presentation, an acute onset of neurological deficit, should clearly raise the possibility of stroke. The most appropriate initial investigation however, is a bedside finger prick for glucose. Hypoglycaemia can cause a wide constellation of symptoms including neurological deficit, frequently mimicking an acute stroke. Current stroke assessment tools, such as the ROSIER scale (see further reading), advise treating a BM of less than 3.5 mmol/l and then re-evaluating the patient's neurology in the context of normoglycaemia. If the patient's BM is normal (or the neurological deficit remains after correction of hypoglycaemia) the next most appropriate test would be an urgent CT scan of the patient's head. The predominant reason for this is to exclude intracranial haemorrhage ahead of consideration for thrombolysis with alteplase. Patients with AF may well be warfarinized so an INR would clearly also be a useful test. In younger patients presenting with stroke an ESR is a useful test as a screening tool for cerebral vasculitides. In patients with a patient foramen ovale a so-called 'paradoxical embolus' may occur when thrombus formed in the deep venous system is able to traverse the heart and enter the left-sided circulation. It is therefore a rare cause of strokes.

NICE Guidance [CG68], Stroke and transient ischaemic attack in over 16s: diagnosis and initial management. https://www.nice.org.uk/guidance/Cg68

48. A. Inclusion body myositis

This man has the characteristic pattern of weakness found in inclusion body myositis. As with all myopathies, the pattern of weakness tends to be proximal, but in addition finger flexors and knee extensors are often profoundly affected. The waddling gait is a reflection of the proximal weakness in the legs. Pharyngeal muscles are also often disproportionately affected. Motor neurone disease would cause upper motor neurone signs such as extensor plantars in addition to weakness. Multifocal motor neuropathy would cause a predominantly distal pattern of weakness, and the gait would be high-stepping due to foot drop. A syrinx would typically cause a dissociated sensory loss before any motor involvement.

Collins MP, Inclusion body myositis, *Medscape*, 2015. http://emedicine.medscape.com/article/ 1172746-overview

49. A. Ovary

Paraneoplastic syndromes are incredibly rare non-metastatic neurological or endocrine syndromes associated with an underlying (often occult) tumour. They are caused either by the production of hormones by the tumour, or by the autoimmune response triggered by it. Paraneoplastic syndromes include: cerebellar degeneration (anti-Yo—ovary, lung breast; and anti-Hu—lung, prostate; anti-CV2—lung, thymoma), dermatomyositis (anti-Mi2 or anti-Jo—lung, pancreas, ovary, bowel), Lambert–Eaton myasthenic syndrome (anti-voltage-gated Ca^{2+} channel antibodies—lung, prostate), peripheral neuropathy (anti-Hu—lung, prostate; and anti-CV2—lung, thymoma), encephalitis (anti-Hu—lung, prostate; anti-CV2—lung, thymoma; anti-amphiphysin—breast, lung; and anti-Ma2—testis), ectopic hormone secretion (SIADH or Cushing's—small cell lung cancer; malignant hyperparathyroidism (parathyroid-related protein)—squamous cell lung cancer, breast, renal cell carcinoma).

Longmore M et al., *Oxford Handbook of Clinical Medicine*, Eighth Edition, Oxford University Press, 2010, Chapter 11, Oncology and palliative care: Tumour markers.

50. C. Intact accommodation reflex

Argyll Robertson pupils are typically small (2 mm), irregular in shape, and react poorly or not at all to light. The response to both accommodation and convergence remains intact. Visual acuity is usually normal. Dilation with mydriatic agents is typically poor. The dysfunction begins unilaterally and becomes bilateral with time. Horner's syndrome typically results in ptosis, miosis, and anhidrosis. Central scotoma is caused by lesions in the retinal fovea and is not a feature of Argyll Robertson pupils. Characteristics of the latter are as follows: (1) Syphilitic disease must be present. (2) There must be zero to trace reaction when stimulated by light. (3) The response to near objects should appear intact. (4) The pupil is frequently quite miotic. (5) The pupil often has an irregular shape. (6) The Argyll Robertson pupil is recalcitrant to pharmacologic dilation.

Manji H et al., *Oxford Handbook of Neurology*, Oxford University Press, 2006, Chapter 2, Neuroanatomy, the cranial cavity.

51. A. Medial longitudinal fasciculus

Ataxic nystagmus (i.e. nystagmus greater in contralateral abducting eye, with impaired adduction of the ipsilateral eye) is due to damage to medial longitudinal fasciculus causing an internuclear ophthalmoplegia: the lesion lies within the pons. Nystagmus is often bilateral in cerebellar, labyrinth, and vestibular disorders. Temporal lobe lesions are not associated with nystagmus.

Kennard C, Examine eye movements, *Practical Neurology* 2007;7:326–330.

52. E. Advice regarding the teratogenic risk of anti-convulsants to an unborn child

All of the answers are important things to discuss with patients newly diagnosed with epilepsy, except that of course the patient in this case is male, and so there is no risk to an unborn child in the way that there would be if the patient were female. Safety is of prime importance when counselling patients with seizures, avoiding situations where loss of consciousness would put them or others at risk. This includes not driving (a legal requirement), not swimming alone, standing back from the edge of train platforms, taking a shower instead of a bath, and avoiding unsecured heights such as ladders. Patients who take regular medications for epilepsy are exempt from prescription charges, and it is often forgotten that patients who are unable to drive due to their epilepsy are eligible to receive a Freedom Pass for public transport.

epilepsy action, Benefits for people with epilepsy. http://www.epilepsy.org.uk/info/entitlements/england

53. D. Gelineau syndrome

Demyelinated neurons rely on Na^+ channels to conduct impulses across demyelinated segments. These channels are very temperature sensitive, and cease to function properly as temperatures rise (e.g. with exercise or in a hot bath) causing slowing or even conduction block in affected neurons. This can temporarily worsen any MS symptom, but most characteristically causes Pulfrich's effect, where stereoscopic depth perception is lost due to delayed conduction in an affected optic nerve, and Uhthoff's phenomenon, where vision becomes blurred, again due to impaired conduction in the optic nerve. Lhermitte's sign is positive when flexion of the neck causes parasthesiae down the back or in the arms/legs. Lhermitte's sign is not specific to MS, and may also be positive in cervical stenosis. Spinal claudication can also cause exercise-induced leg symptoms. Marcus Gunn sign describes a relative afferent pupillary defect (RAPD), caused by poor light perception through one optic nerve relative to the other (i.e. if both are equally damaged there will not be an RAPD). Each pupil constricts normally to direct light stimulation, but when alternating light stimulation directly from one eye to the other and back again the pupil on the affected side continues to dilate when the light shines on it. This is because the consensual relaxation response predominates over the direct constriction response, which is reduced due to impaired conduction in the optic nerve on that side. Gelineau syndrome is of course the eponym associated with narcolepsy.

Longmore M et al., *Oxford Handbook of Clinical Medicine*, Eighth Edition, Oxford University Press, 2010, Chapter 10, Neurology, Multiple sclerosis.

54. D. Cerebrovascular disease

This man presents with typical features of, and risk factors for, vascular parkinsonism, caused by an infarct in the basal ganglia. Parkinson's Plus syndromes present with a variable degree of parkinsonism, and a variety of other features that are not found in the early stages of idiopathic Parkinson's disease. Lewy body dementia: visual hallucinations, marked fluctuation in cognition from day to day. Multiple system atrophy: autonomic features (postural hypotension, bladder dysfunction), cerebellar and pyramidal signs, rigidity > tremor. Progressive supranuclear palsy: supranuclear gaze palsy, no tremor, truncal rigidity, symmetrical onset, postural instability, dysphagia. Cortico-basal degeneration: asymmetrical akinetic rigidity, apraxia, alien limb phenomenon, cortical sensory loss (e.g. astereognosis). Vascular parkinsonism: legs more affected than arms, apraxic gait (marche à petit pas), pyramidal signs.

Longmore M et al., *Oxford Handbook of Clinical Medicine*, Eighth Edition, Oxford University Press, 2010, Chapter 10, Neurology: Parkinson's disease.

55. A. Cyanosis

The two most reliable pointers to true epileptic seizures are cyanosis and stertorous breathing, both due to tonic overactivity of the respiratory muscles during a seizure. Hip-thrusting and opisthotonus are more commonly associated with psychogenic seizures, while confusion, urinary incontinence, and even tongue biting cannot be wholly relied on.

Sen A et al., Stertorous breathing is a reliably identified sign that helps in the differentiation of epileptic from psychogenic non-epileptic convulsions: an audit, *Epilepsy Research* 2007;77:62–64. http://www. epires-journal.com/article/S0920-1211%2807%2900219-7/abstract

56. C. Central venous sinus thrombosis

The most likely diagnosis is cerebral venous sinus thrombosis (CVST). Of patients 75–95% of patients tend to present with a subacute onset of a global headache with the remainder suffering from a thunderclap type headache. The headaches of CVST are persistent and are exacerbated by transient increases in intracranial pressure that occur during coughing, sneezing, or other Valsalva manoeuvres. Headaches can also worsen when in the recumbent position and upon awakening. Most patients will present with complications of CVST which include seizures, papilloedema, altered level of consciousness, and focal neurological symptoms or signs. Of patients 15–30% present with an isolated headache. CVST is more common during puerperium. CT brain is normal in about 25% of patients and as such patients should have CT with contrast which will demonstrate venous filling defects as a first-line investigation. In those with focal neurological deficits, there are CT abnormalities in about 90% and can include venous infarcts, evidence of oedema or hyperdensity within the occluded sinus. CSF analysis reveals a high red blood cell count, high protein, and lymphocytic pleocytosis, or high opening pressure. MRI with venography is commonly needed for the diagnosis of CVST and should be considered whenever there is clinical suspicion for this disorder.

Manji H et al., *Oxford Handbook of Neurology*, Oxford University Press, 2006, Chapter 3, Common neurological presentations, Acute headache.

57. A. Anti-Yo

Paraneoplastic syndromes are incredibly rare non-metastatic neurological or endocrine syndromes associated with an underlying or even occult tumours. They are caused either by the production of hormones by the tumour, or by an autoimmune response triggered by it. Paraneoplastic syndromes include: cerebellar degeneration (anti-Yo—ovary, lung breast; and anti-Hu—lung, prostate; anti-CV2—lung, thymoma), dermatomyositis (anti-Mi2 or anti-Jo—lung, pancreas, ovary, bowel), Lambert Eaton myasthenic syndrome (anti-voltage-gated Ca^2? channel antibodies—lung, prostate), peripheral neuropathy (anti-Hu—lung, prostate; and anti-CV2—lung, thymoma), encephalitis (anti-Hu—lung, prostate; anti-CV2—lung, thymoma; anti-amphiphysin—breast, lung; and anti-Ma2—testis), ectopic hormone secretion (SIADH or Cushing's—small cell lung cancer; malignant hyperparathyroidism (parathyroid-related protein)—squamous cell lung cancer, breast, renal cell carcinoma).

Longmore M et al., *Oxford Handbook of Clinical Medicine*, Eighth Edition, Oxford University Press, 2010, Chapter 11, Oncology and palliative care: Tumour markers.

58. B. Non-REM sleep disorder

The non-motor symptoms of idiopathic Parkinson's disease include: depression, hallucinations (late stage), psychosis (late stage), REM behavioural sleep disorder (not non-REM sleep disorder, as in the question), dementia (late stage), falls, autonomic disturbance (bladder/bowels), pain (late stage), fatigue, and olfactory disturbance (often the very first symptom, prior to the onset of motor symptoms).

Longmore M et al., *Oxford Handbook of Clinical Medicine*, Eighth Edition, Oxford University Press, 2010, Chapter 10, Neurology: Parkinson's disease.

59. B. Miller Fisher syndrome

Miller Fisher syndrome is a variant of Guillain–Barré syndrome, occurring in approximately 5% of cases, associated with anti-GQ1b antibodies. It typically presents with progressive ataxia, ophthalmoplegia, and areflexia. The gait and truncal ataxia is characteristically disproportionate to the degree of limb ataxia. Power and sensation are usually not affected. Management is the same as for Guillain–Barré syndrome.

Andary MT et al., Guillain-Barre Syndrome, *Medscape*, 2016. http://emedicine.medscape.com/article/315632-overview

60. B. Left arm apraxia

This woman presents with features of cortico-basal degeneration, one of the Parkinson's Plus syndromes, including good descriptions of an apraxic left arm and the 'alien limb' phenomenon, where one limb appears to have a mind of its own and interferes with the actions of the other. Parkinson's Plus syndromes present with a variable degree of parkinsonism, and a variety of other features that are not found in the early stages of idiopathic Parkinson's disease. Lewy body dementia: visual hallucinations, marked fluctuation in cognition from day to day. Multiple system atrophy: autonomic features (postural hypotension, bladder dysfunction), cerebellar and pyramidal signs, rigidity > tremor. Progressive supranuclear palsy: supranuclear gaze palsy, no tremor, truncal rigidity, symmetrical onset, postural instability, dysphagia. Cortico-basal degeneration: asymmetrical akinetic rigidity, apraxia, alien limb phenomenon, cortical sensory loss (e.g. astereognosis). Vascular parkinsonism: legs more affected than arms, apraxic gait (marche à petit pas), pyramidal signs.

Longmore M et al., *Oxford Handbook of Clinical Medicine*, Eighth Edition, Oxford University Press, 2010, Chapter 10, Neurology: Parkinson's disease.

61. A. Failure of downgaze that corrects with the doll's head manoeuvre

This man presents with a number of the features of progressive supranuclear palsy, one of the Parkinson's Plus syndromes. The name comes from the characteristic vertical supranuclear gaze palsy—the patient is unable to make volitional upward or downward eye movements, but the intactness of the muscle and lower motor neuron is demonstrated using the vestibulo-ocular reflex (doll's head manoeuvre). Parkinson's Plus syndromes present with a variable degree of parkinsonism, and a variety of other features that are not found in the early stages of idiopathic Parkinson's disease. Lewy body dementia: visual hallucinations, marked fluctuation in cognition from day to day. Multiple system atrophy: autonomic features (postural hypotension, bladder dysfunction), cerebellar and pyramidal signs, rigidity > tremor. Progressive supranuclear palsy: supranuclear gaze palsy, no tremor, truncal rigidity, symmetrical onset, postural instability, dysphagia. Cortico-basal degeneration: asymmetrical akinetic rigidity, apraxia, alien limb phenomenon, cortical sensory loss (e.g. astereognosis). Vascular parkinsonism: legs more affected than arms, apraxic gait (marche à petit pas), pyramidal signs.

Longmore M et al., *Oxford Handbook of Clinical Medicine*, Eighth Edition, Oxford University Press, 2010, Chapter 10, Neurology: Parkinson's disease.

62. E. Multiple system atrophy

This man presents with features suggestive of multiple system atrophy, one of the Parkinson's Plus syndromes. As the name suggests, it is a degenerative disease that affects multiple cortical and subcortical systems, and therefore there are pyramidal, extrapyramidal, cerebellar, and autonomic signs. Parkinson's Plus syndromes present with a variable degree of parkinsonism, and a variety of other features that are not found in the early stages of idiopathic Parkinson's disease. Lewy body dementia: visual hallucinations, marked fluctuation in cognition from day to day. Multiple system atrophy: autonomic features (postural hypotension, bladder dysfunction), cerebellar and pyramidal signs, rigidity > tremor. Progressive supranuclear palsy: supranuclear gaze palsy, no tremor, truncal rigidity, symmetrical onset, postural instability, dysphagia. Cortico-basal degeneration: asymmetrical akinetic rigidity, apraxia, alien limb phenomenon, cortical sensory loss (e.g. astereognosis). Vascular parkinsonism: legs more affected than arms, apraxic gait (marche à petit pas), pyramidal signs.

Longmore M et al., *Oxford Handbook of Clinical Medicine*, Eighth Edition, Oxford University Press, 2010, Chapter 10, Neurology: Parkinson's disease.

63. C. Finger–nose ataxia

This man presents with features suggestive of multiple system atrophy, one of the Parkinson's Plus syndromes. As the name suggests, it is a degenerative disease that affects multiple cortical and subcortical systems, and therefore there are pyramidal, extrapyramidal, cerebellar and autonomic signs. Parkinson's Plus syndromes present with a variable degree of parkinsonism, and a variety of other features that are not found in the early stages of idiopathic Parkinson's disease. Lewy body dementia: visual hallucinations, marked fluctuation in cognition from day to day. Multiple system atrophy: autonomic features (postural hypotension, bladder dysfunction), cerebellar and pyramidal signs, rigidity > tremor. Progressive supranuclear palsy: supranuclear gaze palsy, no tremor, truncal rigidity, symmetrical onset, postural instability, dysphagia. Cortico-basal degeneration: asymmetrical akinetic rigidity, apraxia, alien limb phenomenon, cortical sensory loss (e.g. astereognosis). Vascular parkinsonism: legs more affected than arms, apraxic gait (marche à petit pas), pyramidal signs.

Longmore M et al., *Oxford Handbook of Clinical Medicine*, Eighth Edition, Oxford University Press, 2010, Chapter 10, Neurology: Parkinson's disease.

64. C. Single-fibre EMG

The gold standard for myasthenia is single-fibre EMG recording, which shows 'jitter' in repeat recordings. However, it is a very painstaking and time-consuming test, and repetitive stimulation EMG is the first-line electrophysiological test. This would be expected to show decremental amplitudes of muscle response as the muscle fatigues. Anti-ACh receptor antibodies are only positive in around 80–90% of myasthenics. The edrophonium test should be performed as a double-blinded test (with saline as a control) to see if the patient responds to an IV bolus of a potent short-acting acetylcholinesterase inhibitor. It requires that the patient has a quantifiable deficit so that objective improvement can be measured. Intravenous edrophonium can cause cardiac bradyarrhythmias, so the patient should have cardiac monitoring during the test and for ten minutes after, and there should be atropine available immediately should the patient become bradycardic.

Skeie GO et al., European Federation Guidelines on treatment for myasthenia, *European Journal of Neurology* 2010, doi:10.1111/j.1468-1331.2010.03019.x. http://www.efns.org/fileadmin/user_upload/guidline_papers/EFNS_guideline_2010_autoimmune_neuromuscular_transmission_disorders.pdf

65. E. Progressive multifocal leukoencephalopathy

Progressive multifocal leukoencephalopathy (PML) is a disease of widespread central nervous system demyelination that arises from a lytic infection of glial cells. The causative virus is the neurotropic human DNA polyomavirus JC. Prior to the HIV epidemic, PML was a rare disease only seen in immunocompromised patients (i.e. those with haematological malignancies and transplant patients). Recently, there has been an increase in cases in those patients undertaking immunosuppression therapy with biological agents including natalizumab for mutliple sclerosis and Crohn's disease, rituximab for lupus, and efalizumab for psoriasis. Patients present with demyelination and so the presenting symptoms vary accordingly but can include: weakness, sensory deficits, hemianopias, cognitive dysfunction, aphasic ataxia syndromes, and gait disturbance. MR imaging demonstrates hyperintensities on T2 images. Diagnosis can be confirmed with the presence of JC virus DNA following CSF PCR.

Tan CS, Koralnik IJ, Progressive multifocal leukoencephalopathy and other disorders caused by JC virus: clinical features and pathogenesis, *Lancet Neurology* 2010;9:425–437.

66. A. CSF analysis

This patient presents with a picture of encephalitis. The most important diagnosis to exclude, because of its treatability, is an infective process such as viral encephalitis. The absence of a fever does not preclude viral encephalitis. CSF would typically show a lymphocytosis and raised protein. This would help differentiate it from a tumour, such as a glioma, or ADEM (acute disseminated encephalomyelitis), which would also show white matter predominant lesions, but in which CSF would generally show normal white cell counts. Acute serum and CSF is useful for PCR if empirical treatment with acyclovir does not work, and consideration should be given to limbic encephalitis, which is an autoimmune encephalitis typically with positive anti-voltage-gated K+ channel antibodies or anti LGI-1 antibodies. Treatment is immunomodulatory, for example with plasma exchange. Venous thrombosis and ischaemic infarcts can cause seizures, but would not have imaging findings like this.

de Assis Aquino Gondim F, Viral encephalitis, *Medscape*, 2016. http://emedicine.medscape.com/article/1166498-overview

67. A. Protein >4 g/dl, 2 x 10⁶/l white blood cells, glucose consistent with serum glucose

The diagnosis here is Guillain-Barré syndrome (GBS). The most frequent antecedent symptoms in GBS and related disorders were fever (52%), cough (48%), sore throat (39%), nasal discharge (30%), and diarrhoea (27%). In most GBS studies, symptoms of a preceding infection in the upper respiratory tract or gastrointestinal tract predominate. The most frequently identified cause of infection is *Clostridium jejuni*. Other well-defined types of infection related to GBS are cytomegalovirus, Epstein–Barr virus, *Mycoplasma pneumoniae*, and *Haemophilus influenzae*. Symptoms suggestive of GBS include: progression of symptoms over days to four weeks, relative symmetry of symptoms, mild sensory symptoms or signs, cranial nerve involvement, especially bilateral weakness of facial muscles, autonomic dysfunction, pain (often present), high concentration of protein in CSF, or typical electrodiagnostic features. Features suggestive of an alternate diagnosis are: severe pulmonary dysfunction with limited limb weakness at onset, severe sensory signs with limited weakness at onset, bladder or bowel dysfunction at onset, fever at onset, sharp sensory level, slow progression with limited weakness without respiratory involvement (consider sub-acute inflammatory demyelinating polyneuropathy or CIDP), marked persistent asymmetry of weakness, persistent bladder or bowel dysfunction, increased number of mononuclear cells in CSF (>50×10?/l) or polymorphonuclear cells in CSF.

van Doorn PA et al., Clinical features, pathogenesis, and treatment of Guillain-Barré syndrome, *Lancet Neurology* 2008;7:939–950.

68. B. Spinal cord infarct

The time course of the progression of this man's symptoms is over days rather than hours or minutes. This could be consistent with Guillain–Barré syndrome, transverse myelitis (caused for example by MS or a viral infection such as CMV, HIV, VZV, or EBV) or a disc prolapse. Indeed, approximately 10% of HIV presents with a neurological syndrome, such as transverse myelitis, at the time of seroconversion. However, a spinal cord infarct would cause symptoms over minutes or perhaps hours, and therefore it is not compatible with the history given.

Andary MT et al., Guillain-Barre Syndrome, *Medscape*, 2016. http://emedicine.medscape.com/article/315632-overview

69. C. Giant cell arteritis

The previous history of polymyalgia rheumatica, raised ESR and CRP in the absence of any rise in WBC makes giant cell arteritis the most likely cause of seizures. Meningitis and encephalitis are excluded by the normal CSF results and absence of antiglial antibodies makes paraneoplastic encephalitis unlikley. Intracerebral tumour and cerebrovascular disease, as a cause of recurrent seizures, are excluded by the normal head CT. Generalized cerebral atrophy in the absence of infarcts or focus of irritation is not associated with seizures. The patient's weight loss can be explained by the giant cell arteritis and this along with a normal CXR and absence of any other features to suggest malignancy with negative antiglial antibodies makes a paraneoplastic syndrome unlikely, and therefore malignancy unlikely.

Shlamovitz GZ et al., Lumbar puncture, *Medscape*, 2016. http://emedicine.medscape.com/article/80773-overview

70. D. Transient global amnesia

This man had classical picture of transient global amnesia (TGA) by sudden onset of inability to form new memories which lasted for less than 24 hours with associated retrograde amnesia. He was acutely disorientated but did not have any obvious precipitant for delirium and lacked the fluctuating course and inattention necessary for a diagnosis of delirium. Absence of neurological deficit renders transient ischaemic attack and seizure unlikely, and subdural haematoma is ruled out by normal CT scan. The aura of migraine is typically a 'positive' symptom of perceptual disturbance—usually visual fortification spectra. Interestingly, there is a correlation between those with a history of migraine and transient global ischaemia, and some centres postulate that TGA results from basilar artery migraine.

Sucholeiki R, Transient global ischaemia, *Medscape*, 2016. http://emedicine.medscape.com/article/1160964-overview

71. E. Vascular parinsonism

The most likely cause of her tremor is vascular parkinsonism. Calcium channel blocking drugs may cause tremor but this would not be the most likely cause in this case as they usually produce symmetrical tremor. Patients with essential tremor often have a family history of tremor and earlier age of onset (not always); tremor is commonly bilateral from onset. The rapidity of progression to bilateral tremor and deterioration in physical function would be unusual in idiopathic Parkinson's disease. Tremor in a patient with atrial fibrillation should raise the possibility of thyrotoxicosis and older patients may present atypically without weight loss or other features of this condition.

Parkinson's Disease—Diagnosis & Management in Primary and Secondary Care: NICE.

http://www.nice.org.uk/nicemedia/live/10984/30088/30088.pdf

72. B. Toxoplasmosis

Cerebral toxoplasmosis remains a prevalent disorder of the central nervous system, particularly among severely immunosuppressed human immunodeficiency virus (HIV) infected patients. Toxoplasmosis is a zoonotic infection in humans caused by the protozoal intracellular parasite *Toxoplasma gondii*. Cats are the primary hosts. It is generally acquired via eating undercooked or raw meat infected with tissue cysts or via ingestion of food or water contaminated with infected cat faeces. Most cases of toxoplasmosis in immunocompromised patients are a consequence of latent infection and reactivation. In patients with AIDS, *T. gondii* tissue cysts can reactivate with CD4 counts less than 200 cells/microlitre. Findings on MRI and CT scans are not pathognomonic for toxoplasmic encephalitis. Primary CNS lymphoma cannot be distinguished from toxoplasmosis solely on the basis of neuroradiologic criteria (both present as contrast-enhancing lesions with mass effect). However, the presence of hyperattenuation on nonenhanced CT scans and subependymal location suggests the possibility of lymphoma. Meningitis is rarely associated with intracerebral lesion. AIDS-related Kaposi's sarcomas would cause darkish purple tinged or brown spots all over the body. Such spot formations could be noted over the skin's surface or the oral region. Kaposi's sarcoma could additionally impact other body regions (lungs, spleen, liver, digestive system) or the lymph nodes; it rarely affects the brain.

Montoya JG, Remington JS, Toxoplasma gondii. In: Mandell GL et al., *Principles and Practice of Infectious Diseases*, Churchill Livingstone, 2000, pp. 2858–2888.

73. D. Wernicke's encephalopathy

This young woman presents with diabetic ketoacidosis (DKA) and probable hyperemesis gravidarum. Her condition is appropriately treated overnight and her pH, glucose, and electrolytes are in normal ranges. Unfortunately she goes on to develop an acute confusional state, nystagmus, opthalmoplegia, and ataxia. This combination of neurological signs should alert you to the possibility of Wernicke's encephalopathy. This rare neurological condition is caused by thiamine (vitamin B1) deficiency and, if not promptly recognized and treated with thiamine replacement, can in fact be fatal. Wernicke's encephalopathy is frequently considered in malnourished patients with a background of alcohol excess but it may occur in other conditions that cause poor nutritional states. Hyperemesis gravidarum and diabetic ketoacidosis with administration of intravenous glucose have been associated with its development (see reference). It has also been reported in association with malnourished thyrotoxic patients. Thiamine's relatively short half-life (~2 weeks) means stores can be easily depleted with poor nutrition. Note that the encephalopathy is often precipitated by a carbohydrate load, be it intravenous dextrose or supplemental feeding via a naso-gastric tube. Cerebral oedema may occur in patients with DKA who experience rapid intracellular fluid shifts when blood sugars are corrected too rapidly. Cerebral oedema typically appears as hypodense areas on CT. The other three options listed may present with some of the neurological features described but are incorrect in this question.

Selitsky T et al., Wernicke's encephalopathy with hyperemesis and ketoacidosis, *Obstetrics and Gynaecology* 2006;107(Suppl. 2, Part 2):486–490.

74. A. Acute on chronic confusion

The most likely cause of the patient's presentation is delirium due to recent urinary tract infection. The MMSE of less than 23 and CLOX-1 of less than 11 indicates cognitive impairment, and the positive CAM and IQCODE of more than 3.41 indicate both acute and chronic deficits according to British Geriatrics Society document 'Delirious about dementia'. Although the patient was agitated initially, she does not show any signs of depression. She is not manifesting any psychotic symptoms and so this could not be a psychotic depression, which would also be unusual to present for the first time at this age.

Blazer DG, Depression in late life: review and commentary, *Journals of Gerontology Series A: Biological Sciences and Medical Sciences* 2003;58A(3):249–265.

75. A. Voltage-gated calcium channel (VGCC) antibodies

Lambert–Eaton myasthenic syndrome is a disease of the neuromuscular junction. It is an autoimmune condition and is often paraneoplastic, associated with conditions such as small cell lung cancer. Symptoms are similar to myasthenia gravis, and the patient complains primarily of muscle weakness. However, there are some subtle differences. For example, strength may improve after repetitive activity, unlike myasthenia gravis, and electrophysiological features are not the same. It is associated with VGCC antibodies.

Honnorat J, Antoine J-C, Paraneoplastic neurological syndromes, *Orphanet Journal of Rare Diseases* 2007;2:22. http://www.ncbi.nlm.nih.gov/pmc/articles/PMC1868710/?tool=pubmed

76. D. 40%

The rate of recurrence for unprovoked seizures is much greater at around 30–50%, versus only 3–10% where there is a clear provoking factor such as a minor head injury, or metabolic disturbance. This drives the necessity for a period of anti-epileptic medication, with most patients with a provoked seizure not taking prophylaxis, but those with an unprovoked seizure basing their decision on other factors such as driving, lifestyle, etc.

NICE Guidance [CG137], Epilepsies: diagnosis and management, January 2012. https://www.nice.org.uk/guidance/cg137/chapter/1-guidance

Sharma S, Dixit V, Epilepsy: a comprehensive review, *International Journal of Pharma Research & Review* 2013;2:61–80.

77. A. Guillain-Barré syndrome

Guillain-Barré syndrome does not typically involve the extraocular muscles. There is a variant of this condition called Miller Fisher syndrome which can affect the extra ocular muscles, although it tends to compromise more than just one muscle. Myasthenia may present as a sixth nerve palsy although fatiguable ptosis is a frequent feature in those patients with ocular involvement. Duane syndrome may cause limited ocular adduction or sometimes abduction which may simulate a sixth nerve palsy. It will have been present from birth and globe retraction with narrowing of the eyelids occurs on attempted abduction of the eye. Retinoic acid medication may cause a sixth nerve palsy as a localizing sign due to drug-induced 'idiopathic' intracranial hypertension. Multiple sclerosis may cause a nuclear sixth nerve palsy.

Jackson TL (ed), *Moorfields Manual of Ophthalmology*, Elsevier, 2008, Neuro-ophthalmology chapter.

78. B. Herpes simplex encephalitis

The symptoms described here are typical of those seen in herpes simplex encephalitis, where changes in the frontal and temporal lobes are most commonly seen. The use of a course of prednisolone may have served to precipitate reactivation of latent viral infection. Diagnosis is based around demonstrating herpes simplex virus with the use of PCR, although commencement of IV acyclovir should not wait for the diagnosis to be confirmed. Treatment is usually given IV for ten days, with further oral treatment up to 21 days in total.

Ramrakha PS et al., *Oxford Handbook of Acute Medicine*, Third Edition, Oxford University Press, 2010, Chapter 6, Neurological emergencies.

79. E. Short-lasting unilateral neuralgiform headache attacks with conjunctival injection and tearing (SUNCT)

The diagnosis here is that of short-lasting unilateral neuralgiform headache attacks with conjunctival injection and tearing (SUNCT). SUNCT is one of the trigeminal autonomic cephalalgias, which are characterized by intense neuropathic pain associated with the distribution of the trigeminal nerve and often have prominent autonomic symptoms (e.g. tearing, nasal congestion, facial flushing). Each TAC has different presentations which are important for potential treatment choices. SUNCT is a rare primary headache syndrome which is characterized by strictly unilateral, severe neuralgic attacks centred on the ophthalmic trigeminal distribution that are brief in duration and occur in association with both conjunctival injection and lacrimation. The attacks last between 5 and 240 seconds and occur with a frequency ranging between 3 and 200 per day. It may be associated with cutaneous trigger points as well. Treatment options are limited but lamotrigine may be of some benefit to most patients. Imaging is required in most patients to investigate for structural lesions.

Cittandini E, Matharu MS, Symptomatic trigeminal autonomic cephalalgias, *Neurologist* 2009;15:305–312.

80. B. Non-contrast MRI brain

The likely diagnosis is multiple sclerosis—which is best diagnosed with an MRI of the brain, and the non-contrast sequences are the most important. MRI of the spine can be performed to assess for cord demyelination, but the first investigation should be of the brain.

Osborn A et al., *Diagnostic Imaging: Brain*, Amirsys, 2004, Multiple sclerosis 1, pp. 8–77.

81. B. CT head with contrast

The most likely diagnosis is cerebral venous sinus thrombosis (CVST) and as such the most appropriate initial investigation should be a CT head with contrast. If contrast is contraindicated then the patient should have an urgent CT head. Between 75% and 95% of patients tend to present with a subacute onset of a global headache with the remainder suffering from a thunderclap-type headache. The headaches of CVST are persistent and are exacerbated by transient increases in intracranial pressure that occur during coughing, sneezing, or other Valsalva manoeuvres. Headaches can also worsen when in the recumbent position and upon awakening. Most patients will present with complications of CVST which include seizures, papilloedema, altered level of consciousness, and focal neurological symptoms or signs. Between 15% and 30% of patients present with an isolated headache. CVST is more common during puerperium. CT brain is normal in about 25% of patients and as such patients should have CT with contrast which will demonstrate venous filling defects as a first-line investigation. In those with focal neurological deficits, there are CT abnormalities in about 90% and these can include venous infarcts, evidence of oedema, or hyperdensity within the occluded sinus. CSF analysis reveals a high red blood cell count, high protein, and lymphocytic pleocytosis, or high opening pressure. MRI with venography is commonly needed for the diagnosis of CVST and should be considered whenever there is clinical suspicion of this disorder.

Schwedt TJ et al., Thunderclap headache, *Lancet Neurology* 2006;5:621–631.

82. C. Dilatation of the third and lateral ventricles

The history suggests that the patient has suffered either another TIA or a stroke. Both may be associated with a normal CT, and loss of grey–white differentiation may be the only manifestation on CT of a stroke at this stage. Acute thrombus can be seen as high attenuation (brightness) within an artery, and a stroke can be due to either thrombus/embolus or intra-parenchymal haemorrhage. The answer is C because although a stroke can cause mass effect, it is rare of the severity to cause ventricular dilatation, especially in the acute phase.

Osborn AG et al., *Diagnostic Imaging: Brain*, Amyrsis, 2004, Stroke I, pp. 4–107.

83. D. Contrast-enhanced MRI of the brain

Suspected pituitary lesions (prolactinoma in this case) are best assessed by dynamic, contrast-enhanced MRI of the brain, centred on the pituitary fossa. This is the most sensitive way to assess for a micro/macro-adenoma. X-rays and CT may show the consequent bone changes, but only if the pituitary tumour is of sufficient size.

Segu VB et al., Prolactinoma, *Medscape*, 2016. http://emedicine.medscape.com/article/124634-diagnosis

84. E. Hyperosmolar non-ketotic coma

Hyperosmolar non-ketotic coma (HONK) is characterized by hyperglycaemia and high serum osmolality with no significant acidosis or ketonuria (best thought of as not enough insulin, but enough to prevent ketosis). As in this case, HONK is often associated with very high serum glucose levels, whereas diabetic ketoacidosis tends to occur with much lower glucose levels. It most commonly affects elderly type 2 diabetics, and can occur in patients who are previously undiagnosed. The clues here are that the question provides you with the sodium, potassium, bicarbonate, and chloride values. If this appears in MRCP exams it is vital you calculate the anion gap using the following formula; anion gap = $(Na^+ + K^+)$—$(Cl^- + HCO^-)$ In this case the anion gap is 15; this excludes the presence of significant ketoacidosis. Likewise the presence of the urea and glucose levels should prompt you to calculate serum osmolality using the following formula $(2[Na^+ + K^+] + urea + glucose)$. In this case the serum osmolality is calculated as 360 mosmol/kg.

Umpierrez GE et al., Diabetic ketoacidosis and hyperglycaemic hyperosmolar syndrome, *Diabetes Spectrum* 2002;15(1):28–36. http://spectrum.diabetesjournals.org/content/15/1/28.full.pdf+html

85. E. Lamotrigine

Given this woman has suffered three seizures already in the course of her pregnancy, it seems unwise to put her at further risk by not starting her on seizure prophylaxis. Data from pregnancy registries appears to support use of lamotrigine as having a low rate of reported malformations associated with its use. This is in contrast to sodium valproate which is associated with significant malformations at a dose of above 1 g/day.

Longmore M et al., *Oxford Handbook of Clinical Medicine*, Eighth Edition, Oxford University Press, 2010, Chapter 10, Neurology, Epilepsy: management.

86. D. Change to clopidogrel 75 mg

NICE guidance is clear that in cases of completed stroke on aspirin, a switch to clopidogrel is most appropriate. There is little benefit in using aspirin and clopidogrel in combination. For recurrent TIAs on aspirin, NICE guidance recommends addition of dipyridamole MR, as per the ESPS 2 study. On the information provided, there is little to support warfarinization here.

NICE guidance [TA210], Clopidogrel and modified-release dipyridamole for the prevention of occlusive vascular events. http://publications.nice.org.uk/clopidogrel-and-modified-release-dipyridamole-for-the-prevention-of-occlusive-vascular-events-ta210

87. B. Thiamine deficiency

Thiamine deficiency is common in patients with chronic alcoholism, and the picture seen here with nystagmus, conjugate gaze palsy, and confusion (which may include evidence of confabulation) supports the diagnosis. An urgent step in management, to prevent/limit permanent short-term memory loss, is therefore to instigate intravenous thiamine replacement. Hypoglycaemia is also a possibility and glucose monitoring is an important part of management of these patients, but would not cause the constellation of symptoms seen. Subdural again is a possibility in an alcoholic patient (who usually has alcohol-related brain atrophy and is at increased risk of falls), but there is no history or evidence of falls. Delerium tremens results in hallucinations and agitation. B12 deficiency can be associated with chronic features of memory loss, depression, and withdrawal.

Longmore M et al., *Oxford Handbook of Clinical Medicine*, Eighth Edition, Oxford University Press, 2010.

88. B. Tissue plasminogen activator (TPA) should be given within three hours if possible

Thrombolysis treatment with recombinated-tissue plasminogen activator (r-tPA) leads to 44 fewer dead or dependent patients per 1000 treated if given within six hours, and 126 fewer dead or dependent patients per 1000 if given within three hours. This translates to a number needed to treat (NNT) of approximately eight if patients are treated within three hours. Because of this, r-tPA delivery within three hours is advisable. Delivery of r-tPA is via a peripheral cannula. The risks of r-tPA are of haemorrhagic transformation of the stroke, where there is a five-fold increase in risk versus placebo. More recent surgery may be a contraindication to thrombolysis, but not abdominal surgery six months previously.

Bowker L et al., *Oxford Handbook of Geriatric Medicine*, Second Edition, Oxford University Press, 2012, Chapter 8, Stroke.

89. C. Posterior communicating artery aneurysm

Against a background of hypertension, a posterior communicating artery aneurysm as a cause of third nerve palsy, the clinical presentation here, carries a high probability. Where there is a compressive aetiology, pupil dilatation is often seen first, as here. Given the fasting glucose is to the upper end of the impaired fasting glucose range, diabetes mellitus as a cause of the nerve palsy is very unlikely. In the presence of a normal MRA with no signs of aneurysm, an idiopathic third nerve palsy would be considered.

Denniston AKO, Murray PI, *Oxford Handbook of Ophthalmology*, Second Edition, Oxford University Press, 2009.

90. E. *Listeria monocytogenes*

The scenario given here, of an elderly person having eaten a number of soft cheeses, raises the possibility of Listeria meningitis, which is more common in pregnant women, those who are immunocompromised, and the elderly. Intravenous amoxycillin is the treatment of choice. Intravenous ceftriaxone is effective against *Escherichia coli*, *Haemophilus influenzae* type b, *Streptococcus pneumoniae*, and *Neisseria meningitidis*, but not *Listeria monocytogenes*.

Torok E et al., *Oxford Handbook of Infectious Diseases and Microbiology*, Oxford University Press, 2009, Chapter 5, Clinical syndromes, Bacterial meningitis.

91. D. Chronic inflammatory demyelinating radiculoneuropathy (CIDP)

The symptoms and signs suggest a progressive peripheral neuropathy. The time course of the progression of this man's symptoms is over several weeks. Guillain–Barré syndrome is defined as an acute inflammatory demyelinating radiculoneuropathy (AIDP) that reaches its nadir within four weeks. In contrast, a chronic inflammatory demyelinating radiculoneuropathy (CIDP) reaches its nadir at greater than eight weeks. The prodromal upper respiratory tract infection that might precede Guillain–Barré is in this case a distractor. A diabetic neuropathy would typically evolve over months or years, and so the ten-week history makes this rather less likely. CIDP, as the name suggests, is chronic and relapsing, and so regular treatment with IVIg every 2–3 months is usually necessary for symptom control. In contrast, AIDP (Guillain–Barré syndrome and other variants such as Miller Fisher syndrome) is monophasic, and so only one course of IVIg is needed.

Lewis RA, Chronic inflammatory demyelinating polyradiculoneuropathy, *Medscape*, 2016. http://emedicine.medscape.com/article/1172965-overview

92. A. Glucose tolerance test

The clinical scenario is consistent with bilateral foot drop. The commonest causes of foot drop result in unilateral pathology. These include sciatic or common peroneal nerve trauma or nerve root compression (e.g. disc herniation or nerve root exit foramina narrowing). Bilateral foot drop implies either dual pathology or a systemic cause. Spinal or CNS pathologies may cause bilateral weakness and sensory changes, but are likely to be associated with increased tone and hyperreflexia. An MRI spine is therefore unlikely to be diagnostic in this instance. Similarly, nerve conduction studies would likely confirm the clinical diagnosis, but not further elucidate the cause. Tertiary syphilis is a recognized cause of foot drop, but is becoming increasingly uncommon owing to the widespread use of antibiotics. The commonest cause for bilateral foot drop would be a peripheral neuropathy. The chronicity and sensory disturbance discount Guillain–Barré syndrome. Hereditary conditions (e.g. Charcot–Marie–Tooth) are unlikely to present in the ninth decade. The clinical history and normal B12 assays render alcohol excess or B12 deficiency as a cause. Diabetes mellitus is often unrecognized and patients may present with complications of under-treatment. The normal fasting glucose initially appears to discount this. However, the European Union Geriatric Medicine Society recognize that reliance on fasting glucose for diagnosis may be misleading in the elderly, and advocate formal glucose tolerance testing if clinical suspicion persists despite a normal fasting glucose. A significantly raised HbA1c may also be useful in supporting a diagnosis (e.g. if formal glucose tolerance testing is not feasible), but should not be relied on for diagnosis.

NICE guidance [NG28]. Type 2 diabetes in adults: management, December 2015. http://www.nice.org.uk/guidance/ng28

93. C. Anti-voltage-gated calcium antibodies

This is Lambert–Eaton myasthenic syndrome and is associated with anti-voltage-gated calcium channel antibodies. Patients usually present with a proximal weakness, autonomic dysfunction (dry mouth, male impotence, dry eyes, constipation) and reduced tendon reflexes. Approximately half will have a mild ptosis. Given this is a neuromuscular problem, imaging and cerebrospinal fluid analysis are usually normal. Electromyography is the investigation of choice and shows a reduced compound muscle action potential with a 100–1000-fold increase following maximum voluntary contraction. This can be induced with direct stimulation at a frequency of 20 Hz. This disease is almost exclusively associated with small cell lung cancer.

Gozzard P, Maddison P, Which antibody and which cancer in which paraneoplastic syndromes? *Practical Neurology* 2010;10:260–270.

94. B. Guillain–Barré syndrome

The diagnosis here is Guillain–Barré syndrome (GBS). The most frequent antecedent symptoms in GBS and related disorders were fever (52%), cough (48%), sore throat (39%), nasal discharge (30%), and diarrhoea (27%). In most GBS studies, symptoms of a preceding infection in the upper respiratory tract or gastrointestinal tract predominate. The most frequently identified cause of infection is *Clostridium jejuni*. Other well-defined types of infection related to GBS are cytomegalovirus, Epstein–Barr virus, *Mycoplasma pneumoniae*, and *Haemophilus influenzae*. Symptoms suggestive of GBS include: progression of symptoms over days to four weeks, relative symmetry of symptoms, mild sensory symptoms or signs, cranial nerve involvement, especially bilateral weakness of facial muscles, autonomic dysfunction, pain (often present), high concentration of protein in CSF, or typical electrodiagnostic features. Features suggestive of an alternate diagnosis are: severe pulmonary dysfunction with limited limb weakness at onset, severe sensory signs with limited weakness at onset, bladder or bowel dysfunction at onset, fever at onset, sharp sensory level, slow progression with limited weakness without respiratory involvement (consider subacute inflammatory demyelinating polyneuropathy or CIDP), marked persistent asymmetry of weakness, persistent bladder or bowel dysfunction, increased number of mononuclear cells in CSF (>50×10?/l), or polymorphonuclear cells in CSF.

van Doorn PA et al., Clinical features, pathogenesis, and treatment of Guiilain-Barré syndrome, *Lancet Neurology* 2008;7:939–950.

95. B. Sporadic Creutzfeldt–Jakob disease

Sporadic Creutzfeld–Jakob disease (CJD) is the most likely diagnosis in this case, whilst the others all form part of the differential diagnosis. Although Alzheimer's disease could present this young, the time course of the symptoms is somewhat rapid (although not unheard of). Huntington's disease is a possibility but the patient is older than expected and startle myoclonus is unexpected. Depression is a cause of pseudo-dementia and should be considered as a cause of dementia. Sporadic CJD affects men and women equally with an average age at onset of approximately 60 years. It is rare to see in those younger than age 40 years or over age 80 years. Initial symptoms in about a third of cases are systemic complaints of fatigue, disordered sleep, and decreased appetite; a third of patients present with behavioural or cognitive changes; and the final third have focal signs such as visual loss, cerebellar ataxia, aphasia, or motor deficits. The disease progresses rapidly with prominent cognitive decline and the development of myoclonus, particularly startle-sensitive myoclonus. The median time to death from onset is only five months, and 90% of patients with sporadic CJD are dead within one year. There are no diagnostic investigations for sporadic CJD (other than brain biopsy) but several investigations are useful when considered together: characteristic basal ganglia changes on MRI, the synchronized biphasic or triphasic sharp-wave complexes on the electroencephalogram, and the finding of 14-3-3 protein in CSF all support the diagnosis of CJD. 14-3-3, a normal neural protein released with rapid neuronal loss, is present in CSF after strokes or during encephalitis. The pathological findings in CJD are limited to the brain and spinal cord. There is neuronal loss, and vacuolization within cell bodies and dendrites that gives a spongiform appearance to the cortex and deep nuclei. The pathogenic isoform of prion protein can be demonstrated in the brain by immunocytochemical staining and by western-blot analysis.

Johnson RT, Prion diseases, *Lancet Neurology* 2005;4:635–642.

96. E. Charcot–Marie–Tooth disease

The most likely diagnosis here is that of Charcot–Marie–Tooth (CMT) disease (also known as hereditary sensory and motor neuropathy). CMT is subdivided into two main groups: (1) a demyelinating form (CMT1 if autosomal-dominant, CMT4 if autosomal-recessive), characterized by slowed nerve-conduction velocities and myelin abnormalities (i.e. onion-bulb formations) at nerve biopsy; and (2) an axonal form (CMT2), with preserved or only mildly slowed nerve conduction velocities and pathological evidence of chronic axonal degeneration and regeneration. Motor symptoms start from the feet, which develop high arches, hammer toes, and intrinsic muscle weakness and wasting; subsequently, the disease gradually affects the leg and then the lower third of the thigh, producing the typical distal atrophy of the lower limbs. The hands usually become affected at this stage, progressing to the forearms. Sensory loss follows the same pattern with decreased sensation of vibration, touch, and pain. Proprioceptive sensory loss can cause a sensory ataxia. Deep-tendon reflexes are reduced or absent following the same distal to proximal gradient. Symptoms and signs indicative of CMT include: pes cavus (or pes planus, often later progressing to cavus deformity); hammer toes; difficulty in running; twisting of the ankle and tripping; difficulty in walking; foot drop; high-stepping gait; wasting, weakness, and sensory loss of distal segments of lower and then upper limbs; and reduced or absent deep-tendon reflexes. Other common symptoms and signs are hand tremors, muscle cramps (particularly of the foot and leg), cold feet, foot callosities, and acrocyanosis. Positive sensory symptoms such as paraesthesias are rare, but pain is common, particularly in the feet, lower limbs, and lumbar spine. The disease onset usually occurs in the first two decades of life and subsequently shows a slow progression over decades. CMT is more commonly transmitted as an autosomal-dominant trait; X-linked transmission is not uncommon; and autosomal-recessive inheritance is generally uncommon. The disease is associated with a variable penetrance. Treatment options are limited but mild to moderate exercise is effective and safe for patients with CMT and leads to a significant improvement in walking ability and lower-limb strength. Intervention aimed at improving posture and balance is also considered to be useful. Shoe modifications, plantars, orthoses, and assistive devices can be of help. Ankle–foot orthoses are often uncomfortable and poorly tolerated. Bracing orthotics are also useful when upper limb involvement is severe.

Pareyson D, Marchesi C, Diagnosis, natural history, and management of Charcot–Marie–Tooth disease, *Lancet Neurology* 2009;8:654–667.

97. C. Lacunar stroke

This patient has suffered a lacunar stroke. The Bamford stroke classification is as follows: (1) Total anterior circulation stroke (TACS). All three of: unilateral motor or sensory deficit (two or three of face, arm and leg), higher function dysfunction (receptive or expressive dysphasia, inattention/neglect), and homonymous hemianopia. (2) Partial anterior circulation stroke (PACS). Two out of three of the features for a TACS. (3) Lacunar infarct. Five lacunar syndromes exist: pure motor weakness (presenting with unilateral motor weakness with the thrombus within the corona radiate as it passes through the basal ganglia), pure sensory loss (lesion to the contralateral thalamus), mixed sensorimotor (lesion to the thalamus and adjacent internal capsule), ataxic hemiparesis (lesion within the internal capsule and pons), and dysarthria or clumsy hand (pons lesion). (4) Posterior circulation stroke (POCS). This may be associated with any of the following: cranial nerve palsy, and contralateral motor/sensory defect, bilateral motor or sensory defect, eye movement problems (e.g. nystagmus), cerebellar dysfunction, and isolated homonymous hemianopia. The MRC power grades are as follows: (0) No movement. (1) A flicker of movement or fasciculations are present. (2) Movement with the force of gravity. (3) Anti-gravity power is present. (4) Reduced muscle strength but the muscle is able to move against resistance. (5) Muscle contracts normally against resistance.

Manji H et al., *Oxford Handbook of Neurology*, Oxford University Press, 2006, Chapter 4, Neurological disorders, Cerebrovascular disease: stroke.

98. A. Anti-acetylcholine receptor antibodies

The diagnosis here is myasthenia gravis (MG). Eighty-five percent of patients with MG will present with ocular weakness (fluctuating ptosis, diplopia). The remaining 15% will tend to present with bulbar weakness (dysarthria including nasal speech, dysphagia, dysphonia or masticatory weakness) and/or facial weakness (eyelid weakness against forced opening or lower face weakness). The absence of ocular signs might lead to a misdiagnosis of motor neuron disease which is the main differential diagnosis. Disease progression to generalized weakness usually occurs within two years of disease onset. Rarely patients may present with a prominent limb-girdle or axial distribution of weakness, focal weakness in single muscle groups, exertional dyspnoea, orthopnoea, or even respiratory failure if severe. Generalized MG can be divided into early-onset and late-onset disease, with early-onset MG occurring before 40. Early-onset patients tend to be female, have anti-AChR antibodies, and a thymoma. These patients might also be affected by other autoimmune diseases, most commonly autoimmune thyroid disease. Late-onset patients are more often male and usually have normal thymic histology or thymic atrophy. Late-onset MG can present with ocular or generalized weakness and a more severe disease course. Spontaneous remissions are rare. If weakness remains limited to the ocular muscles after two years, there is a 90% likelihood that the disease will not generalize. Investigations for MG include the edrophonium or ice-pack tests, electrophysiology, and serum autoantibodies. Chest CT or MRI should be done in all patients with confirmed MG to exclude the presence of a thymoma. Mainstays of treatment should include: pyridostigmine titrated to side effects (diarrhoea, stomach cramps) for weakness and long-term immunosuppression with steroids or steroid-sparing agents (e.g. azathioprine, mycophenolate moeftil, ciclosporin, tacrolimus). Other treatment options include plasma exchange and intravenous immunoglobulin. Thymectomy should be considered for those with a thymoma.

Meriggioli MN, Sanders DB, Autoimmune myasthenia gravis: emerging clinical and biological heterogeneity, *Lancet Neurology* 2009;8:475–490.

99. C. Cluster headache

The diagnosis here is cluster headache. Cluster headache is located mainly around the orbital and temporal regions, although any part of the head can be affected. The headache usually lasts 45–90 minutes but can range between 15 minutes and three hours. Typically, this syndrome has a male:female ratio of 5:1 and is characterized by a striking circannual and circadian pattern, hence the term cluster. Eighty to ninety percent of patients have an episodic form whereby they have bouts that last for approximately one week, which then remits for more than a month. The remaining 10–20% have a chronic form, with no remission within one year or remission periods that last less than a month. The autonomic system is implicated in cluster headache (indeed cluster headache is one of the trigeminal autonomic cephalalgias—headaches associated with the trigeminal nerve and autonomic features), and so patients will get features of autonomic dysfunction that include: ipsilateral ptosis, conjunctival injection, and tearing and lacrimation. Treatments aim at aborting the acute headache or a preventative measure. Acute treatments include inhaling 100% oxygen for 10–15 minutes or taking ergotamine. Intranasal sumitriptan may be of benefit. Preventative measures include: verapamil or high-dose steroids for three days. Lithium and methysergide have also been used but have potential harmful side effects and complications. Imaging is usually undertaken to rule out structural lesions causing a compressive neuropathy.

Manji H et al., *Oxford Handbook of Neurology*, Oxford University Press, 2006, Chapter 4, Neurological disorders, Cluster headache.

100. D. Normal serum creatine kinase

Duchenne muscular dystrophy (DMD) should be considered irrespective of family history and is usually clinically suspected by the observation of abnormal muscle function in a male child, an increase in serum creatine kinase, or the discovery of increased transaminases (aspartate aminotransferase and alanine aminotransferase). The diagnosis of DMD should thus be considered before liver biopsy in any male child with increased transaminases. DMD is typically diagnosed at around 5 years of age but might be suspected much earlier because of delays in attainment of developmental milestones, such as independent walking or language. The presence of Gowers' sign (inability to rise from the floor without using the body to 'walk' up) in a male child is suspicious for

DMD. In the presence of a positive family history of DMD, there should be a low threshold for testing creatine kinase, although this will be influenced by the age of the child. In a child less than 5 years of age, suspicion of DMD probably cannot be excluded completely by a normal muscle examination. Mutations responsible for DMD occur in the dystrophin gene which is on the X chromosome, hence the male propensity. About one-third of patients will have a de novo mutation. Muscle biopsy may be required to stain immunohistochemically for the absent dystrophin protein. Management is multidisciplinary in nature but life might be prolonged with early non-invasive ventilation. Respiratory failure may occur in adolescence with death in the third decade of life.

Manji H et al., *Oxford Handbook of Neurology*, Oxford University Press, 2006, Chapter 4, Neurological disorders, Duchenne muscular dystrophy.

101. B. Contralateral loss of temperature sensation

Spinal cord hemisection is associated with ipsilateral spastic paralysis below the level of the lesion and ipsilateral Babinski sign. There is also ipsilateral loss of fine touch, position sense, and vibration sense. Contralateral pain and temperature sensation are also lost. During the early stages of the injury the Babinski sign may be absent.

Manji H et al., *Oxford Handbook of Neurology*, Oxford University Press, 2006, Appendix 3: Neurological eponyms.

102. A. 14

Presenilin-1 is encoded by the PSEN1 gene located on chromosome 14. Presenilin-1 is a gamma secretase which cleaves the amyloid precursor protein (APP). Mutations cause an accumulation of the neurodegenerative amyloid-beta to form the amyloid plaques associated with Alzheimer's disease. PSEN1 mutations are associated with early-onset dementia (i.e. those presenting <60 years, usually 35–55 years). Presenilin-2 mutations are found on chromosome 1.

Rossor MN et al., The diagnosis of young-onset dementia, *Lancet Neurology* 2010;9:793–806.

103. B. Urgent CT head

The most likely diagnosis here is a subarachnoid haemorrhage (SAH), which would certainly need to be excluded. The incidence is approximately 8 per 100,000 and would normally account for 3% of the patients presenting to emergency departments with headache. The prognosis is poor with up to half of patients dying and a third of survivors remaining dependent. Early diagnosis and treatment is key. The headache of SAH typically peaks within seconds to minutes and lasts for more than one hour. It may be associated with meningitic features such as nuchal rigidity, nausea and vomiting, and light intolerance/photophobia. SAH should also be considered in the differential diagnosis of someone presenting with an acute deterioration in GCS. SAH is more common in those who have pre-exisiting cardiovascular disease and who smoke, are hypertensive, and drink more than recommended quantities of alcohol. Subarachnoid haemorrhage is graded in various ways but the most common is the WFNS classification which utilizes the GCS. The grades are: grade I: GCS 15 with no focal neurological deficits; grade II: GCS 13–14 with no focal neurological deficits; grade III: GCS 13–14 with focal neurological deficit; grade IV: GCS 7–12 with or without focal neurological deficit; grade V: GCS <7 with or without focal neurological deficit. Management requires an urgent CT scan. If negative, a 12-hour lumbar puncture should be performed for haemoglobin breakdown products in the CSF (xanthochromia). SAH patients should be transferred to a neurosurgical unit for ongoing treatment but initial treatments should include oral nimodipine 60 mg every four hours and intravenous fluids (both to prevent cerebral vasospasm). Endovascular aneurysmal coiling is preferred to clipping in most circumstances. The differential diagnosis could include meningitis but the history is usually quite suggestive of a SAH.

Al-Shahi R et al., Subarachnoid haemorrhage, *British Medical Journal* 2006;333:235–240.

104. D. Myotonic dystrophy

The diagnosis is myotonic dystrophy. The predominant symptom in myotonic dystrophy is distal muscle weakness which causes a reduction in manual dexterity and foot drop. The characteristic 'hatchet' facies is caused by weakness and wasting of the facial, levator palpebrae, and masticatory muscles giving rise to ptosis. The neck, finger, and wrist flexors are also commonly involved. The weakness is slowly progressive, but an added axonal peripheral neuropathy may contribute to the weakness. The myotonia may interfere with daily activities and can be elicited by percussion of the thenar eminence. Myotonic dystrophy is notable for its systemic complications which include: posterior subcapsular cataracts; cardiac conduction system fibrosis leading to conduction disturbances (prolonged PR interval, widened QRS, second- and third-degree heart blocks), brady- and tachyarrhythmias that may culminate in ventricular tachycardia and fibrillation; cardiomyopathy; minor intellectual deficits; daytime sleepiness (probably due to serotonergic neuron loss in the dorsal raphe and superior central nucleus of the brainstem); cholecystitis and biliary spasm; dysphagia secondary to reduced hypopharyngeal peristalsis; constipation and slow gastric emptying; multiple endocrinopathies of the thyroid, hypothalamus, and gonads; insulin resistance; early frontal balding; and a risk of hypoventilation and respiratory arrest under general anaesthesia. The average age of death is 48–60. Electromyography demonstrating a combination of myotonic discharges and myopathic-appearing motor units within distal muscles and the face is suggestive of myotonic dystrophy. The characteristic myotonic discharges occur as bursts of repetitive potentials on insertion of the needle, and the potentials vary in both amplitude and frequency. When played over a loudspeaker they resemble a 'dive bomber', hence 'dive bomber potential'. Myotonic dystrophy is caused by CTG trinucleotide expansion in the gene DMPK (myotonic dystrophy protein kinase) which codes for a myosin kinase expressed in skeletal muscle. The gene is located on chromosome 19q13.3. Normal individuals have between five and 37 CTG repeats where repeat lengths exceeding 37 are abnormal. Patients with between 38 and 49 CTG repeats are asymptomatic but are at risk of having children with larger, pathologically expanded repeats (this disease is associated with anticipation). Full penetrance alleles occur with repeats greater than 50 CTGs and are nearly always associated with symptomatic disease. CTG repeat sizes in patients range from 50 to 4000. Molecular genetic testing detects mutations in 100% of affected individuals.

Turner C, Hilton-Jones D, The myotonic dystrophies: diagnosis and management, *Journal of Neurology, Neurosurgery & Psychiatry* 2010;81:358–367.

105. E. Anti-NMDA receptor antibodies

This is anti-NMDA receptor antibody-mediated disease. A more recently described condition, it presents with a predominantly psychiatric picture with rapid neurological decline. Given the most common tumour type is ovarian it tends to be a disease of women. Where it does occur in men it is usually associated with teratomas.

Manji H et al., *Oxford Handbook of Neurology*, Oxford University Press, 2006, Chapter 4, Neurological disorders, Paraneoplastic syndromes: Central nervous system.

106. A. Friedreich's ataxia

The diagnosis here is Friedreich's ataxia. Friedreich's ataxia is the most common of the autosomal recessive ataxias and the most common hereditary ataxia overall with a prevalence of approximately 1 person in 30,000 to one in 50,000 in most populations and a carrier frequency of approximately 1 in 85 in white people. Age at presentation is typically age 5–25 years. Friedreich's ataxia is characterized by early-onset progressive gait and limb ataxia, dysarthria, loss of vibration and proprioceptive sense, areflexia, abnormal eye movements (such as fixation instability), and pyramidal weakness of the feet with upgoing plantars. Friedreich's also has a number of systemic complications including cardiomyopathy, diabetes, scoliosis, and pes cavus. The pathology in Friedreich's is a loss of large sensory neurons in the dorsal root ganglia initially with subsequent deterioration of the spinocerebellar tract, pyramidal tract, and dorsal columns. Typically, neuroimaging does not show progressive cerebellar degeneration. Various atypical phenotypes exist and include late-onset presentations after age 25 years, which are commonly associated with lower limb spasticity, retained reflexes, and mild cerebellar atrophy. In 98% of patients the disease is caused by a triplet GAA expansion within the first intron of the frataxin gene found on chromosome 9q13. The size of repeat expansion has an inverse correlation with the age of onset, severity of the disease, and associated systemic symptoms with the size of the repeat expansions. Point mutations constitute the remainder of the genetic mutations underlying Friedreich's ataxia. Treatment options have been directed at antioxidant protection as the loss of the frataxin gene is believed to result in the impairment of mitochondrial function and the formation of antioxidants thereafter. A recent four-year pilot study of ten patients on a combination of coenzyme Q10 and vitamin E reported improvement in cardiac function and suggested possible stabilization or reduced decline in certain neurological symptoms, but no drugs have led to any improvement in ataxia or other associated neurological features in patients, and treatment for this disease remains symptomatic.

Manji H et al., *Oxford Handbook of Neurology*, Oxford University Press, 2006, Chapter 4, Neurological disorders, Hereditary ataxias.

107. E. Dominant-hemispheric partial or total anterior circulation stroke

Dysphonia is a redution in the volume of speech. Lesions to the dominant hemisphere will cause a dysphasia in which the quality of the speech should be normal. The dysphonia of myasthenia gravis should be intermittent in nature in keeping with the pathophysiology of myasthenia gravis (i.e. weakness of the muscles of articulation in particular the laryngeal muscles). Cerebellar disease is said to have a dysphonia with a scanning quality.

Manji H et al., *Oxford Handbook of Neurology*, Oxford University Press, 2006, Chapter 4, Neurological disorders, Myasthenia gravis (management).

108. D. Progressive supranuclear palsy

Progressive supranuclear palsy (PSP) is most often misdiagnosed as Parkinson's disease early in the course of the illness. Memory problems and personality changes may also lead a physician to mistake PSP for depression. The key to diagnosing PSP is identifying early gait instability and reduced vertical movements of the eyes, the hallmark of the disease, as well as ruling out other similar disorders, some of which are treatable. Both PSP and Parkinson's disease cause rigidity, bradykinesia, and clumsiness. However, people with PSP usually stand straight or occasionally even tilt their heads backward (and tend to fall backward), while those with Parkinson's disease usually bend forward. Problems with speech and swallowing are much more common and severe in PSP than in Parkinson's disease, and tend to develop earlier in the course of the disease. Eye movements are abnormal in PSP but usually normal in Parkinson's disease. Both diseases share other features: onset in late middle age, bradykinesia (slow movement), and rigidity. Tremor, almost universal in individuals with Parkinson's disease, is rare in PSP. Although individuals with Parkinson's disease benefit considerably from the drug levodopa, people with PSP respond poorly and only transiently to this drug. Extrapyramidal signs are not characteristic features of multiple sclerosis, motor neuron disease, or Alzheimer's disease.

Williams DR, Lees AJ, Progressive supranuclear palsy: clinicopathological concepts and diagnostic challenges, *Lancet Neurology* 2009;8(3):270–279.

109. B. Impulse control disorders such as hypersexuality

Dopamine agonists can be effective at treating the symptoms of Parkinson's disease. They are often the first treatment initiated, particularly in the younger patient. There may be slightly fewer motor complications than with levodopa. However, another important side effect is the development of impulse control disorders.

As you can imagine, conditions such as this can seriously damage quality of life for the patient and their families. It is therefore vital to ask about symptoms such as this, however sensitive it may be.

BNF, Dopamine-receptor agonists, 4.9.1, Dopamine drugs used in Parkinson's disease. http://www.evidence.nhs.uk/formulary/bnf/current/4-central-nervous-system/49-drugs-used-in-parkinsonism-and-related-disorders/491-dopaminergic-drugs-used-in-parkinsons-disease/dopamine-receptor-agonists

110. C. One year

If a patient has epilepsy, then they must be seizure-free for a year before they are allowed to restart driving. The DVLA has strict requirements regarding whether patients are able to drive if they suffer from health conditions. It is very important to advise patients of this if you see them, and it is our responsibility to ask about this if they present to us. If you are in doubt, then you can refer to the DVLA guidance.

gov.uk, Assessing fitness to drive: a guide for medical professionals. http://www.dft.gov.uk/dvla/medical/ataglance.aspx

111. E. No further diagnostics or treatments and review in six months

Diagnosis should be clinical. Levodopa or apopmorphine challenges are not diagnostic, although the pattern of response when treatment is initiated may further support the diagnosis. Neuroimaging may be useful in investigating Parkinsonian syndromes (e.g. vascular parkinsonism) but does not have a role in routine diagnosis. DaT scans identify the distribution of striatal dopaminergic neurones, which can further support a clinical diagnosis and help to differentiate idiopathic disease from Parkinsonian syndromes. In early idiopathic Parkinson's disease, there is likely to be uneven reduction between the left and right basal ganglia, whereas the reduction may be more symmetrical in Parkinsonian syndromes. However there is marked variability in test results, rendering the DaT scan a tool to be used to support diagnosis in light of the clinical picture, rather than diagnostic in its own right. As discussed, treatment should only be initiated when symptomatic and the benefits of treatment outweigh the side effects.

Parkinson's Disease—Diagnosis & Management in Primary and Secondary Care: NICE

http://www.nice.org.uk/nicemedia/live/10984/30088/30088.pdf

112. E. 1 in 100

Epilepsy is the most common neurological disease in the UK. It has a prevalence often quoted at about 1%, but is more likely to be between 0.5 and 1%. It is often managed by neurologists, but it important for all physicians to be able to recognize features of a seizure on taking a history so that they are not misdiagnosed, and can be managed appropriately.

NICE Guidance [CG20], The epilepsies: the diagnosis and management of the epilepsies in adults and children in primary and secondary care. http://guidance.nice.org.uk/CG20/Guidance/pdf/English

113. C. Neuromyelitis optica

The diagnosis is neuromyelitis optica (NMO) or Devic's disease. The main differential diagnosis here is that of multiple sclerosis (MS). Typical features of NMO are: ocular pain with loss of vision, myelitis with severe symmetric paraplegia, sensory loss below the lesion, and bladder dysfunction. Other symptoms typical of spinal cord demyelination that are seen in both neuromyelitis optica and multiple sclerosis include paroxysmal tonic spasms (recurrent, stereotypic painful spasms of the limbs and trunk that last 20–45 seconds) and Lhermitte's symptom (spinal or limb dysaesthesias caused by neck flexion). Cervical myelitis extending into the brainstem causes nausea, hiccoughs, or acute neurogenic respiratory failure. NMO has a female to male ratio of 9:1 (MS 2:1) with a median age of onset of 39 (MS is 29). Eighty to ninety percent of NMO patients experience a relapsing-remitting disease. Cerebrospinal fluid findings in NMO are variable and include: occasional prominent pleocytosis with pleomorphic or mononuclear cells and oligoclonal bands in 15–30%. MR brain may be normal or have non-specific white-matter lesions, a unique hypothalamic, corpus callosal, periventricular or brainstem lesion. MR spine should normally show a longitudinally extensive lesion (at least 3 vertebral segments). Investigative diagnosis can usually be confirmed with at least two of three laboratory findings: longitudinally extensive cord lesion, a brain MRI that is non-diagnostic for multiple sclerosis at presentation, or aquaporin 4 antibodies (99% sensitive and 90% specific). There can be a clinical overlap with Sjögren's syndrome when patients with Sjögren's are positive for aquaporin antibodies. Treatment is with high-dose steroids and plasmapheresis.

Wingerchuk DM et al., The spectrum of neuromyelitis optics, *Lancet Neurology* 2007;6:805–815.

114. C. Fat embolism

Fat embolism may complicate major trauma and the condition usually manifests some 24–48 hours following the trauma. Embolization to the lungs causes hypoxia (hence the confusion in this patient), cough, haemoptysis, and the characteristic rash of fat embolization. Occasionally, fat embolism may be seen in the retina and examination of the urine will show presence of fat.

Ramrakha PS et al., *Oxford Handbook of Acute Medicine*, Third Edition, Oxford University Press, 2010, Chapter 1, Cardiac emergencies, Fat embolism.

115. B. Carbamazepine

This woman's history is entirely consistent with trigeminal neuralgia. The mainstay of therapy is carbamazepine which carries the greatest evidence base with respect to therapeutic intervention.

Lesley Bowker et al., *Oxford Handbook of Geriatric Medicine*, Second Edition, Oxford University Press, 2012, Chapter 7, Neurology.

116. B. Consider stopping her valproate

The recommendation is to stop the valproate completely if possible, which should be an option if patients have remained fit-free for two years or more. Otherwise, starting folic acid supplementation for at least 12 weeks prior to conception is essential. Switching to another anti-epileptic associated with a low risk of malformation such as lamotrigine may also be an option. If fits occur relatively commonly, in the post-partum period it is important to give advice to women about safe bathing and feeding of the child to reduce the risk of harm from maternal seizures.

Sally Collins et al., *Oxford Handbook of Obstetrics and Gynaecology*, Third Edition, Oxford University Press, 2016, Chapter 5, Medical disorders in Pregnancy.

117. C. Lhermitte's sign

Demyelinated neurons rely on Na$^+$ channels to conduct impulses across demyelinated segments. These channels are very temperature-sensitive, and cease to function properly as temperatures rise (e.g. with exercise or in a hot bath) causing slowing or even conduction block in affected neurons. This can temporarily worsen any MS symptoms, but most characteristically causes Pulfrich's effect, where stereoscopic depth perception is lost due to delayed conduction in an affected optic nerve, and Uhthoff's phenomenon, where vision becomes blurred, again due to impaired conduction in the optic nerve. Lhermitte's sign is positive when flexion of the neck causes parasthesiae down the back or in the arms/legs. Lhermitte's sign is not specific to MS, and may also be positive in cervical stenosis. Spinal claudication can also cause exercise-induced leg symptoms. Marcus Gunn sign describes a relative afferent pupillary defect (RAPD), caused by poor light perception through one optic nerve relative to the other (i.e. if both are equally damaged there will not be an RAPD). Each pupil constricts normally to direct light stimulation, but when alternating light stimulation directly from one eye to the other and back again, the pupil on the affected side continues to dilate when the light shines on it. This is because the consensual relaxation response predominates over the direct constriction response, which is reduced due to impaired conduction in the optic nerve on that side.

Longmore M et al., *Oxford Handbook of Clinical Medicine*, Eighth Edition, Oxford University Press, 2010, Chapter 10, Neurology, Multiple sclerosis.

1. **A 46-year-old woman has a GCS score of 10/15. Ambulance staff report that they found several empty diazepam packets on her kitchen table, prescribed by her GP due to difficulty sleeping triggered by a difficult marital breakdown. Which is the *single* most appropriate medication to administer initially?**
   A. Adrenaline (epinephrine)
   B. Flumazenil
   C. N-acetylcysteine
   D. Naloxone
   E. Naltrexone

2. **A 73-year-old man has Alzheimer's dementia with an MMSE®-2™ of 24/30. He lives with his wife, although is largely independent, having only recently retired from teaching. He has never been lost or disorientated whilst away from home. He asks for advice about driving as his wife never learnt and relies on him. Which is the *single* most appropriate advice to give?**
   A. He should arrange to undergo a driving assessment test
   B. He should inform the DVLA and his insurance company
   C. He should inform the DVLA who will retract his licence until he passes an assessment
   D. He should stop driving immediately
   E. His doctor should inform the DVLA on his behalf

3. **A 29-year-old man has had spasms in his neck and rolling of his tongue for the last day. He started taking haloperidol 10 mg once daily one week ago. Which is the *single* most appropriate description of this common side effect?**
   A. Acute dystonia
   B. Akathisia
   C. Tardive dyskinesia
   D. Tics
   E. Parkinsonism

4. An 18-year-old man is admitted to a psychiatric ward. For the last two weeks he has felt people were following him and has overheard strangers talking about him. He has ideas of reference, vivid auditory hallucinations, but with no clouding of consciousness. His family report social withdrawal, unusual behaviour over the last year, and that he has recently dropped out of college. He reports smoking joints almost daily for the last 12 months. Which is the *single* most appropriate diagnosis?

    A. Acute schizophrenia-like psychotic disorder
    B. Mental and behavioural disorders due to cannabis: amnesic state
    C. Mental and behavioural disorders due to cannabis: psychotic disorder, schizophrenia-like
    D. Mental and behavioural disorders due to cannabis: withdrawal with delirium
    E. Paranoid schizophrenia

5. A 30-year-old woman comes to the emergency department with palpitations and an associated tension headache. Her ECG is normal. A full history reveals that she has been worrying almost daily for several months for no apparent reason and with no subjective precipitators. She feels constantly nervous and jumpy. She has no other symptoms. Which is the *single* most likely diagnosis?

    A. Acute stress disorder
    B. Generalized anxiety disorder
    C. Panic disorder
    D. Phaeochromocytoma
    E. Thyrotoxicosis

6. A 75-year-old woman appears confused and forgetful for one week. She has told her family that her neighbours are stealing things from her fridge. She says she can see them hiding in the garden. She is labile in mood, distracted, and drowsy. Which is the *single* most appropriate first investigation?

    A. CT brain scan
    B. Dipstick mid-stream urine (MSU)
    C. FBC and differential white cell count (WCC)
    D. MSU culture and sensitivity
    E. Vitamin B_{12} and folate serum level

7. A 26-year-old woman tried to remove an electronic bug from under her skin and has a deep forearm wound requiring suturing. She is, however, very agitated, pacing, and aggressive to treating staff, who are unable to finish the job. It is decided that rapid tranquillization is appropriate in this case. Which is the *single* most appropriate medication to use initially?

    A. Diazepam 10–20 mg IM
    B. Diazepam 10–20 mg PO
    C. Lorazepam 1–2 mg IM
    D. Lorazepam 1–2 mg PO
    E. Olanzapine 10–20 mg IM

8. **A 25-year-old man seeks protection in the emergency department from the 'shadow men' following him. He is hot, tachycardic, and sweaty. He admits indulging in a three-day drug binge at a festival. Which *single* drug is most likely to have caused these symptoms?**
   A. Amphetamines
   B. Cannabis
   C. Cocaine
   D. Ketamine
   E. Mushrooms

9. **A 46-year-old man with alcohol dependence presents with confusion. Neurological examination reveals nystagmus and opthalmoplegia. Which is the *single* most likely other finding in this case?**
   A. Ascites
   B. Asterixis
   C. Ataxia
   D. Jaundice
   E. Pyrexia

10. **A 29-year-old woman has dizziness, headaches, nausea, and sensations in her legs which she describes as being like 'electric shocks'. She was prescribed psychotropic medication four months ago but recently stopped taking it as she felt a lot better. She did not consult her GP or taper off her dosage. Which is the *single* most likely medication she was prescribed?**
    A. Lithium
    B. Paroxetine
    C. Propranolol
    D. Quetiapine
    E. Temazepam

11. **A 23-year-old woman sustains a minor limb injury while intoxicated with alcohol. This is her third emergency department visit in a month. She is treated and is assessed as sober and safe for discharge. She scores 4 out of 16 on the Fast Alcohol Screening Test (FAST). Which is the *single* most appropriate initial management?**
    A. Advise complete abstinence from alcohol
    B. Follow-up bloods, including FBC and LFTs
    C. Inpatient admission
    D. Offer a brief intervention
    E. Outpatient detoxification

12. **A 78-year-old woman has recently been diagnosed with depression. She has started using St John's wort remedy to help improve her low mood. Which is the *single* most relevant advice to give her?**
    A. It has not been shown to be particularly effective in depression
    B. It is not licensed for treating depression
    C. She cannot take it with her prescribed SSRI antidepressant
    D. She should not take it
    E. There may be significant interactions with her other medications

13. **A 24-year-old woman is dependent on heroin, confirmed by two positive urine drug screens. She wants help to stop injecting and 'sort her life out', and would like to have a 'clear head'. Which is the *single* most appropriate drug to prescribe?**
    A. Injectable diamorphine
    B. Injectable methadone
    C. Oral buprenorphine
    D. Oral lofexidine
    E. Oral methadone

14. **A 35-year-old woman is transferred from an inpatient psychiatric unit with a fever, rigid muscles, sweats, tremor, and fluctuating BP. She started a depot antipsychotic three days ago. Which is the *single* most appropriate initial blood investigation?**
    A. Creatine kinase (CK)
    B. C-reactive protein (CRP)
    C. Magnesium
    D. Sodium
    E. Thyroid stimulating hormone (TSH)

15. **An 83-year-old woman with Alzheimer's dementia who has recently started taking donepezil is reviewed in the memory clinic. Which is the *single* most appropriate observation to review?**
    A. Abbreviated mental test score
    B. Blood pressure
    C. Geriatric Depression Scale
    D. Pulse
    E. Respiratory rate

16. **A 51-year-old man is unwell on day 2 of an attempted home detox from alcohol. He is brought to the emergency department by his partner, who is seeking help. A diagnosis of delirium tremens is suspected. Which *single* feature is most suggestive of this diagnosis?**
    A. Clouding of consciousness
    B. Jaundice
    C. Suicidal thoughts
    D. Sweating
    E. Tremor

17. **An 83-year-old woman with severe Alzheimer's dementia lives in a nursing home. Staff report that she is stable and presents no problems to them. Her MMSE®-2™ score is 9/30. Her list of medications is being reviewed. Which *single* medication is the most appropriate to stop first?**
    A. Co-codamol 8/500 PRN maximum qds
    B. Donepezil 10 mg once daily
    C. Olanzapine 5 mg at night
    D. Simvastatin 20 mg at night
    E. Temazepam 10 mg at night as needed

18. **A 54-year-old man is found on the streets, drowsy and vomiting. He is unkempt with a strong odour of alcohol, is ataxic, verbally aggressive, and slurring his words. His temperature is 37.5°C, heart rate 96 bpm, and BP 115/87 mmHg. Which is the *single* most appropriate diagnosis to exclude?**
    A. Alcohol intoxication
    B. Alcohol withdrawal
    C. Aspiration pneumonia
    D. Head injury
    E. Psychotic episode

19. **A 74-year-old man feels tired during the day but doesn't know why. His wife says he is up overnight fighting with the bedsheets and at these times tells her he can see snakes. They have put padding on the bedside table to prevent injury. Which is the *single* most likely diagnosis?**
    A. Alzheimer's dementia
    B. Delirium
    C. Harmful use of alcohol
    D. Psychosis
    E. REM sleep disorder

20. **A 55-year-old woman with BPAD has a seizure. She has never fitted before. Her husband reports she had a three-day history of tremor, nausea, vomiting, muscle twitches, and bloody diarrhoea before they boarded their flight home from a holiday in Egypt. Which is the *single* most likely cause?**
    A. Acute confusional state secondary to acute infection
    B. Lithium toxicity
    C. Pulmonary embolus
    D. Thyrotoxicosis
    E. Traveller's diarrhoea

21. **A 74-year-old woman became increasingly confused over a period of six months. Before a formal diagnosis could be made, she died of a heart attack. A provisional diagnosis of Alzheimer's dementia was made, and her daughter would like to know if this was the case. She agrees to an autopsy. Which *single* neuropathological finding would be most likely to confirm this diagnosis?**
    A. Cytoplasmic inclusion bodies
    B. Extracellular neurofibrillary tangles
    C. Extracellular senile plaques
    D. Knife-edge atrophy
    E. Pick's bodies

22. **A 23-year-old man has acute chest pain and palpitations which came on suddenly while he was shopping. He is sweaty and feels as though he is dying. His ECG and physical examination were normal and systemic enquiry revealed no other significant symptoms. Which is the *single* most likely diagnosis?**
    A. Asthma
    B. Delusional disorder
    C. Depression
    D. Hyperthyroidism
    E. Panic attack

23. **A 56-year-old man is admitted to a substance misuse unit for alcohol detoxification. Thirty-six hours after his last drink he develops ataxia, nystagmus, ophthalmoplegia, memory impairment, agitation, and severe tremor. Which is the *single* most appropriate medication combination to prescribe?**
    A. Acamprosate, chlordiazepoxide (reducing regime), oral B vitamins
    B. Acamprosate, chlordiazepoxide (reducing regime), parenteral B vitamins
    C. Chlordiazepoxide (reducing regime), disulfiram, parenteral B vitamins
    D. Chlordiazepoxide (reducing regime), haloperidol, oral B vitamins
    E. Diazepam (reducing regime), haloperidol, parenteral B vitamins

24. **A 68-year-old woman was admitted 24 hours earlier with headache, nausea, and anxiety. She now has a new tremor, is sweating, and has become agitated and rude to staff, demanding her medication. It is believed she is showing signs of drug withdrawal. Which is the *single* most likely medication responsible for this?**

    A. Fluoxetine
    B. Levothyroxine
    C. Lorazepam
    D. Quetiapine
    E. Zopiclone

25. **A retired 76-year-old man with a UTI is septic and dehydrated. He has become aggressive and agitated, and is demanding to leave the emergency department as he says he has to go to work. Which is the *single* most appropriate management?**

    A. Admit him to the medical ward under the Mental Capacity Act
    B. Ask him to complete a 'discharge against medical advice' form
    C. Detain him under Section 5(2) of the MHA
    D. Discharge him with a course of antibiotics with GP follow-up
    E. Organize an MHA assessment

26. **A 40-year-old man was an alcoholic and heroin addict. He has now completed an alcohol detox and is receiving methadone maintenance treatment. He has an established diagnosis of emotionally unstable PD, borderline type. He would like to continue with his methadone treatment and to reduce the risk of alcohol relapse; he is particularly concerned about alcohol cravings. Psychosocial intervention is initiated. Which is the *single* most appropriate medication to prescribe?**

    A. Acamprosate
    B. Disulfiram
    C. Fluoxetine
    D. Haloperidol
    E. Naltrexone

27. **A 79-year-old man has short-term memory loss, non-troublesome visual hallucinations, and has had some stiffness and tremor for nine months. His MMSE®-2™ score is 23/30. Which is the *single* most appropriate medication to slow cognitive decline?**

    A. Donepezil
    B. Galantamine
    C. Levodopa
    D. Memantine
    E. Rivastigmine

28. **An 18-year-old woman took an overdose five hours ago. Blood tests reveal a serum paracetamol level above the treatment line. Which is the *single* most appropriate treatment to initiate?**

   A. Activated charcoal
   B. Alkaline diuresis
   C. Gastric lavage
   D. IV Pabrinex®
   E. IV Parvolex®

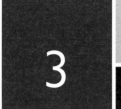
1. B. Flumazenil

Flumazenil is a gamma-aminobutyric acid (GABA) antagonist, available for injection only, which can be used as an antidote in the treatment of benzodiazepine overdoses. Long-acting benzodiazepines such as diazepam may require repeated administration of flumazenil due to its short half-life. Diazepam is a benzodiazepine medication commonly used for short-term relief of anxiety and sleeping problems. Adrenaline has various uses in emergency medicine, but reversal of benzodiazepine overdose is not one of them. Many generic drug names have been changed following recommended International Non-Proprietary Name (rINN) rules. However, adrenaline (epinephrine), and noradrenaline (norepinephrine) will continue to be called by both names because it was believed to be too risky given their widespread use in emergency medicine. N-acetylcysteine is used in the management of paracetamol overdose. Naloxone is an opioid inverse agonist drug, used to counter the effects of opiate overdose. Naltrexone is an opioid receptor antagonist used primarily in the management of alcohol dependence and opioid dependence.

British National Formulary—emergency treatment of poisoning. www.bnf.org→ www.toxbase.org.

2. B. He should inform the DVLA and his insurance company

Once informed, the DVLA would then ask for consent to contact his GP or specialist for medical information and, based on this, may ask him to undertake a driving assessment. Then he may be issued with a licence for a shorter period and need regular reassessments, or he may be asked to stop driving. Option A is partly correct but he should be advised to inform the DVLA and his insurance company. He may wish to undergo an assessment for his own information and reassurance or the DVLA may ask him to. He should inform the DVLA but they will not automatically retract his licence (option C). He may have to complete a driving assessment. Stopping driving immediately (option D) may be advisable if the doctor is very worried about the patient's driving safety, but based on the history given in this question, there is no evidence to suggest he needs to be told to stop driving immediately. That his doctor should inform the DVLA on his behalf (option E) is not the best initial piece of advice. However, if a patient refuses to contact the DVLA, a doctor may do this without the patient's consent if the doctor is concerned for the safety of that person or other road users. If a doctor does decide to breach confidentiality and inform the DVLA, the doctor has a professional duty to try to inform the patient of their intentions, and should confirm in writing once this disclosure has been made.

Alzheimer's Society, Driving and dementia. http://alzheimers.org.uk/site/scripts/documents_info.php?documentID=144

3. A. Acute dystonia

Acute dystonia is a reaction following exposure to antipsychotic medication with sustained, often painful muscular spasms. Most frequent are neck dystonias, followed by tongue and jaw. Incidence is 3–10% of patients exposed to antipsychotics (up to 30% with high-potency drugs). Younger age group, males, and high-potency antipsychotics confer higher risk. Ninety percent of the onset of symptoms occurs within the first five days of exposure. Akathisia is a subjective feeling of inner restlessness and objective psychomotor agitation (such as pacing) associated with antipsychotic medication. Tardive dyskinesia is characterized by involuntary, repetitive, and purposeless movements occurring with long-term antipsychotic exposure of months to years. A tic s a sudden, repetitive, non-rhythmic motor movement or vocalization involving discrete muscle groups. Tics are not a common side effect of antipsychotic medication. Parkinsonism is a frequent adverse effect in around 20% of patients treated with antipsychotic medication. Parkinson's disease is a progressive neurological condition not associated with antipsychotic medication per se.

YouTube video of acute dystonia. http://www.youtube.com/watch?v=Gjiy1rDZpp8.

4. C. Mental and behavioural disorders due to cannabis: psychotic disorder, schizophrenia-like

Drug-induced psychoses are characterized by a cluster of psychotic phenomena that occur during or immediately after psychoactive substance use and are characterized by vivid hallucinations (typically auditory, but often in more than one sensory modality), ideas of reference (often of a paranoid or persecutory nature), psychomotor disturbances, and other psychosis-like symptoms. The sensorium is usually clear, but some degree of clouding of consciousness may be present. While on the ward he should ideally have no access to illicit drugs (confirmed by repeat urine testing), and the symptoms should resolve at least partially within one month and fully within six months. Particular care should be taken to avoid diagnosing a more serious condition like schizophrenia when a diagnosis of drug-induced psychosis is more appropriate. A diagnosis of psychotic disorder should not be made merely on the basis of perceptual distortions or hallucinatory experiences when substances having primary hallucinogenic effects (e.g. LSD, mescaline, cannabis at high doses) have been taken. In acute schizophrenia-like psychotic disorder the psychotic symptoms are comparatively stable and justify a diagnosis of schizophrenia but have lasted for less than about one month. The polymorphic unstable features (variable psychotic features and mood) are absent. If the schizophrenic symptoms persist for more than one month the diagnosis should be changed to schizophrenia. While the patient is using cannabis, as in this scenario, one cannot be certain that the psychotic features are not due to direct intoxication or drug induced. False diagnosis in such cases may have distressing and costly implications for the patient and for the health services. Cannabis and alcohol can induce amnesia, but there is no mention of memory impairment in this case. There is some debate on whether cannabis produces dependence and withdrawal. Either way there are no symptoms here to suggest a withdrawal state, including no evidence of physiological changes, or clouding of consciousness, which are typical in withdrawal states. The diagnosis of schizophrenia is supported by the clinical symptoms (restricted affect, ideas of reference, vivid auditory hallucinations, psychomotor agitation) and possible prodromal symptoms (social withdrawal, unusual behaviour). However, he is still using cannabis, which complicates the picture, and the psychotic symptoms are short-lived (only two weeks). Many psychoactive substance-induced psychotic states are of short duration (e.g. amphetamine and cocaine psychoses). ICD-10 requires at least one month of either one of the FRSs, bizarre delusions, or two or more symptoms including persistent hallucinations, thought disorder, catatonic behaviour, negative symptoms, or significant and persistent behavioural change. ICD-10 recognizes that there may be a prodromal phase associated with schizophrenia, which is not included in the one-month time requirement.

World Health Organization, ICD-10, Mental and behavioural disorders due to psychoactive substance use. http://www.who.int/substance_abuse/terminology/ICD10ClinicalDiagnosis.pdf

5. B. Generalized anxiety disorder

The most likely diagnosis is generalized anxiety disorder. This has been described by NICE as 'a very common but under-recognized condition characterized by endless worrying, which results in substantial disability for many sufferers, affecting their capacity to work and to live fulfilled and meaningful lives'. Its symptoms are hard to define as they are a near-constant free-floating anxiety about everything, with some somatic symptoms but with no clear causative or alleviating behaviours. People with generalized anxiety disorder may appear outwardly 'ordinary' but are actually managing significant worries. There is often an acute-on-chronic element to the disorder with symptoms changing over time to have more, or less, effect on activities of daily living. Acute stress disorder would arise following a significant trauma. Without this event it would be unlikely this would be the diagnosis. There is an overlap of symptoms with a generalized anxiety disorder, as both can include agitation and anxiety, or with a panic disorder: where there is autonomic arousal, tachycardia, sweating, etc. It is important to always ask about events occurring before the symptoms start and any clear precipitating factors. Panic disorder, or panic attack, involves periods of acute anxiety or fear which start suddenly and can last from minutes to hours, usually peaking at about ten minutes. There are associated features of depersonalization, dizziness, and fears of losing control or dying. Many people describe them as intensely frightening and in themselves a traumatic experience. For a panic disorder to be diagnosed there should be a discrete period of anxiety, with a peak and fall, and at least four symptoms of sympathetic nervous system response: palpitations, sweating, shortness of breath, nausea, paraesthesias, dizziness, etc. In this scenario, the anxiety is more free-floating, constant, and without a start or stop. Phaeochromocytoma is a neuroendocrine tumour of the medulla of the adrenal glands where high levels of catecholamines are secreted, leading to sympathetic nervous system hyperactivity as described above. Most worryingly there is a rise in blood pressure which can be dangerous, and is poorly controlled with anti-hypertensive medication. It is an organic condition which should be considered when 'psychiatric' symptoms are present, as missing it can be fatal. Diagnosis is by plasma or 24-hour urinary measurements of catecholamines. Thyrotoxicosis can be confused with generalized anxiety disorder as both have increased subjective anxiety with palpitations, and headaches. However, in thyrotoxicosis there would be characteristic signs of a tremor, weight loss, and heat intolerance. These are associated with an overactive thyroid resulting in excessive concentrations of free thyroid hormones in the blood. A simple bedside test is to examine the hands; in thyrotoxicosis they are likely to be sweaty, tremulous, and warm, rather than cold and clammy in anxiety (where there is peripheral vasoconstriction). Routine TFTs would confirm the diagnosis.

Iacovides A et al., Difference in symptom profile between generalized anxiety disorder and anxiety secondary to hyperthyroidism. *International Journal of Psychiatry in Medicine* 2000;30:71–81.

Phaeochromocytoma, *BMJ* 2012;344:e1042.

6. B. Dipstick mid-stream urine (MSU)

UTIs are a very common cause of delirium in the elderly. Dipstick urinalysis is an easy and useful first test in any setting. A CT brain scan is an important part of a full dementia screen, especially if there are any atypical features (e.g. short history or sudden decline, younger age at onset of symptoms, focal neurological signs). However, in this case, because of the short onset of symptoms, visual hallucinations, and associated drowsiness, the more likely diagnosis in this patient is delirium. Remember, for a diagnosis of dementia you need a history of symptoms for at least six months in clear consciousness. FBC is an important part of the dementia screen. The differential WCC might help point towards a diagnosis of delirium, although it is not as quick or specific a result as a urine dipstick. MSU culture and sensitivity would be an important next step if the dipstick is positive. Testing vitamin B_{12} and folate is an essential part of a dementia screen, as low levels of either can masquerade as dementia or exacerbate an existing dementia. However, this appears to be a presentation of delirium and this would not be the best immediate investigation.

Gelder M et al., *New Oxford Textbook of Psychiatry*, Second Edition, Oxford University Press, Oxford, 2012, 4.1, Delirium.

NICE Guideline [CG103], Delirium: prevention, diagnosis, management, July 2010. https://www.nice.org.uk/guidance/cg103.

7. D. Lorazepam 1–2 mg PO

Local protocols for rapid tranquillization and control and restraint should be followed. However, it is important to use the least restrictive measure and work with the patient as far as possible to reduce risk of harm to patient and others. Oral (PO) medication should be offered first line, with escalation to IM medication only where oral medication has failed, been refused, or is not indicated. Oral lorazepam 1–2 mg should be offered first line in this case. IV medication should only be used in exceptional circumstances where immediate tranquillization is necessary. Thus diazepam 10–20 mg IM is not the correct answer. Diazepam 10–20 mg PO is not recommended for rapid tranquillization because of its slower onset of action and longer duration compared with shorter-acting benzodiazepines. Lorazepam is the benzodiazepine of choice for rapid tranquillization, 1–2 mg both for PO and IM dosing. This may be combined with haloperidol if psychosis is present. Olanzapine IM (E) may be considered second line for moderate disturbance, but must not be given within one hour of IM lorazepam.

Semple D, Smyth R, *Oxford Handbook of Psychiatry*, Third Edition, Oxford University Press, 2013, Chapter 24, Difficult and urgent situations.

8. A. Amphetamines

Amphetamines are stimulant drugs used recreationally to make users feel alert and chatty, hence the street name 'speed'. Acute harmful effects include tachycardia, hyperpyrexia, and a quasi-psychotic state with visual, auditory, and tactile hallucinations. Acute amphetamine intoxication can mimic schizophrenia but needs to be differentiated; a careful history here is helpful. Cannabis intoxication can cause mild tachycardia and mild paranoia, but delusions and hallucinations would not be seen as an acute effect. Chronic cannabis use, especially from an early age, is a risk factor associated with development of schizophrenia. Cocaine is a stimulant drug causing increased energy, confidence, and euphoria. Acute harmful effects include arrhythmias, anxiety, and hypertension. Acute psychosis is not seen. Ketamine is a hallucinogenic anaesthetic used recreationally for dissociative experiences. Common acute side effects are nausea, ataxia, and slurred speech. Magic mushrooms in small doses can cause euphoria, while large doses can cause perceptual abnormalities such as visual distortions, synaesthesia, and distorted body image. Harmful effects include nausea, vomiting, and diarrhoea.

Semple D, Smyth R, *Oxford Handbook of Psychiatry*, Third Edition, Oxford University Press, 2013, Chapter 15, Substance misuse.

9. C. Ataxia

This man presents with the tetrad of symptoms seen in Wernicke's encephalopathy: acute confusional state, ataxia, and nystagmus and opthalmoplegia. Wernicke's encephalopathy is caused by thiamine deficiency, often from prolonged alcohol consumption. Untreated, it may progress to Korsakoff psychosis, coma, and death. Ascites is a feature of decompensated liver disease. Liver disease may be associated with chronic alcohol dependence but is not a diagnostic feature of Wernicke's encephalopathy. Ascites is confirmed on physical examination. There is a visible abdominal bulge with 'shifting dullness'—a difference in percussion which shifts when the patient turns onto their side. Asterixis, or liver flap, is a gross motor tremor of the hand. It is seen when the wrist is extended then bent upwards with the arm outstretched. It is caused by abnormal function of the diencephalic motor centres in the brain, which regulate the muscles involved in maintaining position. It is a feature of decompensated liver disease and can also be seen in Wilson's disease or carbon monoxide toxicity. Jaundice is often seen in hepatitis or in other liver disease, such as liver cancer, or obstruction of the biliary tract. It is present in many people with alcoholic liver disease but is not a diagnostic feature of Wernicke's encephalopathy. Pyrexia is unrelated to Wernicke's encephalopathy. It may be related to an untreated infection, such as a urinary tract infection (UTI), which in turn could lead to delirium.

Alzheimer's Society, What is Korsakoff's syndrome? http://www.alzheimers.org.uk/site/scripts/documents_info.php?documentID=98

10. B. Paroxetine

This question asks about the symptoms associated with antidepressant discontinuation syndrome (often called SSRI withdrawal syndrome). Paroxetine is the SSRI with the shortest half-life and hence is associated with the highest risk of withdrawal symptoms from stopping use. Lithium withdrawal may bring common problems such as feeling anxious, irritable, tense, restless, highly emotional, or confused. There do not seem to be any physical 'rebound phenomena'. Stopping propranolol can cause irregular heartbeat and a rebound anxiety on withdrawal. Withdrawal psychosis and tardive dyskinesia are two of the most serious problems caused by withdrawal from antipsychotics such as quetiapine. Temazepam is an intermediate-acting benzodiazepine. Benzodiazepine withdrawal symptoms include anxiety, confusion, hallucinations, insomnia, cold sweats, heart palpitations, tremor, tinnitus, and detachment.

NICE guidelines [CG90], Depression in adults: recognition and management, October 2009. http://guidance.nice.org.uk/CG90

11. D. Offer a brief intervention

The most appropriate management is to offer a brief intervention. The FAST is a quick screening tool with a sensitivity of 93% and a specificity of 88% for detection of hazardous drinking (compared to the CAGE questionnaire with 40% and 98% respectively). The cut-off for clinical significance is 3/16 points on the FAST. By scoring 3+ the patient falls into the 'hazardous drinking' category at least. There is good evidence for 'screening and brief intervention' in an ED or primary care setting reducing hazardous drinking by 17% (NICE guideline on preventing alcohol use disorders). Brief alcohol interventions as short as five minutes have been shown to be effective in reducing alcohol consumption within primary care settings (Poikolainen 1999; Wilk et al. 1997). There is no evidence that recommending abstinence works, especially in this age group. Follow-up bloods, including FBC and LFTs, are a good option to assess for alcohol-related damage, but not as important as the initial management option in this case. NICE does not recommend use of biochemical measures 'as a matter of routine' to screen for harmful or hazardous use. There is no evidence that this woman is suffering from a mental or physical illness that would necessitate admission. Although admission is the 'safest' possible management it is not cost-effective or pragmatic in most instances. The FAST does not detect alcohol dependence specifically. The CAGE is considered more useful for detecting severe alcohol dependence (with a cut-off of 2/4). In this case we do not know yet if the patient is alcohol dependent, and therefore detoxification may not be appropriate.

Health Development Agency, FAST manual. http://alcoholresearchuk.org/downloads/finalReports/AERC_FinalReport_0005.pdf

NICE guidelines [ph24[, Alcohol-use disorders: prevention. https://www.nice.org.uk/guidance/ph24

Poikolainen K, Effectiveness of brief interventions to reduce alcohol intake in primary health care populations: a meta-analysis, *Preventive Medicine* 1999;28:503–509.

Wilk AI et al., Meta-analysis of randomized control trials addressing brief interventions in heavy alcohol drinkers. *Journal of General Internal Medicine* 1997;12:274–283.

12. E. There may be significant interactions with her other medications

The most important thing a patient should know about St John's wort is that there may be significant interactions with other medications. It induces the cytochrome P450 enzyme and therefore can cause significant interactions with important medications such as warfarin, antiretrovirals, and the contraceptive pill. Evidence shows that St John's wort could be effective in the treatment of mild or moderate depression but there is less evidence for its use in severe depression. Most preparations are not licensed in this country. It is used more in some other countries (e.g. Germany). It is not absolutely contraindicated with SSRIs. Helping the patient to make an informed decision is more professional and respectful than forbidding her to take the remedy. Patients will, of course, ultimately do what they think is best for them, and this approach could significantly jeopardize the doctor–patient relationship.

Komoroski BJ et al., Induction and inhibition of cytochromes P450 by the St. John's wort constituent hyperforin in human hepatocyte cultures, *Drug Metabolism and Disposition* 2004;32:512–518.

Lynch T, Price A, The effect of cytochrome p450 metabolism on drug response, interactions, and adverse effects, *American Family Physician* 2007;76:391–396.

13. C. Oral buprenorphine

Buprenorphine, an opioid receptor partial agonist, is licensed for the treatment of opiate dependency. Substitute opioid treatment reduces illicit opioid use, overdoses, criminal activity, and drug-related deaths. Due to its partial agonist properties, buprenorphine prevents opioid withdrawal and also blocks the effects of additional opioids, and so discourages drug use 'on top'. Unlike methadone, buprenorphine allows patients more of a clear head with less sedation. Injectable diamorphine (heroin) is a recognized treatment but is rarely used, and is certainly not first line. It is sometimes used for intractable opioid injecting, where first-line treatments have been unsuccessful and where the risks of ongoing illicit use (overdose, blood-borne viruses, death) outweigh the risks of prescribing injectable heroin. The Randomised Injectable Opiate Treatment Trial (RIOTT) found that treatment with supervised injectable heroin leads to significantly lower use of street heroin than does supervised injectable methadone or optimized oral methadone. Methadone can also be injected where oral methadone or buprenorphine are insufficient (e.g. intractable injectors). However, like injectable diamorphine, it requires supervision, is resource intensive, and is not popular with patients. Lofexidine is a central alpha-adrenoreceptor agonist licensed for the treatment of opioid withdrawal. Lofexidine is given to relieve the symptoms associated with opioid withdrawal including chills, sweating, piloerection, stomach cramps, muscle pain, and rhinorrhoea. The patient is not specifically requesting a detoxification, and opioid substitute prescribing (methadone or buprenorphine) is therefore a better option. There is good evidence of methadone's efficacy in opioid dependency syndrome, and methadone is commonly prescribed. Methadone is an opioid, usually taken orally in liquid form. Methadone reduces drug-related injecting, overdoses, deaths, and criminal activity. However, many patients find it sedating and that it takes the edge off their emotions. As this patient wanted a 'clear head', methadone would not be the best option.

King's College London, RIOTT trial. http://www.kcl.ac.uk/iop/depts/addictions/research/drugs/riott.aspx

Department of Health, Drug misuse and dependence: UK guidelines on clinical management. http://www.nta.nhs.uk/uploads/clinical_guidelines_2007.pdf

14. A. Creatine kinase (CK)

This question tests appropriate investigation for neuroleptic malignant syndrome (NMS). NMS is a rare, life-threatening, idiosyncratic reaction to antipsychotic (and other) medications characterized by fever, muscular rigidity, altered mental status, and autonomic dysfunction. High-potency antipsychotic and depot preparations are known risk factors. Raised serum CK is associated with NMS. CRP is produced by the liver. The level of CRP rises when there is inflammation throughout the body. CRP might well be raised in infection leading to delirium (altered mental state) and fever, but this is unlikely here. Deficiency of magnesium (causes muscle cramps, tremors (due to increased irritability of the nervous system), and confusion. However, it is usually a chronic condition caused by poor diet, diarrhoea, or medication such as diuretics. It is unlikely to appear within three days. It can be seen within a psychiatric setting, as hypomagnesaemia occurs in a third of alcoholics, and almost all delirium tremens inpatients, due to malnutrition and chronic diarrhoea. Deficiency of sodium is unlikely in this presentation but something to consider in a patient with new-onset altered mental state. Symptoms of hyponatraemia include muscle weakness, spasms, seizures, and lethargy. Symptom severity is associated with serum sodium levels: the lower the serum sodium the more prominent and serious the symptoms. Neurological symptoms typically occur only with very low levels of serum sodium (<115 mEq/L). Here excess water entering brain cells causes them to swell, which results in encephalopathy which is life-threatening. TSH testing will reveal underlying hypothyroidism and hyperthyroidism. Although hyperthyroidism will produce a tremor, sweats, and raised BP, it would not account for the rigidity or fever. As NMS (a more likely diagnosis) is life-threatening, this is something that should be investigated and ruled out first.

Adnet P et al., Neuroleptic malignant syndrome, *British Journal of Anaesthesia* 2000;85:129–135.

15. D. Pulse

Donepezil and other acetylcholinesterase inhibitors have been shown in clinical trials to slow the heart rate by on average 1–2 bpm. They may also increase the heart rate interval. If a patient has first-degree heart block, this medication may cause arrhythmia, syncope, and collapse. It is good practice to obtain an ECG prior to prescribing the medication and to monitor a patient's pulse during treatment. Abbreviated mental test scores, usually the MMSE®-2™, are used to monitor progress. This should be recorded prior to starting medication, and then at approximately six-monthly intervals, as well as measures of functioning and behaviour. BP is not known to be significantly impacted by donepezil. The Geriatric Depression Scale would be a useful tool if concerns about low mood were present. It is not routinely used in monitoring donepezil in dementia. Respiratory rate is not known to be affected by these medications.

Rowland JP et al., Cardiovascular monitoring with acetylcholinesterase inhibitors: a clinical protocol, *Advances in Psychiatric Treatment* 2007;13:178–184.

Bordier P et al., Cardiovascular effects and risk of syncope related to donepezil in patients with Alzheimer's disease, *CNS Drugs* 2006;20:411–117.

16. A. Clouding of consciousness

Delirium tremens is an acute confusional state secondary to alcohol withdrawal and is an emergency medical condition requiring inpatient care. In addition to the features of uncomplicated alcohol withdrawal there is clouding of consciousness, disorientation, retrograde amnesia, psychomotor agitation, hallucinations, and marked fluctuations. It occurs in 5% of those with alcohol withdrawal, with a peak incidence at 48 hours. It has a mortality rate of 5–10%. Jaundice is a feature of decompensated liver disease, which may be seen as a complication of chronic alcohol dependence in a case of withdrawal, but is not pathognomic of withdrawal itself. Suicidal thoughts may be present in any altered mental state associated with affective symptoms, though symptoms of fear and paranoia with visual, tactile, and auditory hallucinations tend to be associated with delirium tremens. Sweating is a feature of uncomplicated alcohol withdrawal. Coarse tremor is a feature of uncomplicated alcohol withdrawal. These tremors are usually seen as relatively slow movements which involve larger muscle groups.

Semple D, Smyth R, *Oxford Handbook of Psychiatry*, Third Edition, Oxford University Press, 2013, Chapter 24, Difficult and urgent situations.

17. D. Simvastatin 20 mg at night

Visual hallucinations are one of the three core features of Lewy body dementia: (1) visual hallucinations, typically well formed and not particularly distressing; (2) fluctuating cognition with variations in attention and alertness; and (3) spontaneous features of Parkinson's disease (present for less than a year before cognitive problems). Falls and syncope are often a feature of the presentation of Lewy body dementia but are not very specific for the diagnosis. Falls often occur because the patient's gait and balance are affected by the motor symptoms of Parkinson's. REM sleep disorder is a common symptom of Lewy body dementia which can be very tricky to manage. Patients complain of very vivid dreams and relatives notice disturbed sleep and at times disorientation and wandering at night with associated odd behaviours. However, this is not one of the core symptoms and so this is not the strongest indicator of the diagnosis. Severe neuroleptic sensitivity refers to the common reaction these patients can have to any antipsychotic medication. They can become acutely confused, experience severe extrapyramidal symptoms, and have an increased mortality rate. Word-finding difficulties are often a presenting feature of any dementia and do not indicate Lewy body dementia in particular.

McKeith TG et al., Diagnosis and management of dementia with Lewy bodies, *Neurology* 2005;65:1863–1872.

18. D. Head injury

Head injury is the most important life-threatening complication of alcohol misuse that the doctor must exclude in this challenging but common scenario. Often head injuries have occurred but may not be reported by the patient. Alcohol intoxication might explain the clinical scenario, but it is unlikely to be life-threatening unless there are physical co-morbidities or alcohol has been combined with other drugs. Alcohol withdrawal may explain the patient's odour of alcohol, unkempt appearance, and ataxia (the latter classically as part of Wernicke's syndrome), but in the absence of a tachycardia, sweating and tremor are unlikely. Aspiration pneumonia is not uncommon in heavy drinkers. The patient is afebrile, which makes the diagnosis of infection less likely (although not impossible). Alcohol misuse and aggression are common in acute psychosis. However, in this scenario, organic causes need to be excluded first.

NICE guidelines [CG176], Head injury: assessment and early management, January 2014. https://www.nice.org.uk/guidance/cg176

19. E. REM sleep disorder

People can injure themselves and others without being awake during very vivid dreams when normally atonic muscles become active during REM, dream sleep. It can be a presentation of a Lewy body dementia. Treatment is often clonazepam or other sedatives. It is also important to consider the risk of injury to the patient and their bed partner. People with Alzheimer's dementia do often report sleep disturbance. It is likely that they are more confused in the evenings. A concern is that they may become disorientated overnight and wander. If the man in the scenario above also had other features of dementia, the diagnosis may well be Lewy body dementia. Delirium can present with visual hallucinations and dreams that seem very vivid and merge with reality. There will usually be other features present such as a variable level of consciousness, confusion, and distractibility. It is unlikely to occur only at night. Elderly people are just as susceptible to harmful alcohol use as younger adults, if not more so. Visual hallucinations can be signs of a withdrawal, but this is more likely to occur some days after suddenly stopping or reducing alcohol intake. True psychosis would have a different flavour from this presentation. There would more likely be auditory hallucinations and delusional ideas present or other disorders of thought. Again, these would normally be pervasive and would not occur just at night.

Jacoby R et al., *Oxford Textbook of Old Age Psychiatry*, Fourth Edition, Oxford University Press, 2008.

20. B. Lithium toxicity

Lithium is a mood-stabilizing drug used in BPAD, though also in cases of treatment-resistant depression or psychotic illness with a strong affective component. Lithium has a narrow therapeutic index. Toxicity may be precipitated by inadequate hydration and salt intake. Early signs of toxicity include marked tremor, anorexia, nausea, vomiting, and diarrhoea (sometimes bloody), with associated dehydration and lethargy. As lithium levels rise, severe neurological complications such as hypertonicity and myoclonic jerks can occur. This may progress to ataxia, delirium, cardiac arrhythmias, seizures, coma, and death. Olanzapine is an antipsychotic medication with mood-stabilizing properties that may be prescribed in BPAD. It can cause metabolic syndrome and sedation, but high serum levels are not associated with a toxic syndrome akin to lithium. Acute confusional state secondary to acute infection is unlikely in this case as it does not fit the clinical picture. It includes severe confusion and disorientation, developing with relatively rapid onset and fluctuating in intensity. It is more usual in elderly patients. Recent air travel may be a risk factor for pulmonary embolus, but the symptoms described here are not classical for thromboses. Thyrotoxicosis is characterized by signs of sympathetic overactivity, such as tremor, tachycardia, and sweating, producing weight loss, fatigue, and heat intolerance. Lithium therapy can cause hypothyroidism but not hyperthyroidism. Traveller's diarrhoea could be suspected in a patient with diarrhoea returning from abroad, but seizures and muscle twitches would be unlikely.

Patient.co.uk, Lithium. http://www.patient.co.uk/doctor/lithium-pro

21. C. Extracellular senile plaques

Extracellular senile plaques are found in Alzheimer's dementia. They can also be found in the normal ageing brain to some extent. Their main component is amyloid, formed by abnormal metabolism of a larger amino acid. Inclusion bodies are nuclear or cytoplasmic aggregates of stainable substances, usually proteins. Cytoplasmic inclusion bodies are found with certain viral infections, such as rabies and smallpox, whereas neuronal inclusion bodies are found in diseases like Parkinson's disease and Lewy body dementia. In Alzheimer's disease there are intracellular neurofibrillary tangles, not extracellular. These are abnormal structures that accumulate inside neurons, made principally of hyperphosphorylated tau proteins. Knife-edge atrophy refers to the extreme and global thinning of the gyri of the cerebral cortex seen in the frontal and temporal lobes in Pick's disease. Pick's bodiesare also intracellular neurofibrillary tangles composed of abnormal tau proteins but they differ from those found in Alzheimer's disease as they stain differently and are more straight and fibrous. Those in Alzheimer's are paired and coiled.

Jacoby R et al., *Oxford Textbook of Old Age Psychiatry*, Fourth Edition, Oxford University Press, 2008, Neuropathology.

22. E. Panic attack

Panic attack is the correct answer. A panic attack is a period of intense fear characterized by clusters of symptoms which include palpitations, sweating, trembling, shortness of breath, feeling of choking, chest pain, nausea, dizziness, derealization, and a fear of losing control or dying. They develop rapidly, peak in intensity around ten minutes, and rarely last more than an hour. Community services show co-morbidity with agoraphobia of 30–50%. In this case, the panic attack seems to have been precipitated by social anxiety in a crowded public place. Sufferers may seek help from medical services fearing acute physical illness, such as a heart attack. Asthma would likely be revealed by a patient's previous medical history and wheeze on respiratory examination. Delusional disorder is an uncommon condition where patients present with circumscribed symptoms of non-bizarre delusions, but with an absence of perceptual or mood disorder. They rarely present directly to psychiatrists, more often being seen by other physicians due to somatic complaints, or lawyers and police due to paranoid ideas. Panic attacks have an anxiety basis rather than a delusional construct. Anxiety with panic attacks may be associated with depression, but the features in this case are not of core depressive symptoms. Hyperthyroidism can cause restlessness, nervousness, tremor, and sweating, but the context here is of acute symptoms triggered by a social context.

NHS Choices, Panic disorder. http://www.nhs.uk/conditions/panic-disorder/pages/introduction.aspx

23. B. Acamprosate, chlordiazepoxide (reducing regime), parenteral B vitamins

Acamprosate is a GABA agonist and NMDA antagonist, licensed for treatment of alcohol dependence. Studies show that it reduces cravings, rates of relapse, and severity of relapse. Several studies support use in alcohol withdrawal because it is considered neuroprotective, with few side effects or risks. Use of chlordiazepoxide and parenteral B vitamins is essential, and acamprosate probably helpful, making B the best answer. This patient in alcohol withdrawal has the classic Wernecke's encephalopathy triad which usually presents 24–48 hours after the last drink. Treatment includes a reducing regime of either chlordiazepoxide or diazepam (to reduce CNS overexcitation) and high-potency parenteral (IM or IV) B vitamins. The oral vitamin route, as in option A, is incorrect due to impaired B vitamin absorption in these patients caused by alcoholic villous atrophy. The other medications are usually well absorbed. Under normal metabolism, alcohol is broken down in the liver by the enzyme alcohol dehydrogenase to acetaldehyde, which is then converted by acetaldehyde dehydrogenase to acetic acid. Disulfiram blocks the breakdown of acetaldehyde by antagonizing the enzyme acetaldehyde dehydrogenase. The resultant acetaldehyde build-up produces an unpleasant flushing reaction which may deter people from drinking. A severe reaction may cause cardiovascular instability; therefore it is used only in well-motivated patients. Its use in acute withdrawal is not supported mainly because if there is still alcohol in the patient's bloodstream they will experience an unpleasant, possibly even life-threatening, reaction. Haloperidol, a typical antipsychotic, is often prescribed for acute psychosis or agitation. Haloperidol lowers seizure threshold and increases the risk of alcohol withdrawal seizures; therefore it is not typically used in alcohol withdrawal. Diazepam is a good alternative to chlordiazepoxide. However, use of haloperidol makes this an incorrect option.

Semple D, Smyth R, *Oxford Handbook of Psychiatry*, Third Edition, Oxford University Press, 2013, Chapter 24, Difficult and urgent situations.

24. C. Lorazepam

The constellation of symptoms above are classic for benzodiazepine withdrawal. Lorazepam is one of the shortest-acting benzodiazepines. If taken regularly and for a long enough period to develop dependence, withdrawal symptoms would be expected to be seen if it were suddenly stopped. Fluoxetine is the SSRI antidepressant with the longest half-life, so it would not cause withdrawal effects for many days. Levothyroxine is a treatment for hypothyroidism that does not have side effects of tolerance or dependence. Quietiapine is an atypical antipsychotic, which neither is generally addictive nor causes withdrawal symptoms. Zopiclone is a hypnotic used for night sedation. If relied on for sleep initiation for longer than two weeks, rebound insomnia may occur

Semple D, Smyth R, *Oxford Handbook of Psychiatry*, Third Edition, Oxford University Press, 2013, Chapter 15, Substance misuse.

25. A. Admit him to the medical ward under the Mental Capacity Act

The most appropriate management would be to admit this man to the medical ward under the Mental Capacity Act. He may well be delirious. It is very unlikely that he has capacity to decide to leave hospital. The Mental Capacity Act has replaced what was known as 'common law' and allows treatment of medical conditions against a patient's wishes if in their best interests, and in a least restrictive format if they are assessed to lack capacity concerning treatment decisions. Although sometimes a tempting option in a busy ED, this patient is septic, elderly, and unlikely to be making clear decisions or have the capacity to decide to go home. He would be a great risk if allowed to leave; therefore asking him to complete a 'discharge against medical advice' form is a line of action that would be unsafe and negligent. Section 5(2) of the MHA allows for already admitted patients to be detained in hospital until a full MHA assessment can be arranged, for a maximum of 72 hours. It cannot be used for patients in an ED as they are not yet admitted; therefore C is not the right answer. It is also not appropriate in this case as the patient is likely to lack capacity due to physical illness, and therefore the Mental Capacity Act is the relevant legislation to refer to. Although prescribing antibiotics to take at home is attempting to treat the underlying cause of this man's presentation, it would be unsafe to assume that he will understand and be compliant with this. He may well deteriorate and would certainly be a risk to himself if allowed to leave at this point. This patient would be best served by the Mental Capacity Act as the MHA only allows for treatment of mental illnesses, not physical ones.

Mental Capacity Act Legislation 2005. http://www.legislation.gov.uk/ukpga/2005/9/contents

26. A. Acamprosate

There is good evidence of acamprosate's efficacy in preventing alcohol relapse. Acamprosate is a glutamatergic NMDA receptor antagonist; because alcohol dependence and alcohol withdrawal are associated with a hyperglutamatergic system, acamprosate effectively reduces this. According to NICE, acamprosate should be prescribed as a first-line treatment with an individual psychosocial intervention. Furthermore, there is evidence that acamprosate reduces cravings whereas dilsulfiram, the only other viable option here, does not. Disulfiram is a good option to reduce risk of alcoholic relapse; however, acomprosate, in combination with a psychosocial intervention, is recommended by NICE as first-line therapy for maintenance of abstinence from alcohol. Disulfiram is contraindicated in people with severe PD because of the risk of impulsive drinking on top of disulfiram which could lead to cardiovascular instability and even death. There is no strong evidence that treatment with an SSRI or antipsychotic is effective in reducing alcoholic relapse. Naltrexone was licensed in 2012 in the UK for maintenance of abstinence in alcohol dependence syndrome. However, it is contraindicated here due to its muopioid receptor antagonist properties, which in this patient on methadone maintenance would precipitate acute opioid withdrawal. Therefore, patients using opioids or requiring opioid-based analgesia should not be treated with naltrexone.

NICE guidelines [CG115], Alcohol-use disorders: diagnosis, assessment and management of harmful drinking and alcohol dependence, February 2011. http://guidance.nice.org.uk/CG115/NICEGuidance/pdf/English

27. E. Rivastigmine

Rivastigmine (*Exelon™*) has the biggest body of evidence currently for use in Lewy body dementia. Donepezil (*Aricept™*) is an acetylcholinesterase inhibitor prescribed most readily for patients with Alzheimer's dementia. It would be a reasonable choice but is not the first option as this patient's symptoms point to a diagnosis of Lewy body dementia. Galantamine (*Reminyl™*) is another acetylcholinesterase inhibitor that can be used for dementia. It is more expensive than donepezil and rivastigmine and tends to be used less as a first-line treatment. Levodopa would primarily be used to treat the motor symptoms of Parkinson's and has no significant effects on memory. Memantine (*Ebixor™*) is recommended by NICE to be used to treat moderate to severe dementia. It may also be used in patients who cannot tolerate other antidementia medication due to cardiac arrhythmias as it is a safer option.

NICE technology appraisal [TA217], Donepezil, galantamine, rivastigmine and memantine for the treatment of Alzheimer's disease. https://www.nice.org.uk/guidance/ta217

28. E. IV Parvolex®

The most appropriate treatment is IV Parvolex®. Plasma paracetamol concentrations should be measured in all conscious patients with a history of paracetamol overdose, or suspected paracetamol overdose, as recommended by TOXBASE. They should also be taken in patients with a presentation consistent with opioid poisoning, and in unconscious patients with a history of collapse where drug overdose is a possible diagnosis. Plasma paracetamol levels should be measured for risk assessment no earlier than four hours and no later than 15 hours after ingestion, as results are not reliable outside this time period. IV acetylcysteine (Parvolex®) should be considered as the treatment of choice for paracetamol overdose. When a person who has self-poisoned is in the ED within one hour of ingestion and is fully conscious and able to protect his or her own airway, ED staff should consider offering activated charcoal at the earliest opportunity. In this scenario the patient has presented too late for this to be an option. Forced alkaline diuresis is indicated in the treatment of moderate salicylate poisoning only. It should not be used if the patient is in shock, has heart failure, or has impaired renal function. NICE guidelines state that gastric lavage should not be used in the management of self-poisoning unless specifically recommended by TOXBASE or following consultation with the National Poisons Information Service. Pabrinex® is the brand name for a high-potency injection containing the water-soluble vitamins C (ascorbic acid), B_1 (thiamine), B_2 (riboflavin), B_3 (nicotinamide), and B_6 (pyridoxine). It is administered during alcohol withdrawal to prevent Wernicke's encephalitis.

NICE guidelines [CG16], Self-harm in over 8s: short-term management and prevention of recurrence, July 2004. https://www.nice.org.uk/guidance/cg16

1. There is a recognized association between cystic fibrosis and the presence of nasal polyps. What percentage of adult CF patients have nasal polyps?
   A. <30%
   B. 40%
   C. 50%
   D. 60%
   E. >75%

2. A 17-year-old girl is admitted acutely breathless. She is too breathless to give much history, but her mother informs you that she is asthmatic, and has become increasingly breathless over the preceding 6 hours. She usually has two inhalers, but may not be good at taking them, and smokes 10 cpd. There is no other past history of note. On examination she is supporting herself on the edge of the bed, with a respiratory rate of 22 per minute, heart rate 160 bpm, SpO_2 97% on oxygen, whilst receiving nebulized salbutamol. Arterial blood gas on oxygen reveals: pH 7.35, PaO_2 18.2 kPa, $PaCO_2$ 6.3 kPa, HCO_3· 24. What is the next step in management?
   A. Intravenous aminophylline
   B. Intravenous hydrocortisone
   C. Intravenous magnesium sulphate
   D. Nebulized ipratropium
   E. Refer to intensive care

3. **A 28-year-old woman presents with cough and pleuritic pain in the right axilla. She is normally fit and well, with no past medical history of note, and on no medications. On examination, her pulse rate is 90 bpm, respiratory rate 19 per minute, oxygen saturations 98% on air, and chest is clear on auscultation. Blood tests reveal a d-dimer level of 800 ng/ml (normal range up to 500 ng/ml). Which of the following investigations should be performed next?**

    A. CTPA
    B. CXR
    C. Thrombophilia screen
    D. Urinary hCG
    E. VQ scan

4. **Which of the following statements about cystic fibrosis is correct?**

    A. CF liver disease, requiring liver transplant, is more common in younger patients
    B. CF lung disease is characterized by a predominantly eosinophillic inflammation
    C. CF patients are usually infertile
    D. CF patients have a high rate of diabetes, and often present in diabetic ketoacidosis when unwell
    E. The carrier frequency is 1:25 and the condition affects approximately 1:600 live births in the UK

5. **A 64-year-old man was diagnosed with adenocarcinoma of the lung. Which paraneoplastic syndrome would you be most likely to find in this patient?**

    A. Syndrome of inappropriate anti-diuretic hormone secretion
    B. Ectopic adenocorticotrophic hormone secretion
    C. Hypercalcaemia
    D. Hyperthyroidism
    E. Hypertrophic pulmonary osteoarthropathy

6. **A 45-year-old woman presents with cough, wheeze, and haemoptysis. On detailed questioning she reports cutaneous flushing and diarrhoea. Her CXR shows a solitary mass, and a cherry red endobronchial lesion is seen at bronchoscopy. Which of the following is most likely to be associated with this condition?**

    A. Syndrome of inappropriate anti-diuretic hormone secretion (SIADH)
    B. Eaton–Lambert myasthenic syndrome
    C. Trousseau's syndrome of hypercoagulability
    D. Cushing's syndrome
    E. Hypertrophic pulmonary osteoarthropathy (HPOA)

7. **You are the Respiratory Core Trainee. You have been asked to do some ABGs on Mr Joe Bloggs who has chronic obstructive pulmonary disease. He is being considered for long-term oxygen therapy (LTOT). Mr Bloggs is clinically stable with no clinical symptoms or signs of pulmonary hypertension. Which is the criteria for determining whether Mr Bloggs should be offered LTOT?**

   A. One ABG sample in which pO_2 < 7 kPa
   B. Two ABG samples in which pO_2 < 7.3 kPa
   C. One ABG sample in which pO_2 < 8 kPa
   D. Two ABG samples in which pO_2 < 7 kPa
   E. Three ABG samples in which pO_2 < 7.3 kPa

8. **A 67-year-old woman presents with shortness of breath. On examination she is tachycardic at 112 bpm with BP 120/80 mmHg, temperature 37.6°C and respiratory rate of 32/min. Her chest was clear and heart sounds were normal. She was given high-flow oxygen. ABG on air revealed: pH 7.5, pCO_2 3.9 kPa, pO_2 7.2 kPa. What would be the next best step to manage this situation?**

   A. Salbutamol nebulizer
   B. Intravenous hydrocortisone
   C. Intravenous fluids
   D. Intravenous co-amoxiclav
   E. Low molecular weight heparin

9. **You are referred a 40-year-old man for investigation of cough and haemoptysis. He has a history of asthma for the last ten years, treated with inhaled corticosteroids and β-agonists. CXR reveals an ill-defined opacity in the right upper lobe. He denies smoking tobacco but is a cannabis user, and smokes 4–5 homemade cannabis cigarettes ('joints') per day. Which of the following is correct?**

   A. A 'joint' typically consists of pure cannabis that is smoked unfiltered
   B. Smoking cannabis is associated with an increased risk of developing tuberculosis
   C. Cannabis smoking is associated with a 15-fold increased risk of lung cancer compared to smoking tobacco alone
   D. Cannabis plants carry fungal spores which may lead to invasive aspergilloma in otherwise healthy cannabis smokers
   E. Cannabis smoking is associated with an increased incidence of adult onset asthma and bronchitis

10. **A 21-year-old attends A&E with right-sided chest pain and breathlessness. He has no past medical problems and was working in his job as a scaffolder at the onset of symptoms. He was distressed by the pain so left work in order to come to A&E. On examination his respiratory rate is 32, his oxygen saturation 93% on air, and breath sounds are slightly reduced on the righthand side. A chest X-ray reveals a 3 cm right-sided pneumothorax. What would be the next step in your management?**

A. Discharge home

B. Analgesia and high-flow oxygen only

C. Needle aspiration

D. Insert a chest drain using the Seldinger technique

E. Insert a chest drain using an open procedure

11. **A 70-year-old man has succeeded in giving up smoking. Unfortunately, he has a 60 pack-year smoking history and severe COPD for which he takes high-dose seretide and tiotropium. His FEV1 is less than 50% predicted. Which of the following correlates most closely with mortality in COPD?**

A. FEV1

B. Peak flow

C. Transfer factor

D. Vital capacity

E. Residual volume

12. **A 40-year-old baker presents to the chest clinic with progressive worsening shortness of breath. It seems to be episodic and he reports it being worse whilst at work. He says he gets wheezy and tends to cough. Which is the most appropriate investigation?**

A. High resolution CT scan of his chest

B. RadioAllergoSorbent Testing (RAST)

C. Patch testing

D. Total Ig E testing.

E. Serial peak flow measurements at work and at home

13. **A 42-year-old woman with a history of obesity presents to the clinic with increasing shortness of breath over the past 1–2 years. She is now unable to mobilize more than a few metres. On examination she has a BMI of 34. Her BP is 155/90, pulse 90 atrial fibrillation, her O_2 sats are reduced at 91% on air. She has extensive varicose veins on both lower limbs and there is bilateral pitting oedema, a murmur of tricuspid regurgitation is heard on auscultation, but there are no signs of pulmonary oedema. Investigations: Hb 14.4, WCC 7.3, PLT 234, Na 139, K 4.3, Cr 110, ECG: atrial fibrillation, no acute changes. Which of the following is the most likely diagnosis?**
    A. Ischaemic right heart failure
    B. Left heart failure.
    C. Primary pulmonary hypertension
    D. Secondary pulmonary hypertension
    E. Ischaemic cardiomyopathy

14. **A 71-year-old man who has been admitted three months earlier for an acute exacerbation of COPD comes to the clinic for review. His medication includes high-dose seretide and tiotropium. He reports to you that he is only able to walk a few metres due to severe shortness of breath. On examination his BP is 166/82, his pulse is 80 and regular. He has bilateral coarse crackles consistent with COPD on auscultation of his chest. Which of the following would be an indication for home oxygen?**
    A. Raised JVP
    B. PaO_2 7.2 kPa
    C. $PaCO_2$ 5.9 kPa
    D. Shortness of breath on exercise
    E. Left heart failure

15. **Which of the following paraneoplastic syndromes is least commonly associated with small cell lung cancer?**
    A. Cerebellar degeneration syndrome
    B. Lambert–Eaton myasthenic syndrome
    C. Ectopic ACTH secretion
    D. Hypertrophic pulmonary osteo-arthropathy
    E. Syndrome of inappropriate ADH

16. **A 20-year-old man presents with a two-week history of cough, fever, and malaise. The chest X-ray shows patchy consolidation in the lower lobe of the right lung. Mycoplasma pneumonia is suspected to be the most likely diagnosis. Which of the following medications is MOST effective in the treatment of this infection?**

    A. Cefuroxime
    B. Metronidazole
    C. Erythromycin
    D. Amoxicillin
    E. Aciclovir

17. **What percentage of patients undergoing lung transplantation for idiopathic pulmonary fibrosis are alive one year post transplantation?**

    A. >95%
    B. >85%
    C. 75%
    D. 50%
    E. <50%

18. **A 16-year-old girl with a history of cystic fibrosis is admitted to the respiratory ward with an infectious exacerbation. On examination she is pyrexial 38°C and has a BP of 110/70; her pulse is 84 and regular. Auscultation reveals coarse crackles throughout both lung fields, worse on the left than the right. Sampling reveals *Pseudomonas* colonization for the first time. Which of the following is the most appropriate intervention?**

    A. Ciprofloxacin for two weeks
    B. Ciprofloxacin and nebulized colistin for six weeks
    C. Intravenous cefotaxime for four weeks
    D. Nebulized tobramycin
    E. Cefotaxime and nebulized tobramycin for four weeks

19. **A 20-year-old woman who is 32 weeks pregnant comes to the emergency department with an exacerbation of asthma. She takes seretide 250 1 puff BD and has had two previous admissions to the emergency department and one to intensive care with exacerbations. After one hour of back-to-back salbutamol nebulizers her peak flow is still only 160 and she is tired. She has also received IV hydrocortisone. Which of the following is the most appropriate next step?**

    A. Intravenous magnesium
    B. Intravenous aminophiline
    C. Intravenous salbutamol
    D. ITU review
    E. BIPAP in the emergency department

20. **A 50-year-old woman presents with flushing, sweats, wheeze, and diarrhoea. Her pulse rate is 104 bpm. She has a five-pack-year smoking history. No recent foreign travel. Twenty-four-hour urinary 5-hydroxyindoleacetic acid (5-HIAA) was greater than 25 mg/24 h. What is the likely diagnosis?**
    A. Asthma
    B. Katayama fever
    C. Lung cancer
    D. Pulmonary carcinoid tumour
    E. Menopausal symptoms

21. **A 25-year-old man with low back pain radiating from the sacroiliac joints to the buttocks that improves towards the end of the day presents to the medical assessment unit with a dry cough and red eyes. A chest X-ray is requested. What would you expect to find?**
    A. Bilateral pneumothoraces
    B. Bilateral lower zone fibrosis
    C. Bilateral upper zone fibrosis
    D. Bilateral lower zone consolidation
    E. Bilateral pulmonary infiltrates

22. **A 35-year-old woman presents with shortness of breath and a cough which have been worsening over one week. She has had diarrhoea for two days. She was previously fit and well. She developed her symptoms whilst on holiday in Spain and returned to the UK four days ago. On admission she is orientated but breathless with a respiratory rate of 32 breaths per minute. She has a temperature of 38.5°C. Her chest examination reveals dullness to percussion and bronchial breathing at the left base. Oxygen saturations are 91% on air. Her pulse is 108 and regular and blood pressure is 98/54 mmHg. Blood tests are as follows: Hb 10.9 g/dl, WCC 16.2 (neutrophils 14.6 x 10^9/l), PLT 198 x 10^9/l, Ur 8 mmol/l, Cr 116 micromol/l, Na 130 mmol/l, K 3.5 mmol/l. Which of the following statements is most accurate?**
    A. The diarrhoea suggests gastroenteritis as the cause of infection. The patient should be admitted for rehydration and no antibiotics are indicated
    B. The patient has a high CURB-65 score and needs senior assessment. She should be treated with IV augmentin and clarithromycin in addition to IV fluids
    C. The patient has a high CURB-65 score and needs senior assessment. She should be treated with oral augmentin and clarithromycin in addition to IV fluids
    D. The patient has a high CURB-65 score and needs urgent admission for treatment with IV amoxicillin and fluids
    E. The patient has a low CURB-65 score and can be discharged home with oral amoxicillin

23. A 28-year-old Indian man who moved to the UK in 2008 presents with left-sided chest pain which is worse on breathing in. He has been feeling unwell for several months and has lost 2 stone in weight. For the past month he has been having fever and night sweats. He has a slight dry cough. Examination shows a thin man who does not look systemically unwell and has a respiratory rate of 18 bpm. There is dullness to percussion and reduced air entry at the left base. Pulse is 98 per minute and BP 110/76. A CXR shows a pleural effusion and a diagnostic tap shows this to have a protein of 38 g/l. The diagnostic tap sample shows lymphocytes and no malignant cells on microscopy. No organisms are seen on Gram or Ziehl–Nielsen stains of pleural fluid or sputum. Which of the following statements is?

    A. The most likely diagnosis is adenocarcinoma and the patient should be warned of this
    B. The most likely diagnosis is SLE. The pleural effusion can be managed with drainage alone
    C. The most likely diagnosis is tuberculosis and, following further investigation, appropriate treatment would be with a combination of rifampicin, isoniazid, ethambutol, and pyrazinamide
    D. The most likely diagnosis is tuberculosis and the patient should be isolated immediately and treatment commenced as soon as possible with rifampicin and isoniazid for three months
    E. The presence of cough and fever suggests the most likely diagnosis is pneumonia. Treatment should be with a five-day course of oral augmentin

24. A 69-year-old woman with a 50 pack-year smoking history and severe COPD comes to the emergency room because of a three-day history of severe cough and shortness of breath. She is managed with high-dose seretide and tiotropium. On examination her PEFR is 210 and the pCO_2 on initial blood gas is 6.5; this does not improve with initial management. There is bilateral poor air entry and coarse crackles consistent with COPD. Which of the following findings would drive a decision to use NIV?

    A. PEFR of 210
    B. pH 7.38
    C. pH 7.30
    D. pO_2 9.4
    E. Unconsciousness

25. A 53-year-old man, who has had to give up work as a coal miner because of chronic rheumatoid arthritis, is found to have anaemia, splenomegaly, and on his chest X-ray a rounded lesion in the periphery of the basal left lung. He has no chest symptoms. What is the likely aetiology of his lung lesion?

    A. Caplan's syndrome
    B. Felty's syndrome
    C. Tuberculosis
    D. Primary lung tumour
    E. Secondary tumour

26. **The following are life-threatening features of severe asthma, except:**
    A. PEF 35% of predicted reading
    B. Saturation of 91%
    C. Arrhythmia
    D. Silent chest
    E. Normal Pa CO_2 (4.6–6.0 kPa)

27. **A 67-year-old man comes to the respiratory clinic for review. He has a 50 pack-year smoking history. Currently he takes PRN salbutamol for shortness of breath but no other respiratory medications. On examination his BP is 155/85. His pulse is 82 and regular. Auscultation of his chest reveals coarse crackles consistent with COPD. His peak flow is 280 (50% of predicted). Which of the following medications is likely to impact most on his exercise tolerance?**
    A. Regular salbutamol
    B. 50 mcg beclomethasone BD
    C. 50 mg salmeterol BD
    D. 18 mcg tiotropium BD
    E. Regular low dose oral corticosteroids

28. **Non-small cell lung cancer is:**
    A. Less common than small cell lung cancer
    B. A cause of hypercalcaemia
    C. A cause of hypernatraemia
    D. A smoking-related condition
    E. Usually disseminated by the time of diagnosis

29. **A 30-year-old man with cystic fibrosis attends for a routine chest X-ray. He reports no recent change in symptoms. Which of these would be an unexpected finding on his chest X-ray?**
    A. Reduced lung volumes
    B. Large pulmonary arteries
    C. Dense tubular structures overlying larger airway
    D. Peri-bronchial cuffing
    E. Multiple round lucencies throughout the lungs

30. **An 18-year-old woman has a chest X-ray during an admission for acute exacerbation of asthma. The formal report describes an ill-defined 25 mm solitary nodule in the left lower lobe. She has never smoked and is otherwise well. What is the most appropriate follow-up investigation?**
    A. Bronchoscopy
    B. Repeat chest X-ray six weeks later
    C. CT thorax with IV contrast
    D. Non-contrast high-resolution CT thorax
    E. Repeat chest X-ray one week later

31. **You are reviewing a chest X-ray of a 50-year-old woman who presented to A&E with sudden onset shortness of breath. There is marked increased lucency of one hemithorax compared to the other. Which of these possible causes is unlikely to account for the chest X-ray findings?**
   A. A pneumothorax
   B. Severe unilateral bullous change in COPD
   C. Asthma
   D. Prior mastectomy
   E. A rotated projection

32. **An 80-year-old coal miner who stopped working 16 years ago has worsening shortness of breath. He has a 30-pack-year smoking history. Spirometry: FEV1 1.4l (predicted 2.5), FVC 2.8l (predicted 3.0). Which is the likely diagnosis?**
   A. Chronic obstructive pulmonary disease (COPD)
   B. Idiopathic pulmonary fibrosis
   C. Hypersensitivity pneumonitis
   D. Silicosis
   E. Simple pneumoconiosis

33. **A 30-year-old woman with pulmonary hypertension complains of shortness of breath. She is in her 36th week of gestation in her first pregnancy. Which of the following is true?**
   A. Chest X-ray is contraindicated
   B. Raised D dimer rules out pulmonary embolism
   C. The dose of enoxaparin should be halved
   D. Nifedipine is contraindicated in pregnancy
   E. The risk of maternal mortality in patients with pulmonary hypertension is 30%

34. **A 68-year-old man has been diagnosed with Parkinson's by the neurology clinic after presenting to his GP with paucity of movement, a tremor, and deterioration of his handwriting. He is not keen to take levodopa, and has read in the papers that some of the medications used for the treatment of Parkinson's may cause problems with lung fibrosis. Which of the following is the most appropriate medication for him?**
   A. Carbidopa
   B. Ropinirole
   C. Selegiline
   D. Pergolide
   E. Entacapone

35. **Which of the following features is consistent with life-threatening asthma?**
    A. SpO_2 91%
    B. PEFR 230 (460 predicted)
    C. PO_2 8.3
    D. PCO_2 3.6
    E. Respiratory rate 19

36. **There are many initial causes of bronchiectasis. Causes do NOT include:**
    A. ABPA (allergic bronchopulmaonary aspergillosis)
    B. Kartagener's syndrome
    C. Whooping cough
    D. Tuberculosis
    E. Pleural plaques

37. **A 71-year-old woman with a history of rheumatoid arthritis comes to the clinic for review after her third course of etanercept. She has been complaining of increasing night sweats and a chronic cough over the past few months. There is a past history of COPD and she continues to smoke 20 cigarettes per day. On examination she has chest signs consistent with the COPD. Investigations: haemoglobin 10.9 g/dl (11.5–16.5), white cells 8.8 x 10^9/l (4–11), platelets 181 x 10^9/l (150–400), sodium 138 mmol/l (135–146), potassium 4.7 mmol/l (3.5–5), creatinine 134 micromol/l (79–118), CXR: right apical calcification. Which of the following is the most likely diagnosis?**
    A. Pulmonary tuberculosis
    B. Bronchial carcinoma
    C. Sarcoidosis
    D. Rheumatoid lung
    E. Hydatid disease

38. **A 68-year-old woman with a history of depression and renal stones on two previous occasions presents to the emergency department complaining of severe lethargy and nausea. On examination she seems drowsy and confused. She is thin with a BMI of 20. Her BP is 138/82. Investigations: haemoglobin 10.4 g/dl (11.5–16.5), white cells 10.1 x10^9/l (4–11), platelets 214 x10^9/l (150–400), sodium 143 mmol/l (135–146), potassium 5.1 mmol/l (3.5–5), parathyroid hormone 0.8 pmol/l (0.9–5.4), calcium 3.62 mmol/l (2.20–2.60), creatinine 162 micromol/l (72–118), CXR: left hilar mass. Which of the following is the most appropriate immediate therapy?**
    A. Intravenous furosemide
    B. Intravenous normal saline
    C. Intravenous calcitonin
    D. Intravenous corticosteroids
    E. Intravenous pamidronate

39. Life-threatening asthma is characterized by all of the following EXCEPT:

A. PEFR <33% predicted/best

B. Bradycardia

C. Confusion

D. pO_2 <10.0 kPa

E. Normal or high pCO_2

40. A clinical diagnosis of asthma is made. Which of the following makes the diagnosis of asthma most likely to be correct?

A. A strong family history

B. 15% diurnal variation on PEFR testing on >3 days per week

C. FEV1 improvement of 15% (or 200 ml) after B-agonist

D. 10% diurnal variation in PEFR on >3 days/week

E. Blood eosinophilia

41. Contraindications to non-invasive ventilation include all of the following EXCEPT:

A. Pneumothorax with intercostal drain in situ

B. Inability to protect own airway

C. Excessive vomiting

D. Patient refusal

E. Severe facial injury

42. Which of the following mortality rates as per CURB-65 score in patients admitted with pneumonia is correct?

A. CURB-65 =0, >5%

B. CURB-65 =2, >25%

C. CURB-65 =3, <10%

D. CURB-65 =4, >50%

E. CURB-65 =5, >50%

43. Which of the following statements about pneumonia is most correct?

A. All patients with CURB-65 score >5 should be cared for on an intensive care unit

B. All patients with a CURB-65 score of >4 should be cared for on a high dependency unit

C. A 25-year-old patient with saturations 90% on high flow oxygen, pyrexia 39°C., bilateral consolidation, and a CURB-65 score of zero can be cared for as an outpatient

D. A 25-year-old patient with saturations 94% on air, unilateral consolidation, and a CURB-65 score of 1 can be cared for as an outpatient

E. A 50-year-old man with a CURB-65 score of zero, known COPD, and saturations 92% on air should be cared for as an inpatient

44. **Causes of pulmonary cavities include all EXCEPT which one of the following?**
    A. Wegener's granulomatosis
    B. Sarcoidosis
    C. Rheumatoid arthritis
    D. Squamous cell cancer
    E. Asbestos-related pleural plaques

45. **Step 3 of the BTS asthma guidelines is:**
    A. Regular inhaled SABA (short-acting B-agonist)
    B. PRN inhaled SABA (short-acting B.-agonist) PRN, regular ICS (inhaled corticosteroids) up to 800 mcg/day
    C. PRN inhaled SABA (short acting B-agonist), regular ICS (inhaled corticosteroids) up to 800 mcg/day, regular inhaled LABA (long-acting B-agonist), +/– oral theophylline S/R or leukotriene antagonist
    D. Long-term oral prednisolone in addition to SABA, LABA, and ICS
    E. Leukotriene receptor antagonist in combination with PRN SABA

46. **In COPD and asthma combination inhalers containing LABA and inhaled corticosteroid are often used. Which of the following contains the highest dose of inhaled corticosteroid?**
    A. Seretide (salmeterol and fluticasone) 500 accuhaler 1 puff BD
    B. Seretide (salmeterol and fluticasone) 250 evohaler 1 puff BD
    C. Symbicort (eformoterol and budesonide) 400/12 1 puff BD
    D. Symbicort (eformoterol and budesonide) 200/6 1 puff BD
    E. Symbicort (eformoterol and budesonide) 400/12 2 puffs BD

47. **The five-year outcome post lung transplant in patients with cystic fibrosis is:**
    A. <30%
    B. 40%
    C. 45%
    D. 55%
    E. >60%

48. **An 18-year-old man with no previous past medical history presents with a 2.5 cm pneumothorax identified on a chest X-ray. He is haemodynamically stable and asymptomatic. What is the best management for this patient?**
    A. Admit for observation
    B. Chest drain insertion
    C. Discharge home
    D. Aspiration of pneumothorax
    E. Discharge home and review in OPD in 2–4 weeks' time

49. **A 56-year-old man with a background of chronic obstructive pulmonary disease (COPD) presents one evening to A&E with sudden onset of worsening shortness of breath and right-sided pleuritic chest pain. On examination he is visibly short of breath with a respiratory rate of 36 breaths per minute. His oxygen saturations are maintained at 98% with an inspired oxygen concentration of 28%. An urgent portable chest radiograph performed in the department reveals a 2.5 cm rim of air consistent with a right-sided pneumothorax. The most appropriate next management step is:**

A. Aspiration of pneumothorax with 16G cannula

B. Insertion of surgical chest drain

C. High flow oxygen (10 l/min) and observation overnight

D. Insertion of intercostal chest drain (8–14 French)

E. Discharge and outpatient review in 2–4 weeks

50. **Which of the following is not a feature associated with Pancoast tumours?**

A. Diaphragmatic palsy

B. Exophthalmos

C. Ptosis

D. Shoulder pain

E. Weakness of the small muscles of the hands

51. **Which of the following is true about the Bacillus Calmette–Guerin (BCG) vaccination?**

A. It is a killed vaccine

B. It is derived from *Mycobacterium kansasii*

C. It is licensed for intra-vesical treatment of bladder carcinoma

D. It provides greater than >90% protection against pulmonary tuberculosis

E. It requires a booster dose after ten years

52. **A 45-year-old alcoholic man is being treated on the ward for aspiration pneumonia. Despite appropriate antibiotic therapy his breathing is increasingly laboured and he fails to maintain his saturations on high-flow oxygen. Which of the following features is not consistent with acute respiratory distress syndrome?**

A. Bilateral CXR infiltrates

B. $PaO_2:FiO_2$ <27 kPa (200 mmHg)

C. Pulmonary capillary wedge pressure ≤18 mmHg

D. Reduced A–a gradient

E. V/Q mismatching

53. **A 40-year-old farmer presents with breathlessness, a dry cough, fever, and myalgia after handling hay bales. On examination he has diffuse crepitations throughout both lungs and desaturates with exercise. Chest X-ray demonstrates widespread infiltrates, and high resolution CT scan demonstrates patchy ground glass change with poorly defined nodules. Which of the following is in keeping with a diagnosis of acute hypersensitivity pneumonitis?**

    A. Exposure to *Micropolyspora faeni* (also known as *Saccharopolyspora rectivirgula*)
    B. Blood eosinophilia
    C. Eosinophilia on bronchoalveolar lavage
    D. Type 1 hypersensitivity
    E. Obstructive pulmonary function tests

54. **A 40-year-old woman presents with exertional dyspnoea and chest pain. On examination she has a raised JVP with giant V waves and a loud pansystolic murmur at the left sternal edge. An arterial blood gas demonstrates hypoxia and hypocapnia and she desaturates on exercise. Which of the following drugs may have contributed to her pulmonary hypertension?**

    A. Bosentan
    B. Eproprostenol
    C. Fenfluramine
    D. Nifedipine
    E. Sildenafil

55. **A 30-year-old man, previously fit and well, presents with left-sided pleuritic chest pain. He has a 10 pack-year smoking history. On examination the left side of his chest has reduced expansion and percussion note is hyper-resonant with reduced breath sounds. A click is heard over the precordium, synchronous with his heart beat (Hamman's sign). Chest X-ray confirms a 3 cm left-sided pneumothorax. What should you now advise him?**

    A. He is safe to go diving after four weeks
    B. He requires an inter-costal drain
    C. He requires genetic screening for Marfan's disease
    D. He requires referral to cardio-thoracic surgeons for consideration of pleurodesis
    E. He should stop smoking

56. **A 21-year-old patient attending the respiratory outpatient department asks about the genetics of cystic fibrosis. Which of the following is true?**

    A. Inheritance is X-linked recessive
    B. Carrier frequency is 1:2500
    C. Delta F508 mutation accounts for >90% of CF alleles
    D. Delta F508 mutation results in the omission of phenylalanine at the 508 residue
    E. Gene mutations affect the cystic fibrosis transmembrane conductance regulator (CFTR), a complex sodium channel

57. **An obese 45-year-old man attends the respiratory outpatient clinic with a history of snoring and waking unrefreshed. Which of the following is not in keeping with a diagnosis of obstructive sleep apnoea?**
    A. Neck circumference greater than 17 inches
    B. Decreased libido with impotence
    C. Nocturnal choking
    D. Poor concentration
    E. Sleep paralysis

58. **A previously fit and well 30-year-old woman presents with breathlessness and pleuritic chest pain. Her only medication is the combined oral contraceptive pill. She reports a family history of recurrent miscarriage affecting her mother. On examination she has a swollen left calf and a pleural rub. CTPA confirms a sub-segmental pulmonary embolism and she is commenced on anticoagulants. Which of the following tests should now be performed?**
    A. Screen for anti-thrombin III deficiency
    B. Screen for Factor V Leiden variant
    C. Screen for protein C deficiency
    D. Tumour markers
    E. Ultrasound abdomen and pelvis.

59. **A 65-year-old retired plumber with a 40-pack-year smoking history presents with a dry cough, gradually worsening dyspnoea, and reduced exercise tolerance. On examination he has fine bibasal end-inspiratory crepitations on auscultation of his chest. Pulmonary function tests demonstrate an FEV1:FVC ratio of 0.90 with a reduced TLCO. Chest X-ray demonstrates bilateral lower lobe reticulo-nodular change. What is the most likely diagnosis?**
    A. Alpha1 antitrypsin deficiency
    B. Asbestosis
    C. Chronic obstructive pulmonary disease
    D. Morbid obesity
    E. Pleural plaque disease

60. **A 25-year-old pregnant woman presents with a pruritic, vesicular rash, cough, pleuritic chest pain, and mild haemoptysis. She maintains adequate oxygen saturations on room air. Chest X-ray demonstrates small nodular infiltrates throughout both lung fields. How should she be treated?**
    A. Aciclovir
    B. Amoxycillin and clarithromycin
    C. Amphotericin
    D. Highly active anti-retroviral therapy
    E. Zoster immune globulin

61. **A 45-year-old Caucasian man presents with shortness of breath, nasal congestion, and epistaxis. On examination there is ulceration of the nasal septum and palpable purpura on the lower extremities. Chest X-ray demonstrates diffuse patchy infiltration, and urinalysis demonstrates haematuria, proteinuria, and red cell casts. What is the most likely diagnosis?**
    A. Goodpasture's disease
    B. Henoch–Schönlein purpura
    C. Malignancy
    D. Tuberculosis
    E. Wegener's granulomatosis

62. **A 40-year-old Irish woman presents with cough, fever, pain, and stiffness affecting the small joints of her hands and feet. On examination she has a tender nodular rash on her anterior shins. Chest X-ray demonstrates hilar lymphadenopathy. What is the most likely diagnosis?**
    A. HIV seroconversion
    B. Lymphoma
    C. Post-infectious polyarthropathy
    D. Reiter's syndrome
    E. Sarcoidosis

63. **A 52-year-old smoker with a history of COPD on maximal medical therapy is increasingly disabled by her condition and is given a life expectancy of two years. FEV1 is 15% of predicted. She is referred to the tertiary referral centre for lung transplant assessment. Which of the following is not a contraindication to transplantation?**
    A. Age >50 years
    B. Cigarette smoking within the preceding six months
    C. Inability to walk
    D. Psychiatric illness
    E. Malignancy within the preceding five years

64. **With regards to pleural fluid drainage:**
    A. Less than 2 litres of pleural fluid should be drained at any one time in case of causing re-expansion pulmonary oedema
    B. Large chest drain >20G should be used for pneumothorax
    C. Large chest drain >20G should be used for empyema
    D. Streptokinase should be used for all loculated pleural effusions
    E. Talc pleurodesis is very effective even if pleural fluid drainage via chest drain is >300 ml per day

65. **A 65-year-old presents with worsening shortness of breath on exertion and a non-productive cough. On examination she has finger clubbing and fine end-inspiratory crepitations bibasally on chest auscultation. You suspect a diagnosis of idiopathic pulmonary fibrosis. Which of the following findings would support your diagnosis?**

    A. A predominantly eosinophilic bronchoalveolar lavage fluid
    B. A predominantly lymphocytic bronchoalveolar lavage fluid
    C. A predominantly neutrophilic bronchoalveolar lavage fluid
    D. A raised serum eosinophil count
    E. An obstructive defect on pulmonary function testing

66. **Alpha 1 antitrypsin levels are lowest in which phenotype?**

    A. PiSS
    B. PiMM
    C. PiZZ
    D. PiMZ
    E. PiSZ

67. **In which of the following patients is long-term oxygen therapy not indicated?**

    A. An 80-year-old man with severe COPD and a pO_2 on air of 6.9 kPa, who is still smoking 20 cigarettes per day
    B. A 72-year-old man in a residential home with moderate COPD, congestive cardiac failure, and a pO_2 on air of 7.6 kPa
    C. A 65-year-old woman with severe COPD with a pO_2 of 8.2 kPa on air
    D. A 45-year-old man with Down's syndrome, primary pulmonary hypertension (no lung disease), and a pO_2 of 7.8 kPa on air
    E. A 56-year-old man with NSIP-type pulmonary fibrosis with a pO_2 of 7.3 kPa on air

68. **A young man with cystic fibrosis comes to see you in clinic for review, and would like to know more about the complications of his condition. Which of these complications is seen much more frequently in men with cystic fibrosis compared to women?**

    A. Osteoporosis
    B. Liver cirrhosis
    C. Diabetes
    D. Infertility
    E. None of the above

69. **A 28-year-old woman with a known history of chronic rhinitis and known nasal polyps develops symptoms of exertional dyspnoea and wheeze. Which of the following medications may have contributed to her asthma symptoms?**

A. Anti-TNF alpha

B. Aspirin

C. Combined oral contraceptive pill

D. Montelukast

E. Omeprazole

70. **A 78-year-old man previously working in a shipyard until 20 years ago presents with gradual onset dyspnoea with no chest pain. His pulmonary function test shows a restrictive picture with reduced lung volumes and transfer factor. Which is the likely diagnosis?**

A. Mesothelioma

B. Idiopathic pulmonary fibrosis

C. Pulmonary asbestosis

D. Silicosis

E. Benign asbestos-related pleural disease

71. **Empyema is characterized by a pleural fluid pH of less than:**

A. 7.5.

B. 7.4.

C. 7.2.

D. 7.1.

E. 6.9.

72. **You are asked to urgently attend a 30-year-old man who has collapsed a few minutes after undergoing his first CT to investigate headaches. He was given IV contrast as part of the CT study. He is semi-conscious, has difficulty breathing, facial swelling, and stridor. Which of the following is least important in his immediate medical management?**

A. High-flow oxygen via a face mask

B. Intra-muscular adrenaline

C. Intravenous anti-histamine

D. Intravenous access and immediate, rapid, intravenous infusion of crystalloid

E. Nebulized beta-2 agonist

73. **An 18-year-old woman with a history of severe asthma comes to the emergency room. She has been ill for the past three days with symptoms of a cough and cold. She is normally maintained with a high-dose symbicort inhaler and montelukast tablets. On presentation she has a peak flow of 220 (normal 510), and severe wheeze on auscultation of both lung fields. She is administered 60% O_2. After 20 mins the following results are obtained: PaO_2 9.1 kPa, $PaCO_2$ 6.2 kPa, pH 7.45, peak flow 320, respiratory rate 23. Which of the following would indicate the need for ITU admission?**

    A. PaO_2 9.1
    B. $PaCO_2$ 6.2
    C. pH 7.45
    D. Peak flow 320
    E. Respiratory rate 23

74. **A 19-year-old woman who has just started work at a factory comes to the clinic complaining of progressive wheeze and a dry cough which builds during the course of a working week, and resolves when she is at home. When she comes to the clinic she has just finished a week on holiday. Her BP is 100/60, her pulse is 65 and regular. Her chest is clear. Which of the following is the correct course of action?**

    A. Reassure her there is nothing wrong
    B. Give her a peak flow meter and diary to compare the working week with time off
    C. Prescribe salbutamol PRN
    D. Prescribe regular salbutamol
    E. Prescribe regular beclomethasone

75. **A 32-year-old nurse is known to have a latex allergy and is absolutely assiduous in her use of nitrile gloves whilst working. She collapses in the staff canteen, however, after eating a fruit salad which she purchased for her lunch. Which of the following is the most likely cause of her anaphylaxis?**

    A. Kiwi
    B. Lemon
    C. Orange
    D. Pear
    E. Grape

76. **A 76-year-old gentleman with chronic obstructive pulmonary disease (COPD) presents acutely breathless, with fever and a cough productive of green sputum. He has been wheezier than normal, which has not settled with his home nebs. He was assessed by the respiratory outreach team and sent to hospital, as the respiratory nurse was concerned about his confusion. His respiratory rate was 32 and oxygen saturation 77% on air at the arrival of the ambulance crew; this improved to a respiratory rate of 24 and an oxygen saturation of 98% with 15 litres oxygen via a non-rebreathing mask. Which of the following statements is correct?**

A. Oxygen should be titrated to SaO_2

B. Arterial blood gas analysis should be done only when you change the oxygen settings

C. COPD patients are acidotic due to chronic carbon dioxide retention

D. Non-invasive ventilation should be started on patients with type 1 respiratory failure who fail to respond to initial management

E. Doxapram is useful once patients are commenced on NIV

77. **An 85-year-old ex-smoker with advanced COPD is referred for assessment for home oxygen. Which of the following is NOT a criterion for long-term oxygen therapy?**

A. PaO_2 <7.3 kPa on air

B. PaO_2 7.3–8.0 kPa with nocturnal hypoxaemia

C. PaO_2 7.3–8.0 kPa with secondary polycythaemia

D. $PaCO_2$ <6 kPa

E. Palliative care for the dyspnoea of lung malignancy or other terminal disease

78. **A 51-year-old nurse comes to see you in the chest clinic. She complains of increased shortness of breath, a chronic cough, and wheezing. She has a 30-pack-year smoking history. On examination she smells strongly of cigarettes. On auscultation, there is coarse wheezing and occasional crackles. A chest X-ray confirms hyperinflation. Which would be the most useful investigation to guide her pharmacological management?**

A. Alpha 1 antitrypsin deficiency testing

B. Bronchoscopy

C. CT scan of her chest

D. Autoimmune profile

E. Spirometry with reversibility

79. **A 36-year-old renal transplant recipient (cadaveric donor some seven months previously) presents with shortness of breath and feeling generally unwell. He is taking prednisone, tacrolimus, mycophenolate, quinapril, aspirin, metroprolol, and simvastatin. His chest X-ray shows asymmetrical diffuse interstitial shadowing in the both lung fields. He is found to be hypoxic. His serum creatinine is 154 micromol/l (112 micromol/l 1 month previously). What is the cause for his chest signs?**

    A. Acute rejection
    B. Cytomegalovirus
    C. Drug-induced changes
    D. *Pneumocystis jirovecii*
    E. Pulmonary oedema

80. **A 60-year-old woman gives a clear history of a cough productive of purulent sputum, fevers, and rigors. Blood pressure is 100/50 mmHg, heart rate 95 bpm, RR 28/min, and SpO$_2$ 92% on air. On examination she has evidence of consolidation confirmed on chest X-ray. Blood tests reveal WBC 20 x 10^9/l, urea 8 mmol/l, and albumin 30 g/l. What is her CURB score?**

    A. 1
    B. 2
    C. 3
    D. 4
    E. 5

81. **A 40-year-old man collapses while in the outpatient department and you are the only medic on the scene. Which of the following is according to ALS guidelines?**

    A. A precordial thump is indicated
    B. Start CPR immediately
    C. Call for help early
    D. Give two rescue breaths prior to your first round of CPR
    E. Chest compressions should be commenced at a rate of 15:2 (compressions:breaths)

82. **Patients diagnosed with idiopathic interstitial pneumonias have a variable prognosis. The prognosis with fibrotic NSIP (non-specific interstitial pneumonitis) is similar to which other condition?**

    A. Idiopathic pulmonary fibrosis (IPF)
    B. Chronic hypersensitivity pneumonitis
    C. Bleomycin-induced pulmonary fibrosis
    D. Collagen vascular disease-associated pulmonary fibrosis
    E. Amiodarone-induced pulmonary fibrosis

83. **A 64-year-old man presents with a progressive increase in shortness of breath over the past six months, and a chronic non-productive cough that he says he has had for years. He looks tired and thin and his BMI is 20. His BP is 115/72, and his pulse is 75, atrial fibrillation. There are bilateral end expiratory crackles on auscultation of the chest. He is clubbed, with bilateral pitting oedema to the mid shins. Investigations: Hb 13.4 g/dl, WCC 9.3 x 10^9/l, PLT 204 x 10^9/l, Na 139 mmol/l, K 4.3 mmol/l, creatinine 134 micromol/l, autoantibodies negative, PaO$_2$ 7.7 kPa, PaCO$_2$ 3.8 kPa, CXR: interstitial shadowing, high resolution CT: pulmonary fibrosis. Which of the following treatments has the most evidence to support its use in this man?**

    A. Low-dose inhaled corticosteroids
    B. High-dose inhaled corticosteroids
    C. High-dose oral corticosteroids
    D. Methotrexate
    E. Home oxygen therapy

84. **A 63-year-old former miner has a complex medical history. He reports two years of increasing shortness of breath. A chest X-ray shows bilateral upper lobe volume loss, elevation of the hila, and interstitial shadowing. Which of the following underlying causes is least likely to account for the upper lobe changes?**

    A. Progressive massive fibrosis from occupational silicone exposure
    B. Rheumatoid arthritis
    C. Prior tuberculosis exposure
    D. Parenchymal changes from pulmonary sarcoid
    E. Ankylosing spondylitis

85. **A 38-year-old woman comes to the respiratory clinic complaining of worsening shortness of breath and wheeze. She has been managed with BD 100 mcg inhaled beclomethasone, but has been using increasing amounts of salbutamol. She also has multiple joint pains and night sweats which have increased over past weeks. She is taking lanzoprazole for reflux. There is a temperature of 37.4°C, a pulse of 75, and marked bilateral wheeze on auscultation of the chest. Investigations: Hb 11.0 g/dl, WCC 12.1 x10^9/l (eosinophils 1.4), PLT 192 x10^9/l, Na$^+$ 138 mmol/l, K$^+$ 4.3 mmol/l, creatinine 141 micromol/l. Which of the following is the most likely diagnosis?**

    A. Systemic lupus erythematosis
    B. Henoch Schonlein purpura
    C. Rheumatoid arthritis
    D. Wegener's granulomatosis
    E. Churg–Strauss syndrome

86. **A 30-year-old man, previously fit and well, attends with a reports a blue tinge to his fingers and lips, headache, lightheadedness, shortness of breath, and palpitations. On the day of his hospital admission, he noticed all of his fingers were blue. In his social history, he is an active smoker. He admits to sniffing 'poppers' (alkyl/amyl nitrite). On examination, he is cyanosed. Respiratory rate is 12 and saturations on air are 84%. Chest is clear. Investigations: Hb 14.3, WCC 15.7, PLT 399, MCV 89.5, CRP 0.8, INR 1.0, Na 143, K 4.1, Cl 107, U 2.9, Cr 86, ALT 22, ALP 58, bilirubin 13, corrected calcium 2. ABG on air demonstrates PaO_2 11.0. Chest X-ray is unremarkable. Which investigation will confirm your diagnosis?**

A. D dimer
B. CTPA
C. V/Q scan
D. Methaemoglobin level
E. Carbon monoxide level

87. **A 30-year-old man, with no significant past medical history, presents with symptoms of headache, lightheadedness, shortness of breath, and muscular weakness following recurrent inhalation of amyl nitrate. On examination he appears cyanotic. Saturations are 87% despite high-flow oxygen via a non-rebreathe mask. Blood gases demonstrate a raised PaO_2 and a normal $PaCO_2$. What would be the next appropriate management step?**

A. Administer intravenous bicarbonate
B. Administer intravenous methylene blue
C. Administer intravenous corticosteroids
D. Commence non-invasive ventilation
E. Transfer to a hyperbaric oxygen centre

88. **A 53-year-old man is diagnosed with lung carcinoma with staging CT showing that it may be amenable to surgical resection. Which one of the following features would be a contraindication to surgery?**

A. Hypercalcaemia
B. FEV1 1.0 l
C. Hyponatraemia
D. Pleural effusion
E. Smoker 10/day

89. **A 72-year-old man is brought to the emergency department after a collapse. On further questioning his family tell you that he smokes 40 cigarettes per day and has had increasing trouble from a cough over the past few months. On examination his BP is 90/70 and is pulse is 88. He looks cachetic and has changes consistent with COPD on auscultation of his chest. Investigations: haemoglobin 9.8 g/dl (13.5–17.7), white cell count 10.2 x 10⁹/l (4–11), platelets 180 x 10⁹/l (150–400), serum sodium 124 mmol/l (135–146), serum potassium 5.5 mmol/l (3.5–5), creatinine 148 micromol/l (79–118). Which of the following is the most likely diagnosis?**

   A. SIADH
   B. Autoimmune adrenal failure
   C. Adrenal metastases
   D. Gastroenteritis
   E. Diuretic use

90. **Regarding lung cancer:**

   A. The majority of lung cancers are classified as small cell lung cancer (SCLC)
   B. 99% of lung cancer is smoking-related
   C. Fluorodeoxyglucose positron emission tomography (FDG-PET) scanning should form part of the routine staging investigation of patients with potentially operable non-small cell lung cancer (NSCLC)
   D. Chemotherapy for metastatic disease offers no benefit to the majority of patients
   E. There is no association between pulmonary fibrosis and the development of lung cancer

91. **A 42-year-old man presents to the respiratory clinic with shortness of breath, wheeze, and recurrent left-sided pneumonia. Over the past few months he has noticed problems with haemoptysis. On examination his BP is 142/82, pulse is 75. There is left-sided wheeze on auscultation. Investigations: CXR–well-demarcated lesion in the left upper lobe; bronchoscopy—well-demarcated, cherry-red lesion encroaching into the bronchus. Which of the following is the most likely diagnosis?**

   A. Small cell carcinoma of the bronchus
   B. Large cell carcinoma of the bronchus
   C. Bronchial adenoma
   D. Bronchial carcinoid
   E. Squamous cell carcinoma of the bronchus

92. **A 39-year-old woman presents to chest clinic with a three-month history of worsening shortness of breath on exertion. There is no history of angina and no significant past medical history. Her weight has been stable over the past three months and there is no history of night sweats or fevers. She has a resting 12-lead electrocardiogram which shows sinus rhythm with a heart rate of 64 bpm. Plain chest radiograph shows bilateral hilar lymphadenopathy with peripheral pulmonary infiltrates. Tuberculin skin test is negative. Sarcoidosis is suspected. Which of the following best describes the radiological findings?**

    A. Stage 0
    B. Stage 1
    C. Stage 2
    D. Stage 3
    E. Stage 4

93. **A 26-year-old woman with a history of brittle asthma comes to the emergency department. She has had increasing shortness of breath, a dry cough, and wheeze over the past few days. She takes regular high-dose seretide and has had three previous admissions to the intensive care unit. By the time you see her she has had three back-to-back nebulizers from the emergency room staff. On examination her BP is 135/70, pulse is 110 and regular. She has poor air entry and wheeze throughout both lung fields. Peak flow is 225 (500 predicted). Investigations (on 60% O2):pH 7.35,PaO2 8.0,PaCO2 3.9. Which of the following is the most appropriate next intervention?**

    A. IV magnesium
    B. IV salbutamol
    C. IV aminophylline
    D. Nebulized terbutaline
    E. IV hydrocortisone

94. **A 22-year-old woman comes to the respiratory clinic. She has recently returned from a holiday to Pakistan where she stayed with her cousin. Unfortunately her uncle who lives in the same house has recently been diagnosed with tuberculosis. On examination she looks well and has a scar on her shoulder consistent with a BCG vaccination. She deals with children in her job as a paediatric nurse, and is worried she may have caught TB. Which of the following is the most appropriate screening test for TB in this patient?**

    A. CXR
    B. Interferon gamma release
    C. Heaf test
    D. Mantoux test
    E. Sputum sampling

95. **A 33-year-old woman presents to the respiratory clinic for review. She has progressively increasing shortness of breath, and has had two syncopal episodes. Previously a keen jogger, she is now unable to walk more than 200 yards without stopping. There is no past medical history of note, she takes no medication, and has no children. On examination her BP is 149/88, pulse is 88 and regular. There is a loud second heart sound, and bilateral swelling of the ankles. Her abdomen is soft and non tender and her BMI is 24. Hb 12.7, WCC 9.0, PLT 196, Na 136, K 4.0, Cr 107, CXR—Normal. Echo—elevated pulmonary artery pressure (no signs of shunt or ASD). CTPA—no changes suggestive of pulmonary emboli. Catheterization—pulmonary artery wedge pressure 40 mmHg. Acute vascular reactivity testing negative. Which of the following is the most appropriate initial therapy?**

    A. Amlodipine
    B. Diltiazem
    C. Isosorbide dinitrate
    D. Bosentan
    E. Ramipril

96. **A 59-year-old man with a history of alcoholic cirrhosis presents via ambulance to the emergency department with increasing shortness of breath and confusion. According to his partner he was drinking up to three bottles of wine per day until six months ago. He was last admitted three months ago, with a variceal bleed. On examination he looks unwell and is cyanosed. Saturation is 91% on air and does not really improve with high-flow oxygen replacement. His BP is 122/72, pulse is 85 and regular. He has ascites and peripheral oedema, although his chest sounds clear. Which of the following treatments is most likely to improve his oxygenation?**

    A. Transjugular intrahepatic portosystemic shunting
    B. Liver transplantation
    C. Furosemide
    D. Spironolactone
    E. Home oxygen therapy

97. **A 38-year-old man is referred to the respiratory clinic with a third episode of respiratory tract infection requiring antibiotic therapy in the last year. Each has needed a prolonged course of co-amoxiclav and he still complains of cough productive of yellow sputum in between episodes. A past history of whooping cough as a child is noted. On examination his BP is 122/72, pulse is 70 and regular, and he is a pyrexial. There are coarse crackles on auscultation of his chest, more marked at the right base than the left. Chest X-ray reveals ring shadowing consistent with bronchiectasis, which is confirmed on high resolution CT. Which of the following is the mainstay of therapy in this man?**

A. Physiotherapy
B. Regular rotating oral antibiotics
C. Regular immunoglobulin infusions
D. Local lung resection of the worst affected area
E. Daily nebulised antibiotics

98. **A 66-year-old man is admitted with a cough productive of rust-coloured sputum. He has a history of hypertension controlled with a combination of ramipril and amlodipine. On examination his BP is 105/65, pulse is 100 and regular, his temperature is 38.8°C. There are signs of right lower lobe consolidation on auscultation and his respiratory rate is 32. White count is raised at 15, urea is 6.9. Which of the following features are markers of pneumonia severity in this patient?**

A. Age 66
B. BP 105/65
C. Pulse 100
D. White count 15
E. Urea 6.9

99. **A 42-year-old man is admitted to the emergency department after a house fire. Whilst in the unit, he deteriorates with progressively worsening shortness of breath. His O_2 saturation falls to 92% on oxygen and there are fine inspiratory crackles on auscultation of the chest. Which of the following features would most support a diagnosis of acute respiratory distress syndrome (ARDS)?**

A. Hypercapnea but normal arterial PO2
B. Pulmonary Capillary Wedge pressure 16mmHg
C. Total thoracic compliance >30ml/cm H2O
D. Evidence of clinical congestive cardiac failure
E. BP 185/100

100. **A 64-year-old man with a 40-pack-year smoking history is referred to the respiratory clinic with worsening shortness of breath and wheeze. He has been using a PRN salbutamol inhaler but feels like his symptoms are getting worse. On examination his BP is 155/90, pulse is 70, atrial fibrillation. There is poor air entry and bilateral wheeze on auscultation. Lung function testing reveals FEV1 45% of predicted. Which of the following is the most appropriate next step?**

A. Regular salbutamol
B. Oral theophylline
C. Inhaled salmeterol/high-dose fluticasone
D. Regular ipratropium
E. Regular salmeterol

101. **A 28-year-old man presents with breathlessness which started suddenly three hours ago whilst playing football. He has hayfever but no other significant past medical or family history, and does not take any regular medications. He is a non-smoker. On examination, you note that he is 1.5 m tall and has decreased expansion and diminished breath sounds on the right side. Which of following puts him at greatest risk of having a pneumothorax?**

A. Hayfever
B. His height
C. His non-smoking status
D. Male sex
E. The history of physical activity

102. **You try to aspirate a 3 cm primary spontaneous pneumothorax in a patient who is short of breath. You use an appropriate technique, but the lung fails to re-expand. What is the next best step in your management?**

A. Admit him for observation alone
B. Discharge him with respiratory outpatient follow up in one week
C. Proceed to small-bore chest drain
D. Re-attempt the needle aspiration
E. Refer to the cardiothoracic surgeon for pleurodesis

103. You diagnose a 23-year-old man with a right-sided spontaneous pneumothorax following an erect inspiratory chest X-ray. You measure this as being 3 cm in size. Clinically he is short of breath. You can find no evidence of tracheal deviation, and he is haemodynamically stable. How should you initially manage his pneumothorax?

A. Aspiration
B. Large-bore chest drain
C. Observation
D. Small-bore chest drain
E. Pleurodesis

104. A 28-year-old woman who is 27 weeks pregnant comes to the emergency department with left-sided pleuritic chest pain of sudden onset which began some 12 hours earlier. It has not been relieved by regular paracetamol. She has no past medical history of note. On examination her BP is 100/60, pulse is 90 and regular. Her O_2 sats are 92% on air. Respiratory rate is 26 but there are no abnormal sounds on auscultation. The left calf is swollen and tender. White count and CRP are normal. Venous ultrasound of the left leg is suspicious of a deep vein thrombosis. Which of the following is the most appropriate next step?

A. Chest X-ray
B. CTPA
C. Digital subtraction angiography
D. V/Q scan
E. Low molecular weight heparin

105. A 62-year-old woman comes to the cardiology clinic for review. She has a history of COPD which is managed with both high-dose seretide and tiotropium, and has had four admissions to the respiratory ward over the past 18 months. She suffered an inferior MI some three years ago and is treated with ramipril, furosemide, aspirin, and atorvastatin. Her most recent complaint is of worsening angina which is limiting her exercise tolerance to only a few yards. On examination her BP is 135/72, pulse is 75 and regular. Auscultation of the lungs reveals scattered crackles and wheeze, coupled with poor air entry. Full blood count and U&E are unremarkable. An ECHO reveals poor LV function with an ejection fraction of 31%. Which of the following is the optimal way to treat her angina?

A. Isosorbide dinitrate
B. Bisoprolol
C. Amlodipine
D. Diltiazem
E. Nicorandil

106. **You are reviewing a 67-year-old man with severe COPD. He has failed to gain control of his symptoms on regular salbutamol and you plan to add in aclidinium bromide. Which of the follow fits correctly with it's mode of action?**

    A. Long-acting beta agonist
    B. Long-acting muscarinic agonist
    C. Long-acting beta antagonist
    D. Long-acting muscarinic antagonist
    E. Long-acting inhaled corticosteroid

107. **A 72-year-old man who has a 40-pack-year smoking history is reviewed in the clinic some three months after a second admission with COPD exacerbation. On examination in the clinic his BP is 145/82, pulse is 78 and regular. There is poor air entry and bilateral wheeze on auscultation of the chest. FEV1 is 45% of predicted. Which of the following is the most appropriate intervention?**

    A. Salmeterol
    B. Seretide
    C. Beclomethasone
    D. Salbutamol
    E. Ipatropium bromide

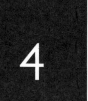

RESPIRATORY MEDICINE

ANSWERS

4

1. C. 50%

Approximately 50% of adult CF patients have nasal polyps. Using endoscopic techniques for diagnosis, the literature suggests frequencies ranging from 32% to 56%. Nasal polyps are initially treated with nasal steroids and if these fail, polypectomy.

Cystic Fibrosis Foundation website. http://www.cff.org/treatments/CFCareGuidelines/

2. E. Refer to intensive care

This patient has acute severe asthma, which has progressed rapidly, and she is starting to tire and decompensate. Raised arterial $PaCO_2$ is an acute emergency in such a patient, and necessitates urgent ICU referral. Her PaO_2 is not reassuring as she is receiving oxygen. Her respiratory rate is low for these blood gases because she is tiring and because it is difficult to maintain a rapid respiratory rate with tightly obstructed airways. All the other treatments are also indicated (and would normally be given in the order: IV hydrocortisone, nebulized atrovent, IV magnesium sulphate, and IV aminophylline), but the priority is to ensure that the ICU are alerted to her and that an anaesthetist is on standby.

British Guideline on the Management of Asthma, *Thorax* 2008;63(Suppl. 4):iv1–121.

3. D. Urinary hCG

Providing the patient is not pregnant, she should then have a CXR. Further investigation beyond this is dependent upon clinical risk scoring for PE, and presence of alternative diagnoses. If her risk is low then a normal D dimer has a sufficiently good negative predictive value for pulmonary embolism to be used to exclude the diagnosis. Patients with additional risk factors require further investigation, regardless of D-dimer level, which could be by VQ scan if her CXR was normal, or CTPA if VQ scan unavailable or CXR not entirely normal. An elevated D dimer is not on its own an indication for CTPA or VQ scanning in a patient with no other risk factors.

British Thoracic Society Guidelines for the Management of Suspected Pulmonary Embolism, *Thorax* 2003;58:470–484.

4. A. CF liver disease, requiring liver transplant, is more common in younger patients

CF liver disease tends to be more fulminant in younger patients. Although many older patients will have some derangement of LFTs or fatty changes on liver ultrasound, progressive liver failure is relatively rare once patients are into their 20s. The inflammation is predominantly neutrophilic. Whilst the majority (>99%) of males are infertile, female patients are usually able to conceive normally. The cervical OS may be obstructed by mucus, resulting in reduced fertility in women, but all female patients should be considered fertile and offered contraception. The consequences of an unwanted pregnancy can be significant for the CF patient. Diabetes is common in CF, with a prevalence of about 50% by 30 years of age. However DKA is rare, since the pancreas usually retains the ability to secrete some insulin. CF diabetes has features of both type 1 and type 2 DM, and is usually treated with insulin. The carrier frequency is 1:25 in those of European descent. Thus there is a 1:25x1:25 chance of a couple both being carriers and, since the disease is autosomal recessive, a 1:4 chance of that couple having a CF child. The birth frequency of CF is therefore 1 in (25x25x4) = 1:2500.

Horsley A et al., *Oxford Respiratory Medicine Library Handbook on Cystic Fibrosis*, Oxford University Press, 2010, Chapter 6, Gastrointestinal disease and nutrition.

5. E. Hypertrophic pulmonary osteoarthropathy

SIADH and ectopic ACTH commonly occurs in small cell lung cancer. Clubbing and hyperthyroidism commonly occur in squamous cell lung cancer. A number of theories are postulated as to the cause of HPO, but the one gaining most credence currently appears to be around a rise in platelet derived growth factor (PDGF). VEGF is also thought to play a role. An alternative theory suggests the condition may be related to vagally mediated changes in blood flow. Removal of the primary tumour can resolve HPOA, although, of course, many patients with bronchial carcinoma present when it is too late for removal of the primary lesion.

Longmore M et al., *Oxford Handbook of Clinical Medicine*, Eighth Edition, Oxford University Press, 2010, Chapter 4, Chest medicine, Lung tumours.

6. D. Cushing's syndrome

This patient has a carcinoid tumour in her lung. Carcinoid tumours are neuroendocrine in origin and have the capability to secrete peptides and hormones, including serotonin, histamine, bradykinin, tachykinin, substance P, VIP, gastrin, insulin, glucagons, ACTH, and parathyroid and thyroid hormones. They typically originate in the gastrointestinal tract (approximately 70% of cases) and the respiratory tract (approximately 30% of cases). The most common endocrine complications associated with pulmonary carcinoid are carcinoid syndrome, Cushing's syndrome, acromegaly, hypercalcaemia, and hypoglycaemia. Carcinoid syndrome occurs very rarely with GI tumours in the absence of liver metastases. Large pulmonary carcinoid tumours may cause carcinoid syndrome by direct release of vasoactive substances (serotonin) into the systemic circulation. SIADH is recognized with pulmonary carcinoid tumors but is more commonly associated with small cell lung carcinoma. HPOA and Trousseau's syndrome are most commonly associated with adenocarcinoma.

Gustafsson BI et al., Bronchopulmonary neuroendocrine tumors, *Cancer* 2008;113(1):5–21. http://www.ncbi.nlm.nih.gov/pubmed/18473355

7. B. Two ABG samples in which pO_2 <7.3 kPa

Assessment for LTOT is done by doing ABG on two occasions at least three weeks apart. These are COPD patients who are stable. If two samples show pO_2 <7.3 kPa, then offer LTOT. However, offer it to patients who have pO_2 7.3 to 8 kPa if they also have any of the following: secondary polycythaemia, peripheral oedema, pulmonary hypertension, nocturnal hypoxaemia.

Chapman S et al., *Oxford Handbook of Respiratory Medicine*, Second Edition, Oxford University Press, 2009, Chapter 58, Oxygen therapy.

8. E. Low molecular weight heparin

Her symptoms and signs fit the diagnosis of a PE. She should be treated with low molecular weight heparin.

Longmore M et al., *Oxford Handbook of Clinical Medicine*, Eighth Edition, Oxford University Press, 2010, Chapter 4, Chest medicine, Pulmonary embolism.

9. E. Cannabis smoking is associated with an increased incidence of adult onset asthma and bronchitis

A number of studies have reported an increase of respiratory symptoms in cannabis smokers, including cough, chronic sputum, and wheeze. In a longitudinal study from New Zealand, cannabis use was associated with an increased decline in FEV1 and FVC. The effects of cannabis and tobacco seem to be additive. Cannabis is most commonly taken by smoking. It is available either as the dried flowers, leaves and stalks of cannabis plants (marijuana), or as concentrated resin produced from the flowers of the female plant (hashish) which is typically mixed with tobacco and smoked unfiltered in a joint. It may also be inhaled through water using a water pipe, or bong. Smoking tobacco is associated with an increased risk of tuberculosis, but there are no studies that suggest the same is true of cannabis. In case reports, it appears that risk of transmission may be increased in those who share apparatus (e.g. water pipes). Because cannabis is typically mixed with tobacco the different effects of the two compounds can be hard to separate. However, in retrospective studies, the odds ratio for developing lung cancer in cannabis smokers, adjusted for tobacco intake, ranges from 1.9 to 5.7. There are case reports in the literature describing invasive aspergilloma in immune-suppressed subjects who smoked cannabis, one of which indicated that the Aspergillus found in the cannabis was the same as that in the lung. However, there are no reports of cannabis being implicated in invasive aspergillosis in otherwise healthy subjects, something that is in any case very rare.

Reid PT et al., Cannabis and the lung, *Journal of the Royal College of Physicians of Edinburgh* 2010;40(4):328–333.

10. C. Needle aspiration

This man has suffered a primary spontaneous pneumothorax. British Thoracic Society guidelines suggest that young fit patients with pneumothoraces of less than 2 cm could be discharged home, provided they are asymptomatic and should reviewed in an outpatient clinic 2–4 weeks later. If the patient is either symptomatic (dyspnoea/low saturations/respiratory compromise) or has a pneumothorax >2 cm needle aspiration is advised. If this is successful discharge may be considered if (1) the pneumothorax is now <2 cm, (2) the volume aspirated is less than 2.5 litres, and (3) symptoms have improved. If any of these criteria are not met, the patient should have a chest drain inserted and be admitted to hospital. If needle aspiration is unsuccessful, a further attempt at aspiration should only be attempted if technical difficulty was encountered during the first attempt (kinked/blocked catheter); otherwise, proceed to chest drain insertion and admission. All patients should have adequate analgesia and oxygen at a flow rate of 10 l/min.

MacDuff A et al., on behalf of the BTS Pleural Disease Guideline Group. Management of spontaneous pneumothorax: British Thoracic Society pleural disease guideline 2010, *Thorax* 2010;65(Suppl 2):ii18eii31.

11. A. FEV1

FEV1 is known to correlate most closely with mortality in COPD; it is the major component of the BODE index, developed by the MRC as a measure of COPD mortality risk. Other components include BMI, shortness of breath, and exercise capacity as assessed in the six-minute walk test. Of course, this man's successful smoking cessation is likely to have the greatest impact on his prognosis.

Longmore M et al., *Oxford Handbook of Clinical Medicine*, Eighth Edition, Oxford University Press, 2010, Chapter 4, Chest medicine, Chronic obstructive pulmonary disease (COPD).

12. E. Serial peak flow measurements at work and at home

The most important diagnosis to rule out initially is occupational asthma. Peak flow measurement is non-invasive and is likely to vary significantly during the working week versus weekends. This can be followed up with a review of likely allergens in the work environment. Treatment involves removal of the precipitant and conventional asthma therapy; continued exposure to the cause of the asthma is not an option. Total IgE measurement is considered if Churg–Strauss is a possibility. RAST testing is used to confirm that a specific allergen is responsible. High-resolution CT might be considered to rule out underlying pulmonary fibrosis. Causes of occupational asthma include: isocyanates (paint spraying), acid anhydrides, metals (welders), glutaraldehyde (health care workers), amine dyes, wood dusts, plant products (bakers), and fluxes (solderers).

Chapman S et al., *Oxford Handbook of Respiratory Medicine*, Second Edition, Oxford University Press, 2009, Chapter 18, Asthma, Occupational asthma.

13. D. Secondary pulmonary hypertension

The suspicion here is that this patient has chronic venous thromboembolism, leading to right heart failure because of pulmonary hypertension related to multiple pulmonary emboli. As such anti-coagulation with warfarin is the intervention of choice. Had she been thinner then an underlying diagnosis of primary pulmonary hypertension would also have been reasonable.

Chapman S et al., *Oxford Handbook of Respiratory Medicine*, Second Edition, Oxford University Press, Chapter 38, Pulmonary hypertension, Non-idiopathic pulmonary hypertension: causes.

14. B. PaO_2 7.2 kPa

Home oxygen therapy should be considered in patients who have FEV1 less than 30% predicted, have cyanosis, peripheral oedema, a raised JVP, or oxygen saturations less than 92% on air. Need for O_2 is assessed by two arterial blood gas measurements at least three weeks apart in a stable patient. LTOT should be offered to patients with a PaO_2 of <7.3 kPa or to those with a PaO_2 7.3–8.0, where there is an associated risk factor such as peripheral oedema or polycythaemia.

NICE Guidance [CG101], Chronic obstructive pulmonary disease in over 16s: diagnosis and management. https://www.nice.org.uk/guidance/cg101/

15. D. Hypertrophic pulmonary osteo-arthropathy

Hypertrophic pulmonary osteo-arthropathy, often associated with clubbing, occurs with any lung cancer cell type but is more common in squamous and adenocarcinoma. Production of parathyroid-hormone-related peptide resulting in hypercalcaemia is more common in squamous cell carcinoma. The other paraneoplastic syndromes listed are all more common in small cell lung cancer.

Patel AM et al., Paraneoplastic syndromes associated with lung cancer, *Mayo Clinic Proceedings* 1993;68(3):278–287.

16. C. Erythromycin

Mycoplasma pneumoniae is a common cause of community-acquired pneumonia, particularly in otherwise healthy young adults. The disease has a prolonged, gradual onset. Macrolide antibiotics (e.g. erythromycin), doxycycline, and second-generation quinolones are effective treatments. Penicillins and cephalosporins are ineffective because the organism lacks a cell wall. Metronidazole is effective against anaerobes. Acyclovir is an anti-viral treatment.

Baum SG, Mycoplasma pneumoniae and atypical pneumonia. In: Mandell GL, Bennett JE, Dolin R, eds. *Principles and Practice of Infectious Diseases*, Seventh Edition, Elsevier Churchill Livingstone, 2009, Chapter 184.

17. C. 75%

Survival rates post lung transplant are lower than for heart and other solid organ transplants. There is an accelerated attrition rate due to the development of chronic graft dysfunction (bronchiolitis obliterans syndrome). Lung transplant recipients are a heterogeneous population, and different diagnostic groups have different survival rates. Survival after lung transplantation for IPF is worse than after other indications for transplantation (e.g. cystic fibrosis, bronchiectasis). Survival at one year is 73%, at three years it is 56%, and at five years it is 44%.

Mason DP et al., Lung transplantation for idiopathic pulmonary fibrosis, *Annals of Thoracic Surgery* 2007;84(4):1121–1128.

18. B. Ciprofloxacin and nebulized colistin for six weeks

The first colonization with *Pseudomonas* should be treated aggressively with the aim of eradication if possible. Standard therapy is ciprofloxacin 750 mg oral BD with nebulized colistin 1 mega unit BD for six weeks. Where chronic colonization exists, patients may benefit from chronic therapy with either colistin or tobramycin. In patients who do not respond to oral therapy, ceftazidime and gentamycin are the treatments of choice.

Torok E et al., *Oxford Handbook of Infectious Diseases and Microbiology*, Oxford University Press, 2009.

19. D. ITU review

This patient has failed to respond adequately to back-to-back nebulizers, and referral to the ITU is the next most appropriate intervention. Whilst IV magnesium is the next most appropriate step according to BTS guidelines, she may be subject to very rapid deterioration given her peak flow and therefore review with respect to ventilatory support is crucial. Pregnancy does not significantly alter her management in this case apart from the fact that the threshold for mechanical ventilation may be lower to prevent damage to the foetus, and obstetric/neonatal teams should of course be closely involved. Foetal monitoring should also be instituted.

BTS/SIGN Asthma Guideline, 2011. https://www.brit-thoracic.org.uk/guidelines-and-quality-standards/asthma-guideline/

20. D. Pulmonary carcinoid tumour

Pulmonary carcinoid tumours can be very similar to small cell lung cancer histologically. Carcinoid syndrome with flushing, tachycardia, sweats, diarrhoea, wheeze, and hypotension occurs in 1% of pulmonary carcinoid. Octreotide can be used to treat these tumours.

Chapman S et al., *Oxford Handbook of Respiratory Medicine*, Second Edition, Oxford University Press, 2009, Chapter 31, Lung cancer, Pulmonary carcinoid tumours

21. C. Bilateral upper zone fibrosis

Five causes of upper zone fibrosis you have to think of in MRCP are: TB, ankylosing spondylitis, allergic bronchopulmonary aspergillosis, extrinsic allergic alveolitis, and sarcoidosis.

Longmore M et al., *Oxford Handbook of Clinical Medicine*, Eighth Edition, Oxford University Press, 2010, Chapter 12, Rheumatology, Spondyloarthritides.

22. B. The patient has a high CURB-65 score and needs senior assessment. They should be treated with intravenous (IV) augmentin and clarithromycin in addition to IV fluids

CURB-65 score: C= confusion; U= urea >7 mmol/l; R= respiratory rate >30 breaths/min; B= Blood pressure <90 systolic or <60 diastolic; 65= Age >65. A CURB-65 score of 3 or more is supportive of severe disease with a high mortality (15–40%). The patient described above appears to have pneumonia with a score of 3 (Urea >7, Resp rate >30/min, diastolic BP<60 mmHg). Admission and intravenous antibiotics are therefore indicated. She has travelled to Spain and has diarrhoea which may indicate Legionnaire's disease as the cause of her pneumonia. Amoxicillin alone would therefore be inadequate treatment.

Nice Guidance [CG191], Pneumonia in adults: diagnosis and management, 2014. http://www.nice.org.uk/guidance/cg191

23. C. The most likely diagnosis is tuberculosis and, following further investigation, appropriate treatment would be with a combination of rifampicin, isoniazid, ethambutol, and pyrazinamide

Tuberculosis is common in recent immigrants from endemic countries. The combination here of fevers, sweats, and weight loss in a new immigrant from India suggests the diagnosis, and the presence of a lymphocytic exudate is supportive. The absence of acid-fast bacilli on Ziehl–Neilsen stain is common in tuberculosis, and the mycobacteria are often only grown on culture, or not found at all. Sputum smears are often negative in pleural tuberculosis, unless there is significant pulmonary disease in association with the pleural disease. Recent NICE guidelines therefore recommend pleural biopsy (closed, USS, CT, or thoracoscope guided) to confirm the diagnosis on culture. Treatment for tuberculosis should be with rifampicin, isoniazid, ethambutol, and pyrazinamide initially and a total treatment duration of at least six months. The treatment can sometimes be reduced to rifampicin and isoniazid after two months of treatment if the organism is obtained from culture and found to be sensitive to all anti-tuberculous agents. Rifampicin and isoniazid alone are given for three months in cases of latent tuberculosis infection, but the case described appears to be active infection and not latent infection. The case described is unlikely to have pneumonia alone in view of the exudative lymphocytic effusion, but a complicated parapneumonic effusion would be in the differential diagnosis. This would usually need more than five days of oral antibiotics for successful treatment. Adenocarcinoma and lymphoma are possible differential diagnoses but epidemiologically less likely in view of the age and travel history of the patient. SLE is possible but less common.

Maskell NA, Butland RJA, BTS guidelines for the investigation of a unilateral pleural effusion in adults, *Thorax* 2003;58:ii8–ii17. http://thorax.bmj.com/content/58/suppl_2/ii8.extract

24. C. pH 7.30

NIV is indicated when the patient is conscious and not confused. Acidosis and CO_2 retention in the presence of hypoxia leads to a vicious circle of progressive CO_2 retention, drowsiness, and respiratory muscle weakness, and so a falling pH below 7.35, and a CO_2 above 6.0 kPa are the major indications for NIV. The patient should of course be managed with maximal bronchodilator therapy and other optimized medical therapy such as corticosteroids in addition.

NICE Guidance [CG101], Chronic obstructive pulmonary disease in over 16s: diagnosis and management. https://www.nice.org.uk/guidance/cg101

25. A. Caplan's syndrome

Caplan's syndrome was first described in Welsh coal miners who developed single or multiple lung nodules. However, they can occur in other dust-exposed occupations. These nodules may appear rapidly and cavitate. Felty's syndrome is characterized by splenomegaly and neutropenia as well as anaemia and thrombocytopenia in patients with chronic rheumatoid arthritis.

Warrell DA et al., *Oxford Textbook of Medicine*, Fifth Edition, Oxford University Press, 2010, Section 18.11.4, The lung in autoimmune rheumatic disorders.

26. A. PEF 35% of predicted reading

The correct answer to this question is predicted PEF of 35%, with the correct value being <33% of predicted value. All the others options are life-threatening features of severe asthma.

Sign, British Guideline on the management of asthma. http://www.sign.ac.uk/guidelines/fulltext/141/index.html

27. D. 18 mcg tiotropium BD

Tiotropium is a long-acting inhaled anti-cholinergic licensed for the treatment of COPD. It has been shown in clinical trials to impact on exercise-induced shortness of breath, measures of the St. Georges Respiratory Questionnaire, and pulmonary function testing. Studies have not, however, shown an impact on mortality. The commonest associated adverse events include those consistent with an anti-cholinergic such as a dry mouth. Some controversy was raised about an association between use of anti-cholinergics and cardiovascular events after publication of a meta-analysis in 2008. A definitive conclusion as not been reached.

emc+, Spiriva 18 microgram inhalation powder, hard capsule, last updated February 2015. http://www.medicines.org.uk/emc/medicine/10039

28. B. A cause of hypercalcaemia

NSCLC is the most common form of lung cancer (75–80% of all lung cancers). NSCLC predominantly comprises squamous cell carcinomas and adenocarcinomas. Adenocarcinoma may not be smoking-related. Recognized paraneoplastic effects with NSCLC include hypercalcaemia (PTHrP secretion) and hypertrophic pulmonary osteoarthropathy, often in association with clubbing. SIADH, causing hyponatraemia, occurs most commonly with small cell lung cancer but is also recognized in NSCLC. Small cell lung cancer is also associated with ectopic ACTH secretion and Cushing's syndrome plus Eaton–Lambert myasthenic syndrome. Small cell lung cancer is more likely to metastasize early than NSCLC.

NICE Guidance [CG121], Lung cancer: diagnosis and management, 2011. http://publications.nice.org.uk/lung-cancer-cg121

29. A. Reduced lung volumes

Cystic fibrosis is one of the few instances where there is fibrosis but preserved or even increased lung volumes. Pulmonary artery enlargement is secondary to chronic pulmonary arterial hypertension. Tubular densities are due to mucus impaction or ABPA. Peribronchial cuffing and cystic lucenies are the hallmarks of bronchiectasis in CF.

Dahnert W, *Radiology Review Manual*, Fifth Edition, Lippincott Williams & Wilkins, 2003, Chest disorders, p. 481.

30. B. Repeat chest X-ray six weeks later

Infection in children and young adults can manifest as a 'round pneumonia'. Given the patient's age, an underlying malignancy is unlikely, hence invasive or high-radiation burden tests are not appropriate. A repeat chest X-ray six weeks later, after antibiotic treatment, should confirm resolution of the focal consolidation. Less likely differentials for this clinical picture and CXR findings would include allergic broncho-pulmonary aspergillosis, cryptogenic organizing pneumonia, eosiniphilic pneumonia, and mucous plugging.

Learning Radiology, Round pneumonia. http://www.learningradiology.com/notes/chestnotes/roundpneumoniapage.htm

31. C. Asthma

It is common to see relative lucency of one hemithorax compared to the other, and a rotated film is the most common cause. Whilst all the other options are possible causes, asthma does not affect one lung preferentially.

Chapman S, Nakielny R, *Aids to Radiological Differential Diagnosis*, Fourth Edition, Saunders, 2003, Chapter 4, Respiratory tract, p. 114.

32. A. Chronic obstructive pulmonary disease (COPD)

The FEV1/FVC ratio is 50%. COPD is the only condition from the options given that results in obstructive pulmonary function tests, and the patient's smoking history and occupation are risk factors to developing COPD.

Chapman S et al., *Oxford Handbook of Respiratory Medicine*, Second Edition, Oxford University Press, 2009, Chapter 21, Chronic obstructive pulmonary disease.

33. E. The risk of maternal mortality in patients with pulmonary hypertension is 30%

A chest X-ray is not contraindicated in pregnancy. The dose of enoxaparin should be doubled in pregnancy because of the increased glomerular filtration rate in pregnancy. A D-dimer value that is not raised is generally used to rule out pulmonary embolism in patients with low clinical probability assessed by the Well's score. It should not be measured in pregnancy as D dimer increases with time in the pregnancy such that most second- and all third-trimester values are significantly elevated. Labetalol and methyldopa are common anti-hypertensives used in pregnancy. Nifedipine is sometimes used in the treatment for pre-eclampsia. Patients with pulmonary hypertension have a high mortality of at least 30%.

Chapman S et al., *Oxford Handbook of Respiratory Medicine*, Second Edition, Oxford University Press, 2009, Chapter 38, Pulmonary Hypertension, IPAH general management.

34. B. Ropinirole

In the absence of levodopa, a dopamine agonist is the next most logical step. The ergot-based compounds such as pergolide are associated with pulmonary fibrosis. Ropinirole, however, is a non-ergot dopamine agonist and is therefore not associated with pulmonary fibrosis, thus it represents the most appropriate choice here. Ropinirole is, however, associated with somnolence and pathological gambling.

emc+, Ropinirole 0.25 mg film-coated tablets, last updated November 2015. http://www.medicines.org.uk/emc/medicine/24870

35. A. SpO_2 91%

A number of features are associated with life-threatening asthma, these include: CO_2 in the normal range, PO_2 below 8.0 kPa, PEFR below 33% predicted, and SpO_2 <92%. Rhythm disturbance and hypotension are also consistent with life-threatening asthma. Candidates should, however, remember that acute asthma is a dynamic situation, and therefore patients who do not initially fit the criteria for acute severe asthma may rapidly deteriorate. Other important factors to take into account when assessing asthma severity include: altered conscious level, exhaustion, cyanosis, presence of silent chest, and poor respiratory effort.

BTS/SIGN, Asthma guidelines. https://www.brit-thoracic.org.uk/guidelines-and-quality-standards/asthma-guideline/

36. E. Pleural plaques

There are congenital and acquired causes of bronchiectasis. Acquired immune deficiency syndrome (AIDS) is the leading cause of bronchiectasis, especially in children. Tuberculosis is another major cause. Bronchiectasis can sometimes be an unusual complication of inflammatory bowel disease, especially ulcerative colitis. Recent evidence has shown an increased risk of bronchiectasis in patients with rheumatoid arthritis who smoke. Other acquired causes of bronchiectasis include respiratory infections, obstructions, pulmonary aspiration, alcoholism, and ABPA. Common congenital causes: Kartagener's syndrome, CF, alpha 1-antitrypsin deficiency. Other less-common congenital causes include primary immunodeficiencies.

Emmons EE, Bronchiectasis, *eMedicine*, 2011. http://emedicine.medscape.com/article/296961-overview

37. A. Pulmonary tuberculosis

Reactivation of old tuberculosis is a well-known adverse event associated with anti-TNF therapy. As such, careful screening is recommended prior to starting treatment with anti-rheumatoid agents such as etanercept. In this case her anti-TNF should be discontinued, sputum sent for AAFB, and once the diagnosis is confirmed, the patient should be commenced on anti-tuberculous chemotherapy.

emc+, Enbrel 25 mg powder and solvent for solution for injection, last updated December 2015. http://www.medicines.org.uk/emc/medicine/3343

38. B. Intravenous normal saline

This patient has severe hypercalcaemia, potentially as a result of a bronchial carcinoma. Initial therapy is with IV rehydration. Bearing in mind that she has chronic renal failure, however, IV furosemide may well be the next step. Intravenous corticosteroids and IV pamidronate may both also help to reduce calcium levels. Hypercalcaemia is associated with squamous cell carcinoma on histology.

Brooks Robey R et al., Does furosemide have a role in the management of hypercalcemia? *Annals of Internal Medicine* 2009;150(2):146–147.

39. D. pO_2 <10.0 kPa

Life-threatening asthma is characterized by PEFR <33%, sats <92%, pO_2 <8 kPa, normal or high pCO_2, cyanosis, exhaustion, confusion, coma, bradycardia, arrhythmia, hypotension, and silent chest.

BTS/SIGN, Asthma guidelines. https://www.brit-thoracic.org.uk/guidelines-and-quality-standards/asthma-guideline/

40. C. FEV1 improvement of 15% (or 200 ml) after B-agonist

Asthma is a clincal diagnosis. The diagnosis is supported by findings of a 20% diurnal variation in PEFR on >3 days/week, an FEV1 decrease >15% after 6 mins exercise, an FEV1 increase >15% after a two-week oral steroid trial or B-agonist trial (spirometry with reversibility). A high serum eosinophil count is not specific for asthma and may indicate allergy, fungal or parasitic infection, or vasculitides including Churg–Strauss. Histamine and methacholine challenge testing may also be used to support the diagnosis of asthma and bronchial provocation is used when occupational asthma is suspected.

BTS/SIGN, Asthma guidelines. https://www.brit-thoracic.org.uk/guidelines-and-quality-standards/asthma-guideline/

41. A. Pneumothorax with intercostal drain in situ

Contraindications include: undrained pneumothorax, facial injury, burns, surgery or deformity, excessive secretions/vomiting, patient refusal, confusion or altered conciousness, severe hypoxia (consider intubation), and cardiac/respiratory arrest.

Roberts CM et al., Non-invasive ventilation in chronic obstructive pulmonary disease: management of acute type 2 respiratory failure, Clinical Medicine, *Journal of the Royal College of Physicians* 2008;8(5):517–521.

42. E. CURB-65 =5, >50%

In patients with pneumonia, risk of death increases with the CURB-65 score: 0—0.6%; 1—3.2%; 2—13.0%; 3—17.0%; 4—41.5%; 5—57.0%. CURB-65 is used as a means of deciding the action that is needed to be taken for that patient. 0–1 can be treated as an outpatient, 2 consider a short stay in hospital or watch very closely as an outpatient, 3–5 requires hospitalization and close monitoring (high mortality rates).

BTS, Pneumonia. https://www.brit-thoracic.org.uk/clinical-information/pneumonia/

43. D. A 25-year-old patient with saturations 94% on air, unilateral consolidation, and a CURB-65 score of 1 can be cared for as an outpatient

CURB-65 is a clinical prediction tool used to risk stratify patients admitted to hospital with community-acquired pneumonia. Thirty-day mortality increases with CURB-65 score. In general, patients scoring 0–1 can be managed in the community, those scoring 2 should be considered for hospital admission and those scoring >3 should be considered for high dependency or intensive care. CURB-65 should always be interpreted in the clinical context, i.e. if a young patient is very unwell with low sats, pyrexia, or multilobar consolidation then despite a low CURB-65, he will still require inpatient care. CURB-65 only GUIDES the clinician as to possible care options. The point of care (hospital ward, HDU, ITU) depends on functional status and co-morbidities.

BTS, Pneumonia. https://www.brit-thoracic.org.uk/clinical-information/pneumonia/

44. E. Asbestos-related pleural plaques

Causes of cavitatory lung masses include lung cancer, infection (*Klebsiella* and *Staphylococcus aureus*), Wegener's granulomatosis, sarcoidosis, TB, aspergilloma, and rheumatoid nodule.

Chapman S et al., *Oxford Handbook of Respiratory Medicine*, Second Edition, Oxford University Press, 2009, Chapter 17, Asbestos and the lung.

45. C. PRN inhaled SABA (short acting B-agonist), regular ICS (inhaled corticosteroids) up to 800 mcg/day, regular inhaled LABA (long-acting B-agonist), +/– oral theophylline S/R or leukotriene antagonist

The BTS guidelines for asthma clearly state: Step 1—PRN SABA. Step 2—add ICS 200–800 mcg. Step 3 suggests add LABA then escalate ICS (to maximum 800 mcg/day) if control inadequate, and consider leukotriene antagonist or theophylline. Symbicort (LABA/ICS) is now suggested at step 3 for regular/rescue use. Step 4—increase ICS up to 2000 mcg/day and add fifth drug (e.g. leukotriene antagonist or theophylline or B-agonist tablet). Step 5—daily oral steroid (use other agents to try to minimize steroid dose).

BTS/SIGN asthma guidelines. https://www.brit-thoracic.org.uk/guidelines-and-quality-standards/asthma-guideline/

46. A. Seretide (salmeterol and fluticasone) 500 accuhaler 1 puff BD

Seretide 500 contains 500 mcg of flixotide. This is the most potent ICS and therefore the answer is as given.

NICE technology appraisal guidance [TA138], Inhaled corticosteroids for the treatment of chronic asthma in adults and in children aged 12 years and over. https://www.nice.org.uk/guidance/TA138

47. E. >60%

Although overall figures vary, the five-year survival for all cystic fibrosis patients with bilateral lung transplantation is in excess of 60%.

Cystic Fibrosis Foundation website http://www.cff.org/treatments/CFCareGuidelines/

48. D. Aspiration of pneumothorax

This is a presentation of a primary pneumothorax in an otherwise healthy young male patient. According to the 2010 BTS guidelines, a pneumothorax >2 cm with or without breathlessness, should undergo aspiration using a 16–18G cannula. If this is successful, with the pneumothorax reducing in size to less than 2 cm or improvement in breathlessness, the patient should be considered for discharge and reviewed in the outpatient clinic in 2–4 weeks.

British Thoracic Society Pleural Disease Guideline Group, BTS Pleural Disease Guideline 2010; 65(Suppl). https://www.brit-thoracic.org.uk/document-library/clinical-information/pleural-disease/pleural-disease-guidelines-2010/pleural-disease-guideline/

49. D. Insertion of intercostal chest drain (8–14 French)

The British Thoracic Society (BTS) has produced guidelines on the management of both primary and secondary pneumothoraces. For both primary and secondary pneumothoraces they advise that breathless patients should not be left without intervention. Placing a patient with COPD on high-flow oxygen overnight could potentially be dangerous given the risk of carbon dioxide retention and respiratory acidosis. BTS advice is that for secondary pneumothorax in a symptomatic patient, with a rim of air greater than 2 cm on chest radiograph, the most appropriate initial management step is insertion of an intercostal drain. The BTS advises that there is no evidence to suggest that larger chest tubes (20–24F) are superior than smaller ones (8–14F). Application of suction to a chest tube should only be considered after 48 hours if there is persistent air leak or failure of the pneumothorax to re-expand.

British Thoracic Society Pleural Disease Guideline Group, BTS Pleural Disease Guideline 2010; 65(Suppl). https://www.brit-thoracic.org.uk/document-library/clinical-information/pleural-disease/pleural-disease-guidelines-2010/pleural-disease-guideline/

50. B. Exophthalmos

Pancoast tumours are found in the superior pulmonary sulcus of the lung apex. They are most commonly non small cell lung cancers, predominantly squamous cell. They invade local structures at the superior thoracic inlet including the chest wall, ribs, lower trunks of the brachial plexus, and the cervical sympathetic nerves. Pancoast's syndrome is defined by the presence of shoulder and arm pain along the distribution of the eighth cervical nerve trunk and first and second thoracic nerve trunks, Horner's syndrome (meiosis, ptosis, enophthalmos, anhidrosis), and weakness and atrophy of the muscles of the hand. Superior vena cava syndrome and involvement of the phrenic and recurrent laryngeal nerves occurs rarely.

Kraut MJ et al., Pancoast (superior sulcus) neoplasms, *Current Problems in Cancer* 2003;27(2):81–104.

51. C. It is licensed for intra-vesical treatment of bladder carcinoma

BCG is a live attenuated vaccine, derived from *Mycobacterium bovis*. Other live attenuated vaccinations are those for yellow fever, measles, mumps, and rubella. BCG is most effective against tuberculous meningitis and miliary tuberculosis, particularly in the paediatric population. Its efficacy against pulmonary TB is between 60% and 80% in the UK. Although protection is believed to wane after around 15 years, repeat vaccinations are not recommended. Vaccination should be offered to previously unvaccinated, heaf test grade zero or one contacts under the age of 16 years and older potential contacts with travel, ethnic or occupational risk.

Chapman S et al., *Oxford Handbook of Respiratory Medicine*, Second Edition, Oxford University Press, 2009.

52. D. Reduced A–a gradient

Acute respiratory distress syndrome occurs typically occurs 24–48 hours after direct or indirect lung injury and is characterized by lung inflammation with increased vascular permeability. Endothelial dysfunction results in fluid and protein leakage into the alveolar spaces. A cardiogenic cause of pulmonary oedema should be excluded. Dysfunction of type II pneumocytes and dilution of alveolar surfactant results in diffuse alveolar collapse and stiff lungs. Massive intrapulmonary shunting develops (right to left), causing arterial hypoxia and large A–a gradients. Intubation and ventilation are almost always required.

Wheeler AP, Bernard GR, Acute lung injury and the acute respiratory distress syndrome: a clinical review, *Lancet* 2007;369(9572):1553–1564.

53. A. Exposure to *Micropolyspora faeni* (also known as *Saccharopolyspora rectivirgula*)

Hypersensitivity pneumonitis, previously known as extrinsic allergic alveolitis, results from the immunological response to inhaled organic antigen in sensitized individuals. Examples include bird fanciers lung (avian proteins), malt workers lung (*Aspergillus clavatus*), and bagassosis (thermophilic actinomycetes). Acute hypersensitivity pneumonitis typically occurs in response to intense exposure over a short period and is characterized by mononuclear infiltrates and non-caseating granulomata, which resolve with cessation of exposure. The chronic form results from prolonged low dose exposure and there is progressive fibrotic change, particularly affecting the upper lobes. The immune response is a combination of type III (immune complex) and type IV (delayed hypersensitivity). In the acute form, there is typically blood neutrophilia and a lymphocytosis on bronchoalveolar lavage. Serum precipitins (IgG antibodies) are found in 90% of patients.

Girard M et al., Hypersensitivity pneumonitis, *Allergy* 2009;64(3):322–334.

54. C. Fenfluramine

Pulmonary endothelial damage can arise as a result of exposure to appetite suppressants such as fenfluramine, dexfenfluramine, cocaine, and amphetamines. Fenfluramine-associated pulmonary arterial hypertension shares clinical, functional, and haemodynamic features with idiopathic pulmonary arterial hypertension, as well as overall survival rates. The onset of the condition may be within days of commencing the drug and progress after drug cessation. The other answers are recognized treatments for pulmonary hypertension.

Souza R et al., Pulmonary arterial hypertension associated with fenfluramine exposure: report of 109 cases, *European Respiratory Journal* 2008;31(2):343–348.

55. E. He should stop smoking

Smoking is a significant risk factor for the development of pneumothorax, and continued smoking increases the chance of recurrence. Initial management of a primary pneumothorax (i.e. in the absence of pre-existing lung disease) >2 cm or associated with breathlessness should be needle aspiration. Aspiration should not exceed 2.5 litres. If there is residual air >2 cm or persistent breathlessness, inter-costal drainage is appropriate. Surgical review is recommended in the event of persistent air leak, first contralateral pneumothorax, second ipsilateral pneumothorax, or bilateral spontaneous pneumothorax. Flight should be delayed for seven days following pneumothorax resolution and diving is absolutely contra-indicated unless the patient has undergone a definitive surgical procedure.

Shrikrishna D, Coker R, Guideline update: managing passengers with stable respiratory disease planning air travel: British Thoracic Society recommendations, *Thorax* 2011;66:831–833.

56. D. Delta F508 mutation results in the omission of phenylalanine at the 508 residue

Cystic fibrosis is an autosomal recessive condition caused by a point mutation of the CFTR gene in the long arm of chromosome 7. More than 1000 different mutations of the CFTR gene exist, of which delta F508 is the most common. Delta F508 accounts for 67% of cystic fibrosis alleles in the UK and Northern Europe. In Caucasians the carrier frequency is 1:25, and 1:2500 live births are affected by the disease. The CFTR is a complex chloride channel.

Goetzinger KR, Cahill AG, An update on cystic fibrosis screening, *Clinics in Laboratory Medicine* 2010;30(3):533–543.

57. E. Sleep paralysis

Obstructive sleep apnoea syndrome results from dynamic upper airway obstruction during sleep causing excessive daytime sleepiness. Upper airway patency depends on the action of dilator muscles. During REM sleep in particular, skeletal muscle tone is markedly reduced, allowing the tongue and soft palate/oropharynx to impede airflow to a degree ranging from mild snoring to complete airway collapse. Narcolepsy also causes excessive daytime sleepiness but is associated with cataplexy (sudden loss of muscle tone in response to emotion or physical exertion), hypnagogic hallucinations (prolific vivid dreams, often at sleep onset), and sleep paralysis (transient global paralysis of voluntary muscles usually on waking that lasts up to a few minutes).

Johns MW, Daytime sleepiness, snoring, and obstructive sleep apnea. The Epworth Sleepiness Scale, *Chest* 1993;103(1):30–36.

58. B. Screen for Factor V Leiden variant

Of patients with venous thromboembolism 25–50% o have an identifiable inherited thrombophilia. Factor V Leiden variant is present in 20% of patients with thrombosis. Routine screening for inherited thrombophilia is not routinely recommended except in patients with recurrent events, those aged younger than 40 years with no obvious risk factors, those with a positive family history in first-degree relatives, thrombosis secondary to pregnancy, the oral contraceptive pill or hormone replacement therapy, and thrombosis at an unusual site (e.g. portal/hepatic/cerebral/mesenteric). All but Factor V Leiden and prothrombin gene mutations must be tested for when the patient is off anti-coagulants. Screening for malignancy is not recommended unless there is clinical suspicion.

Dalen JE, Should patients with venous thromboembolism be screened for thrombophilia? *American Journal of Medicine* 2008;121(6):458–463.

59. B. Asbestosis

This patient has a restrictive lung defect with reduced gas transfer and clinical signs of fibrotic lung disease. His occupation puts him at risk of asbestos exposure. Asbestosis is the most likely diagnosis of those listed, though the differential would include any other interstitial fibrosis such as usual interstitial pneumonitis. Asbestosis is a chronic fibrosis resulting from asbestos inhalation and typically develops around 20 years after exposure. There is a dose–response relationship and smoking increases the severity and rate of progress of the condition. Pleural plaque disease is usually asymptomatic with no effect on lung function.

Bolton C, Richards A, Ebden P, Asbestos-related disease, *Hospital Medicine* 2002;63(3):148–151.

60. A. Acyclovir

This is a case of varicella pneumonia. Risk factors for development of the condition are immunosuppression, steroid therapy, and pregnancy. The diagnosis should be suspected if there is a history of exposure to chicken pox, with rash and chest X-ray features. Diagnosis is confirmed by cytology of skin smears, serology, and viral culture. Treatment is with prompt administration of

IV acyclovir, continued for seven days. Immune globulin is advised for prophylaxis of susceptible individuals exposed to varicella, not for treatment of the condition.

Gogos CA et al., Varicella pneumonia in adults. A review of pulmonary manifestations, risk factors and treatment, *Respiration* 1992;59(6):339–343.

61. E. Wegener's granulomatosis

The age of the patient, in combination with the multi-systemic features of vasculitis suggest a diagnosis of Wegener's. Wegener's is an auto-immune condition in which anti neutrophil cytoplasmic antibodies target small and medium-sized blood vessels. In 90% of cases the disease presents with upper airway involvement. Lung involvement occurs in 85–90% with flitting cavitating nodules, consolidation, pulmonary haemorrhage, effusions, and bronchiectasis. Eighty percent of cases develop renal involvement with rapidly progressive glomerulonephritis or progressive deterioration in renal function leading to end-stage renal failure. Diagnosis is confirmed by biopsy and raised c-ANCA/anti proteinase 3 levels.

Leavitt RY et al., The American College of Rheumatology 1990 criteria for the classification of Wegener's granulomatosis, *Arthritis & Rheumatology* 1990;33(8):1101–1107.

62. E. Sarcoidosis

This is a case of sarcoidosis. The condition is most prevalent in African Americans, West Indians, and the Irish. Features are erythema nodosum (20%) and a transient rheumatoid-like polyarthritis or acute monoarthritis. Hilar lympadenopathy is most often bilateral and symmetrical. The differential diagnoses for hilar lymphadenopathy are lymphoma and TB but these are not commonly associated with arthropathy or erythema nodosum. The diagnosis of sarcoidosis is made clinically, by HRCT, and biopsy, with the finding of non-caseating granuloma. Serum ACE is often raised in active sarcoidosis.

Iannuzzi MC, Rybicki BA, Teirstein AS, Sarcoidosis, *New England Journal of Medicine* 2007;357(21):2153–2165.

63. A. Age >50 years

Suggested age limits for lung transplantation are 65 years for single lung, 60 years for bilateral lung, and 55 years for heart-lung transplant. The other options listed are absolute contraindications to lung transplantation. Additional absolute contraindications are severe extra-pulmonary organ dysfunction (renal/hepatic/cardiac), acute critical illness, and severe malnutrition or obesity (body weight <70% or >130% of ideal weight). Relative contraindications are maintenance prednisolone ≥20 mg/day, pleural thickening (including previous pleurodesis), and mechanical ventilation.

International guidelines for the selection of lung transplant candidates. The American Society for Transplant Physicians (ASTP)/American Thoracic Society(ATS)/European Respiratory Society(ERS)/ International Society for Heart and Lung Transplantation(ISHLT). *American Journal of Respiratory and Critical Care Medicine* 1998;158(1):335–339.

64. A. Less than 2 litres of pleural fluid should be drained at any one time in case of causing re-expansion pulmonary oedema

Streptokinase should be used in selected loculated effusions only, on a case-by-case basis. Smaller drains are often adequate for pneumothorax and empyemas. Larger drains are occasionally needed for empyemas, but regular flushing of small bore drains is often enough. Draining >2 l fluid quickly can cause re-expansion pulmonary oedema. Talc pleurodesis is unlikely to be successful until pleural fluid drainage is at least less than 200 ml per day. Generally smaller chest drains are fine for pneumothoraces except when there is a large air leak, when small bore drains can be inadequate.

British Thoracic Society Pleural Disease Guideline Group, BTS Pleural Disease Guideline 2010;
65(Suppl). https://www.brit-thoracic.org.uk/document-library/clinical-information/pleural-disease/
pleural-disease-guidelines-2010/pleural-disease-guideline/

65. C. A predominantly neutrophilic bronchoalveolar lavage fluid

Idiopathic pulmonary fibrosis is a chronic fibrosing process of unknown cause, limited to the lungs.
Typical radiological findings are bibasal, peripheral, subpleural reticulation with minimal ground glass
change. On histology there are scattered areas of fibroblastic foci and honeycombing. Bronchoalveolar
lavage is often neutrophilic (>4% neutrophils). Pulmonary function tests are restrictive.

Chapman S et al., *Oxford Handbook of Respiratory Medicine*, Second Edition, Oxford University Press,
2009, Chapter 30, Idiopathic interstitial pneumonias, Idiopathic pulmonary fibrosis.

66. C. PiZZ

In PiSS, PiMZ, and PiSZ phenotypes blood levels of A1AT are reduced to 40–60% of normal. This
is usually sufficient to protect the lungs from the effects of elastase in non-smokers. However, in
individuals with the PiZZ phenotype, levels are less than 15% of normal, leading to early-onset
emphysema.

Izaguerre DE, Alpha 1 antitrypsin deficiency, *eMedicine*, 2014. http://emedicine.medscape.com/article/
295686-overview

67. C. A 65-year-old woman with severe COPD with a pO$_2$ of 8.2 kPa on air

Long-term oxygen therapy (LTOT) is indicated for patients with chronic hypoxaemia (pO$_2$ at or below
7.3 kPa). The intention is to raise the waking oxygen tension above 8 kPa. LTOT is usually given for at
least 15 hours daily. Conditions causing chronic hypoxaemia include COPD, severe chronic asthma,
interstitial lung disease, cystic fibrosis, bronchiectasis, pulmonary vascular disease, primary pulmonary
hypertension, and chronic heart failure. LTOT can also be prescribed in chronic hypoxaemia patients
when the clinically stable pO$_2$ is between 7.3 kPa and 8 kPa and there is secondary polycythaemia
or evidence of pulmonary hypertension. Smoking does not prohibit the prescription of LTOT. All
palliative care patients can have LTOT or SBOT (short-burst) for relief of breathlessness.

BTS, Oxygen. https://www.brit-thoracic.org.uk/clinical-information/oxygen/

68. D. Infertility

Cystic fibrosis is a multi-systems disease. In addition to respiratory problems, sufferers are
susceptible to pancreatic insufficiency and diabetes, bowel obstruction, hepatic duct blockage, and
cirrhosis. Males are almost always infertile due to impaired development of the vas deferens and
the seminiferous tubules. Females, on the other hand, have only slightly reduced fertility. Many
females go on to have successful pregnancies. In males, there are now reproductive techniques that
may be used to allow affected men to have children. Sperm can be removed from the epididymis or
the testes by microsurgery or aspiration, and then IVF techniques can be used. Genetic counselling
is important as offspring will carry the cystic fibrosis gene.

Cystic Fibrosis Trust website. https://www.cysticfibrosis.org.uk

69. B. Aspirin

Samter's triad comprises asthma, aspirin sensitivity, and nasal/ethmoidal polyposis. Aspirin and
other NSAIDs precipitate asthma symptoms in up to 20% of asthmatics. Aspirin-induced asthma is
most common in women aged 20–30 years. The mechanism is thought to be via the arachadonic
acid cascade. Inhibition of the cyclo-oxygenase pathway by aspirin results in excess leukotriene
production via the lipo-oxygenase pathway with resultant allergy-like symptoms. Monteleukast is a

leukotriene receptor antagonist and may be given in step 4 of the British Thoracic Society guidelines for the management of asthma.

Babu KS, Salvi SS, Aspirin and asthma, *Chest* 2000;118(5):1470–1476.

70. C. Pulmonary asbestosis

Men with a history of asbestos exposure develop pulmonary asbestosis 15–20 years later. Some can develop it after 40 years. Benign asbestos-related, pleural disease is usually asymptomatic and most studies have failed to demonstrate abnormal lung function in patients who have pleural plaques only. In this case there is evidence of fibrosis, so this would be classified as potentially reimbursable asbestos-related lung disease.

Chapman S et al., *Oxford Handbook of Respiratory Medicine*, Second Edition, Oxford University Press, 2009, Chapter 17, Asbestos and the lung.

71. C. 7.2

Empyema is a collection of infected pleural fluid (fluid contains pus cells) secondary to infection and generally has a pH of less than 7.2. If a pleural effusion is tapped and contains pus cells/white cells and has a pH <7.2, an intercostal drain is required as soon as possible. The exception to a low pleural pH in pleural infection is a *Proteus* infection due to production of ammonia. I would add that pH <7.2 itself can occur in other situations from empyema (e.g. malignant effusions). It is important to base the pH result in the context of an empyema, and NOT all effusions. A low pH in a malignant effusion is a marker of cell turnover and predictive of survival and poor response to pleurodesis.

British Thoracic Society Pleural Disease Guideline Group, BTS Pleural Disease Guideline 2010; 65(Suppl). https://www.brit-thoracic.org.uk/document-library/clinical-information/pleural-disease/pleural-disease-guidelines-2010/pleural-disease-guideline/

72. E. Nebulized beta-2 agonist

The patient is experiencing anaphylaxis to IV contrast. The first four answer options are vital to immediate life-saving treatment. Adrenaline can be given IM or IV. Intramuscular or IV steroids are also given as emergency treatment. The role of nebulized beta-2 agonists in anaphylaxis is debatable, and not part of current guidelines.

Resuscitation Council, UK, Anaphylaxis. http://www.resus.org.uk/pages/anapost1.pdf

73. B. $PaCO_2$ 6.2

Specific criteria exist which recommend admission to ITU, these include: hypoxia (PaO_2 <8 kPa (60 mmHg) despite FiO_2 of 60%; rising $PaCO_2$ or $PaCO_2$ >6 kPa (45 mmHg); exhaustion, drowsiness, or coma; respiratory arrest; failure to improve despite adequate therapy. In this case it is the $PaCO_2$ which dictates ITU admission, and this patient should be reviewed as soon as possible by the ITU outreach team.

SIGN 141, British guideline on the management of asthma 2014. https://www.brit-thoracic.org.uk/document-library/clinical-information/asthma/btssign-asthma-guideline-2014/

74. B. Give her a peak flow meter and diary to compare the working week with time off

This patient may have occupational asthma. As such it is most appropriate to monitor her peak flow during the working week and her time off, and compare the values. It is inappropriate to prescribe asthma medication as, ideally, if she is exposed to a particular allergen then the exposure should be limited first before other intervention. If she still has symptoms once exposure to a potential allergen has been removed/limited, PRN salbutamol would be the first-choice intervention.

BTS/SIGN British guideline on the management of asthma, https://www.brit-thoracic.org.uk/standards-of-care/guidelines/btssign-british-guideline-on-the-management-of-asthma/

75. A. Kiwi

This is an example of latex fruit syndrome which occurs because a number of antigens related to latex allergy are shared by fruits such as kiwi, banana, apricot, mangoes, and passionfruit. Pears are also known to cause the reaction but with less frequency than kiwi or banana. Management of anaphylaxis is the same as for other causes, and the patient should be advised to avoid certain fruits in the future.

Spickett G, *Oxford Handbook of Clinical Immunology and Allergy*, Second Edition, Oxford University Press, 2006, Chapter 3, Allergic disease, Latex allergy.

76. A. Oxygen should be titrated to SaO_2

Patients with severe COPD can be very sensitive to oxygen so it must be tightly regulated to avoid worsening their condition. If required, oxygen should be commenced at 24–28% via a venturi mask, to achieve saturations within the individualized target range (NICE guidelines 2010). The percentage of oxygen administered should be adjusted once blood gas analysis is available. Blood gases should be performed if there are any changes to the oxygen settings or if there is a decline in patient condition. Patients with COPD are not normally acidotic due to renal compensation of a chronically elevated PCO_2, but during an exacerbation this can increase and they can then become acidotic and deteriorate rapidly. In those patients who have type 2 respiratory failure, and are acidotic despite initial therapy (steroids, nebulized salbutamol and ipratropium bromide) non-invasive ventilation is the treatment of choice. Doxapram, a respiratory stimulant, is only used if non-invasive ventilation is unavailable or unsuccessful.

NICE Guidance [CG101], Chronic obstructive pulmonary disease in over 16s: diagnosis and management, 2010. http://guidance.nice.org.uk/CG101

77. D. $PaCO_2$ <6 kPa

When used for a period of at least 15 hours per day, LTOT results in improved survival in COPD patients. LTOT does not, however, influence decline in FEV1. Assessment for LTOT should be performed when the patient is clinically stable, i.e. free from exacerbation for at least four weeks, and ideally should be performed twice. $PaCO_2$ does not influence the prescription of LTOT for COPD although there is a small risk of worsening hypercapnia. Smoking is not an absolute contraindication to LTOT although the benefits are reduced in those who continue to smoke and there is a risk of fire. Palliative care is an indication for home oxygen.

Cranston JM et al., Domiciliary oxygen for chronic obstructive pulmonary disease, *Cochrane Database of Systematic Reviews* 2005(4):CD001744.

78. E. Spirometry with reversibility

The likely diagnosis is chronic obstructive pulmonary disease which is correctly diagnosed with results from 'post-bronchdilator' spirometry. The most effective therapeutic intervention is stopping smoking. Bronchodilator treatment is tailored to symptoms and the most effective intervention to improve symptoms is pulmonary rehabilitation. Assessment of exacerbation freqency is important in determining the role of combination inhalers (see NICE Guidance). In this situation a chest X-ray is of course mandatory to exclude underlying malignancy.

NICE Guidance [CG101], Chronic obstructive pulmonary disease in over 16s: diagnosis and management, 2010. http://guidance.nice.org.uk/CG101

79. D. *Pneumocystis jirovecii*

Renal transplant patients are routinely treated with co-trimoxazole for a period of six months post transplant as prophylaxis against *Pneumocyctis jiroveci* (previously termed *Pneumocystic carinii* and the name changed to honour Dr Otto Jirovec who first isolated the organism from humans). Characteristically, patients develop respiratory failure and the chest X-ray shows fluffy indistinct shadowing in the lung fields.

Warrell DA et al., *Oxford Textbook of Medicine*, Fifth Edition, Oxford University Press, 2010, Section 7.7.5, Pneumocystis jirovecii.

80. B. 2

The CURB score is a severity assessment for community acquired pneumonia. The core features are Confusion (new onset confusion with an AMTS?8), Urea?7 mmol/l, Respiratory rate?30/min and Blood pressure?90 mmHg systolic or?60 mmHg diastolic. If patients have two or more core features they are at high risk of death and should be managed in hospital as having severe community-acquired pneumonia. Age greater than 65 years is also a negative prognostic indicator and is included in the CURB-65 score. Hypoxaemia (PaO$_2$ <8 kPa), albumin?35 g/l, and WBC?4 or?20 x 10?/l predict a poor prognosis but are not included in the scoring assessment.

Lim WS et al., Defining community-acquired pneumonia severity on presentation to hospital: an international derivation and validation study, *Thorax* 2003;58(5):377–382.

81. C. Call for help early

The Resuscitation Council provide extremely good guidelines on adult life support (see further reading). On finding a collapsed patient the first thing you need to do is to assess the patient. Do they have a patent airway, are they breathing, and do they have a cardiac output? Cardiopulmonary resuscitation would only be indicated if there was no respiratory effort or cardiac output. A precordial thump is only advised if the patient is in a monitored bed and there is a witnessed VT/VF arrest and no crash trolley is close to hand; thus, it would be inappropriate in this situation. It is always advisable to call for help early, whether in the pre-hospital or hospital setting, as you are likely to need a competent team to help with the resuscitation which can take time to mobilize. The Resuscitation Council advises that in the adult patient, begin with chest compressions followed by rescue breaths at a rate of 30:2 (compressions:breaths). The next step in management would be to attach a defibrillator and assess the rhythm to determine whether or not a shock is indicated.

Resuscitation guidelines. http://www.resus.org.uk/pages/als.pdf

82. A. Idiopathic pulmonary fibrosis (IPF)

The idiopathic interstitial pneumonias (IIPs) are a group of diffuse parenchymal lung diseases of unknown aetiology with varying degrees of inflammation and fibrosis. IPF has the worst prognosis among the chronic IIPs. Both cellular and fibrotic variants of NSIP are recognized. Fibrotic NSIP appears to follow a similar course to IPF with a median survival of three years. The prognosis in chronic hypersensitivity pneumonitis also depends on whether or not fibrosis is present.

BTS/Thoracic Society of Australia and New Zealand/Irish Thoracic Society, Interstitial lung disease guidelines, *Thorax* 2008;63(Suppl V):v1–v58.

83. E. Home oxygen therapy

This man in all likelihood has idiopathic pulmonary fibrosis, as we are given no previous history which would be consistent with secondary pulmonary fibrosis. Trials of immune-modifying agents including corticosteroids and second-line agents have been universally disappointing in this area, and, as such, given that he has evidence of right heart failure and hypoxaemia, the intervention with the greatest evidence base is home oxygen therapy.

Chapman S et al., *Oxford Handbook of Respiratory Medicine*, Second Edition, Oxford University Press, 2009, Chapter 30, Idiopathic interstitial pneumonias.

84. B. Rheumatoid arthritis

There are multiple causes of upper lobe fibrosis, including prior TB infection, progressive massive fibrosis, previous radiotherapy, ankylosing spondylitis, and chronic extrinsic allergic alveolitis. Other disease processes favour a lower lobe distribution, including rheumatoid arthritis and connective tissue diseases, idiopathic pulmonary fibrosis, and drug-induced fibrotic lung disease. Pulmonary manifestations of rheumatoid arthritis include pleural thickening or an effusion, bronchiectasis, nodules, and fibrosis of either UIP or NSIP pattern.

Chapman S, Nakielny R, *Aids to Radiological Differential Diagnosis*, Fourth Edition, Saunders, 2003, Respiratory tract, p. 151.

85. E. Churg–Strauss syndrome

Worsening acute asthma and marked eosinophila are particularly suggestive of Churg–Strauss, and the history of joint pains and night sweats is further supportive of the diagnosis. ESR, pANCA, and serum IgE would also be helpful markers in confirming Churg–Strauss. Tissue diagnosis can be obtained from skin, lung, or kidney; standard therapy is with the combination of steroids and cyclophosphamide.

Pagnoux C, Guillevin L, Churg-Strauss syndrome: evidence for disease subtypes? *Current Opinion in Rheumatology* 2010;22(1):21–28.

86. D. Methaemoglobin level

This patient has symptoms and signs consistent with methaemoglobinaemia. Methaemoglobin is formed by oxidation of Fe^{2+} to Fe^{3+} thus preventing O_2 carriage. Methaemoglobinaemia is due either to inherited deficiencies of enzymes (cytochrome b5 reductase) that reduce Fe^{3+} to Fe^{2+}, or more commonly due to antioxidant stress from toxic agents (e.g. local anaesthetics (benzocaine), nitrates, nitrites (in 'poppers'), chloroquine, dapsone) that overwhelm this reversal mechanism. Methaemoglobin is slightly left-shifted on the oxygen dissociation curve. Symptoms typically occur with a methaemoglobin level >40%. The typical grey/blue colour of the patient is often mistaken for cyanosis. It would be appropriate to check the methaemoglobin level and treat it.

Chapman S et al., *Oxford Handbook of Respiratory Medicine*, Second Edition, Oxford University Press, 2009, Chapter 48, Toxic agents, Carbon monoxide poisoning.

87. B. Administer intravenous methylene blue

Clinical cyanosis in the presence of normal arterial oxygen tensions is highly suggestive of methaemoglobinemia. Normal methaemoglobin concentrations are 1% (range 0–3%). At concentrations of 3–15%, slight grey-blue discolouration of the skin may be present. At concentrations of 15–20%, patients are typically asymptomatic with detectable cyanosis. In an asymptomatic patient with a methaemoglobin level <20%, no therapy other than cessation of the causative agent may be required (e.g. chloroquine, dapsone, nitrates, nitrites, nitroglycerin, nitroprusside, phenacetin, primaquine, quinones, and sulphonamides). If the patient is symptomatic, or has a methaemoglobin level >20%, therapy with supplemental oxygen and methylene blue is indicated. Hyperbaric oxygen therapy or packed RBC exchange transfusions are alternative therapies for patients who are not candidates for methylene blue (i.e. those with G6PD deficiency, in whom it may precipitate haemolysis).

Chapman S et al., *Oxford Handbook of Respiratory Medicine*, Second Edition, Oxford University Press, 2009, Chapter 48, Toxic agents, Carbon monoxide poisoning.

88. B. FEV1 1.0 l

The correct answer for this is FEV1 1.0 l. An FEV1 <1.5 l is a contraindication to surgery. The nature of the pleural effusion (a transudate or an exudate) is not specified. A malignant pleural effusion would be an absolute contraindication to surgery. Hyponatraemia may suggest SIADH, but would be an absolute contraindication to surgery. Hypercalcaemia may suggest metastatic spread, but the staging CT does not mention this and therefore the most likely cause of the hypercalcaemia is due to the aetiology of the lung carcinoma (squamous cell carcinomas are associated with parathyroid-like hormone production). Smoking and carcinoma of the lung are closely associated. A pre-operative assessment needs to take place, and although smoking history is not an absolute contraindication to surgery, it may be associated with conditions which increase anaesthetic risk.

British Thoracic Society and Society of Cardiothoracic Surgeons of Great Britain and Ireland Working Party, Guidelines on the selection of patients with lung cancer for surgery, *Thorax* 2001;56:89–108. http://www.mccn.nhs.uk/userfiles/documents/BTS%20lungcancersurgery.pdf

89. C. Adrenal metastases

The biggest hint here is the history of weight loss, cough, and symptoms consistent with COPD. Coupled with the smoking history, the low blood pressure, low sodium, and raised potassium, this is highly suggestive of adrenal failure due to metastases from bronchial carcinoma. Clearly, a chest X-ray is important in the patient's work-up, as is steroid replacement, pending imaging of the adrenals and short synacthen testing.

Harvey AM et al., Clinical detection and treatment of adrenal disease, In: Hunt JL and Cagle PT (eds), *Molecular Pathology of Endocrine Diseases*, Springer, Molecular Pathology Library 2010;3(5):197–203.

90. C. Fluorodeoxyglucose positron emission tomography (FDG-PET) scanning should form part of the routine staging investigation of patients with potentially operable non-small cell lung cancer (NSCLC)

World-wide, lung cancer is the most common cause of death from malignancy. Small cell lung cancers account for only around 15% of lung cancer diagnoses. The majority of lung cancers are classified as non small cell lung cancer—approximately 40% of which are adenocarcinomas and 25% of which are squamous cell carcinomas. The remainder comprise less common pathologies including mixed carcinomas (adenosquamous or mixed small cell and non small cell cancers) and neuroendocrine tumours. Up to 90% of lung cancers are due to smoking. However at least 10% occur in patients (particularly women) who have never smoked. Other environmental factors implicated in the aetiology of lung cancer include asbestos exposure, radon, previous thoracic radiotherapy, and pulmonary fibrosis. Complete surgical resection offers patients with early stage (I–II) NSCLC the optimal chance of a cure. Careful pre-operative investigations must be completed to ensure that staging is as complete as possible. This should include clinical examination, bronchoscopy, and CT of the chest and abdomen. However FDG-PET has greater sensitivity and specificity than CT and it is now recommended, under NICE guidelines, for patients who are candidates for surgery or radical radiotherapy on CT, to look for intrathoracic lymph nodes and distant metastases. Integrated PET-CT has been shown to improve the accuracy of staging still further. The majority of lung cancer patients present with advanced disease. Optimal management requires a multi-disciplinary approach with close involvement of an oncologist. Although many patients presenting with SCLC will be poly-symptomatic and of poor performance status at diagnosis, this is a chemo-responsive tumour and the majority of patients will benefit from systemic treatment with chemotherapy. Untreated, median survival for patients with extensive-stage SCLC is only six weeks. Objective response rates to chemotherapy are in the region of 80%, with a greater percentage gaining symptomatic benefit. Chemotherapy can increase survival to 8–12 months. Median survival for patients with advanced NSCLC (IIIb–IV) is around 9–12 months without systemic treatment. Chemotherapy for patients of good performance status with metastatic NSCLC has been shown to improve quality of life and offers symptomatic benefit in >50% of patients, although absolute survival benefit may be small (6–8 weeks). Newer, targeted therapies, such as the oral tyrosine kinase inhibitors (e.g. erlotinib) may also be of benefit in selected patients.

Cassidy J et al., *Oxford Handbook of Oncology*, Third Edition, Oxford University Press, 2010, Chapter 14, Thoracic cancer.

91. D. Bronchial carcinoid

The age at diagnosis, and profile of recurrent pneumonia, wheeze, and haemoptysis over the past few months, fits best with bronchial carcinoid as the most likely diagnosis. Whether to biopsy carcinoid lesions or not is the subject of some debate because of the risk of bleeding after biopsy. The majority of patients with bronchial carcinoid should be considered for surgical excision if possible. Similar to GI carcinoid, bronchial carcinoid does respond to octreotide.

Chapman S et al., *Oxford Handbook of Respiratory Medicine*, Third Edition, Oxford University Press, 2014, Chapter 31, Lung cancer.

92. C. Stage 2

This patient has features of sarcoidosis. The disease can occur in all groups, but is more common in people of Afro-Caribbean backgrounds and more severe than in other groups. Bilateral hilar lymphadenopathy is a common radiological feature, but is not always present on a plain chest radiograph and a high-resolution CT chest scan may be required to gain further information. Tuberculosis should be included in the differential diagnosis.

The mnemonic 'MOXIES' can be used to remember the causes of bilateral hilar lymphadenopathy:

Malignancy: haematological (lymphoma),
Occupational lung disease: Berylloisis, silicosis,
X: Histocytosis X,
Infection: Tuberculosis,
Extrinsic allergic alveolitis,
Sarcoidosis.

The features are more in keeping with sarcoidosis, but a Mantoux test should be considered regarding tuberculosis. Box 4.1 describes the different staging of sarcoidosis according to chest radiograph changes.

Chapman S et al., *Oxford Handbook of Respiratory Medicine*, Third Edition, Oxford University Press, 2014, Chapter 45, Sarcoidosis.

Box 4.1 Radiological changes according to stage	
Stage	**Radiological changes**
0	None
1	Bilateral hilar lymphadenopathy
2	Bilateral hilar lymphadenopathy and peripheral pulmonary infiltrates
3	Bilateral peripheral pulmonary infiltrates only
4	Bullous and cystic changes
	Progressive pulmonary fibrosis
	Involvement of pleura

93. A. IV magnesium

This patient has severe asthma and is hypoxic despite 60% O_2. In this situation BTS/SIGN guidelines support the use of IV magnesium given at a dose of 1.2–2 g over 20 minutes. Aminophylline is less favoured in the treatment of acute asthma because of unfavourable benefit risk (limited efficacy and risk of arrhythmia) versus other therapies. Intravenous salbutamol and nebulized terbutaline are likely to provide little incremental benefit versus the back-to-back nebulizers already given, and IV hydrocortisone will take a few hours to impact on her peak flow. She should, of course, also be reviewed at this stage by the on-call ITU personnel.

BTS/SIGN asthma guidelines. http://www.sign.ac.uk/pdf/qrg101.pdf

94. B. Interferon gamma release

Until recently, the only test available to identify latent tuberculosis was the Mantoux skin test, which is limited by a high negative rate in immunocompromised patients and a high positive rate in patients with prior BCG vaccination. The interferon gamma test uses whole blood and three tuberculous antigens: ESAT-6, CFP-10, and TB7.7. The test is positive if the rise in interferon gamma in response to TB antigen exposure for whole blood is greater than the test cut-off. A negative control is also used. The test is not affected by previous BCG vaccination. A chest X-ray would be the next step in evaluation if the interferon gamma test were positive (latent versus active pulmonary tuberculosis). This approach satisfies the spirit of the recent NICE guidelines on tuberculosis which state: 'recent arrivals from high incidence countries aged 16–34 years old may be screened with inteferon gamma testing'.

Chapman S et al., *Oxford Handbook of Respiratory Medicine*, Third Edition. Oxford University Press, 2014, Chapter 42, Respiratory Infection, mycobacterial.

95. D. Bosentan

Trial of a calcium channel antagonist in primary pulmonary hypertension hinges on acute vasoreactivity testing. If it is positive, then a trial of calcium antagonist is reasonable. If it is negative, then treatment with either an endothelin receptor antagonist, such as bosentan, or a PDE5 inhibitor such as sildenafil is more usual. Combination therapy is often warranted with respect to gaining symptom control.

Chapman S et al., *Oxford Handbook of Respiratory Medicine*, Third Edition, Oxford University Press, 2014, Chapter 38, Pulmonary hypertension.

96. B. Liver transplantation

This patient's presentation is consistent with hepatopulmonary syndrome which is the triad of: chronic liver disease and portal hypertension; abnormal intrapulmonary vasodilatation with decreased pulmonary vascular resistance and subsequent ventilation–perfusion abnormalities (right to left shunt); arterial hypoxia. Patients often demonstrate platypnoea (worsening dyspnoea on sitting from supine) and orthodexia (a drop in saturation/pO_2 on sitting from supine). The condition is poorly responsive to oxygen replacement, which fits with the clinical picture seen here. TIPs is ineffective, as is diuresis. The only treatment known to be effective is liver transplant. Contrast-enhanced ECHO and pulmonary technetium scanning can be helpful in confirming pulmonary shunting.

Chapman S et al., *Oxford Handbook of Respiratory Medicine*, Third Edition, Oxford University Press, 2014, Chapter 27, Gastrointestinal disease and the lung.

97. A. Physiotherapy

The key components of management of bronchiectasis are:

1. Treatment of any underlying medical condition.

2. Prevention of exacerbations and progression of underlying disease by physiotherapy.

   Options for airway clearance include postural or autogenic drainage, active cycle of breathing technique (breathing control with forced expiration 'huffing' using variable thoracic expansion), cough augmentation (using flutter valves/cough insufflator/high-frequency oscillation), and exercise regimes (important to prevent general deconditioning). The physiotherapist is also vital during admission for exacerbations to help clear tenacious sputum. Nebulized hypertonic saline may improve airway clearance, although there is no RCT data to support its use.

3. Reduction of bacterial load and prevention of secondary airway inflammation and damage, with antimicrobial chemotherapy.

4. Supportive treatment—treatment of associated airflow obstruction.

5. Optimize nutrition.

6. Refer for surgery if necessary—localized resection of affected area.

7. Refer for transplantation if indicated, (although in this case it is clearly not indicated).

Chapman S et al., *Oxford Handbook of Respiratory Medicine*, Third Edition, Oxford University Press, 2014, Chapter 19, Bronchiectasis.

98. A. Age 66

The CURB-65 score is used to stratify risk in patients presenting with community-acquired pneumonia. The components of the score are: (1) New onset confusion (abbreviated mental test ≤8). (2) Urea >7mmol/L. 3) Respiratory rate ≥30/min. (4) BP <90/60mmHg). (5) Age ≥65. The score is used to guide management. Total score 0–1 (low severity): home treatment if possible; total score 2 (moderate severity): hospital therapy; total score ≥3 (high severity): consider high-dependency care. Other features increasing the risk of death are co-existing disease, bilateral/multilobar involvement, PaO_2 <8kPa or SaO2<92%.

Longmore M et al., *Oxford Handbook of Clinical Medicine*, Eighth Edition, Oxford University Press, 2010, Chapter 7, Renal medicine, Inherited kidney diseases.

99. B. Pulmonary Capillary Wedge pressure 16mmHg

One consensus on diagnosis of ARDS requires these 4 criteria to exist: (1) Acute onset. (2) CXR:bilateral infiltrates. (3) Pulmonary capillary wedge pressure (pcwp) <18mmHg or a lack of clinical congestive heart failure. (4) Refractory hypoxaemia with PaO_2:FiO_2 <200 for ARDS (<300 for acute lung injury). Others include total thoracic compliance <30mL/cm H_2O. Early ITU assessment and supportive intervention are crucial with respect to outcome.

Longmore M et al., *Oxford Handbook of Clinical Medicine*, Eighth Edition, Oxford University Press, 2010, Chapter 7, Renal medicine, Inherited kidney diseases.

100. C. Inhaled salmeterol/high-dose fluticasone

NICE guidelines on the management of COPD recommend regular inhaled corticosteroids and long-acting beta agonist for COPD with an FEV1<50%. When treating stable COPD, general measures are to stop smoking, encourage exercise, treat poor nutrition or obesity, offer influenza and pneumococcal vaccination, pulmonary rehabilitation/palliative care, and NIPPV. In mild disease, treat with inhaled antimuscarinic (ipratropium) or β-2 agonist (salbutamol) prn. In moderate disease, treat with regular long-acting antimuscarinic (e.g. tiotropium) or long-acting inhaled β-2 agonist (e.g. salmeterol). Add inhaled corticosteroids (e.g. beclometasone) if FEV1 <50% and é2 exacerbations/year (Note Seretide® combines salmeterol and fluticasone; Symbicort® combines formoterol and budesonide). Oral theophylline also has a role. In severe disease, refer to a specialist and consider steroid trial and home nebulizers. If there is evidence of pulmonary hypertension assess the need for LTOT and treat oedema with diuretics.

NICE guidelines [CG101]. Chronic obstructive pulmonary disease in over 16s: diagnosis and management, 2010. http://publications.nice.org.uk/chronic-obstructive-pulmonary-disease-cg101

101. D. Male sex

Male sex, increasing height, and smoking all increase the risk of a pneumothorax. Pneumothoraces are around three times more common in men than in women. This man is relatively short; it is increasing height that increases the risk of pneumothorax. There is no evidence that physical activity increases the risk of developing a pneumothorax. Underlying lung disease increases the risk of having a pneumothorax, but there is no evidence to suggest hayfever does.

BTS guidelines. http://www.brit-thoracic.org.uk/

102. C. Proceed to small-bore chest drain

This patient should not be discharged without further active intervention in view of the size of his pneumothorax (>2cm is significant) and the fact that he remains breathless. You should not repeat needle aspiration unless there were technical difficulties during the first attempt. You should therefore progress to small-bore chest drain insertion following a failed needle aspiration.

MacDuff A et al., Management of spontaneous pneumothorax: British Thoracic Society pleural disease guideline 2010, *Thorax* 2010;65(Suppl 2):ii18–ii31.

103. A. Aspiration

In primary spontaneous pneumothorax, treatment with needle aspiration (using a 16–18 gauge needle) is as effective as chest drain insertion. It may also be associated with a reduced rate of hospital admission and length of stay. You should not aspirate more than 2.5 litres of air, as further re-expansion is unlikely. If there is a persistent pneumothorax >2cm or breathlessness, then you should insert a small-bore chest drain. Initial conservative management is not a good option here because the patient is breathless and has a 3cm-sized pneumothorax (>2cm is considered large).

Ayed AK et al., Aspiration versus tube drainage in primary spontaneous pneumothorax: a randomized study. *European Respiratory Journal* 2006;27(3):477–482.

104. A. Chest X-ray

There is little controlled trial evidence around the diagnosis of PE in pregnancy, so most clinical practice is based around guidelines. These recommend a chest X-ray as the first radiological investigation where clinical suspicion of PE is high, followed by VQ scan where available, then CTPA if VQ is not available or the result is equivocal. In practice in most NHS hospitals CTPA is easier to obtain out of hours versus a VQ scan. Given that warfarin is contraindicated early on and again later in pregnancy, the majority of patients are managed with daily low molecular weight heparin through out the pregnancy.

Leung AN et al., An official American Thoracic Society/Society of Thoracic Radiology clinical practice guideline: evaluation of suspected pulmonary embolism in pregnancy, *American Journal of Respiratory and Critical Care Medicine* 2011 Nov 15;184(10):1200–1208. doi: 10.1164/rccm.201108-1575ST.

105. B. Bisoprolol

The debate in this situation is whether introduction of a beta-blocker will impact significantly on the patient's lung function, as study evidence shows that use of agents such as bisoprolol or carvedilol impacts positively on prognosis in patients with LV dysfunction and a history of ischaemic heart disease. One study looked at use of bisoprolol in patients with COPD, and it showed that any impact on lung function in this situation is likely to be clinically insignificant versus the benefit on cardiac outcomes. Whilst all of the other options are reasonable alternatives for the treatment of angina, only bisoprolol has been shown to have outcome benefits.

Mainguy V et al., Effect of bisoprolol on respiratory function and exercise capacity in chronic obstructive pulmonary disease. *American Journal of Cardiology* 2012 Jul 15;110(2):258–263. doi: 10.1016/j.amjcard.2012.03.019. Epub 2012 Apr 10.

106. D. Long-acting muscarinic antagonist

Aclidinium bromide is a competitive, selective muscarinic receptor antagonist, with a longer residence time at the M3 receptors than the M2 receptors. M3 receptors mediate contraction of airway smooth muscle. Inhaled aclidinium bromide acts locally in the lungs to antagonize M3 receptors of airway smooth muscle and induce bronchodilation. Aclidinium bromide is quickly broken down in plasma; the level of systemic anticholinergic side effects is therefore low. The other treatment strategy employed in the management of COPD is high-dose inhaled corticosteroids, combined with long-acting beta agonist therapy, such as seretide.

emc+, Aclidinium bromide: pharmacodynamic properties. http://www.medicines.org.uk/emc/medicine/27001/SPC#PHARMACODYNAMIC_PROPS

107. B. Seretide

When the FEV1 is less than 50% of predicted, GOLD guidelines recommend beginning therapy with either a long-acting beta agonist (LABA) and inhaled corticosteroid (ICS) in a combination inhaler, or a long-acting muscarininc antagonist (LAMA). As such, seretide is the only possible correct answer from the options given. Studies suggest there is little benefit to be gained in COPD from low-dose inhaled corticosteroids, and short-acting muscarinic antagonists/short-acting beta agonists drive symptomatic improvement only and are not disease modifying. In patients who remain breathless on seretide therapy, a long-acting muscarinic antagonist should be offered.

NICE Guidance [CG101], Chronic obstructive pulmonary disease in over 16s: diagnosis and management, 2010. http://publications.nice.org.uk/chronic-obstructive-pulmonary-disease-cg101/key-priorities-for-implementation

1. **A 35-year-old woman presents with a painful swollen left knee and difficulty in walking for the last three days. She was treated for a sexually transmitted infection two months ago with complete resolution of symptoms. She rarely drinks alcohol and there is no significant past or family history. On examination she has a temperature of 36.1°C. There is a right knee effusion. Knee flexion is painful and restricted to 90°. What is the most likely diagnosis?**
    A. Acute gout
    B. Gonococcal arthritis
    C. Pseudogout
    D. Psoriatic arthritis
    E. Reactive arthritis

2. **You are seeing a 20-year-old man in a rheumatology clinic with recurrent attacks of gout. He comes in with his parents who report that he has mild learning difficulties and as a child he used to harm himself. He is found to be hyperuricaemic. Which of the following conditions is he likely to have?**
    A. X-linked HPRT deficiency (Lesch–Nyhan)
    B. Von Hippel–Lindau
    C. Lambert–Eaton syndrome
    D. Prader–Willi syndrome
    E. Reye's syndrome

3. A 34-year-old woman presents to the clinic with chronic pain. She has had pain over many points on her axial skeleton for up to six months, feels chronically tired, and has had to take long-term sick leave from her job. On examination she has pain on 14 different points widely spread across her skeleton. Her BMI is 23. Investigations: Hb 13.1, WCC 7.2, PLT 203, Na 137, K 4.3, Cr 102, ESR 12. Which of the following is the most likely diagnosis?
    A. Seronegative arthritis
    B. Rheumatoid arthritis
    C. Osteoarthritis
    D. Fibromyalgia
    E. Chondrocalcinosis

4. **Anti-cyclic citrullinated peptide (anti-CCP) antibody is an important marker for the diagnosis of rheumatoid arthritis (RA). Which of the following statements is?**
    A. It has almost 100% sensitivity in early disease
    B. Levels fluctuate with disease activity
    C. Anti-CCP antibodies unlike the RF (rheumatoid factor) have no prognostic value
    D. Higher sensitivity in Sjögren's syndrome than RF
    E. In rheumatoid arthritis it is more specific than the RF

5. A 42-year-old man presents with pain affecting the small joints of his hands and feet, wrists and elbows. He has also had particular problems with stiffness in the morning and found it very difficult to hold down his job as an accountant because of difficulties typing. On examination his BP is 142/72, pulse is 73 and regular. Cardiovascular, respiratory, and abdominal examinations are unremarkable. Musculoskeletal examination reveals evidence of active synovitis. Which of the following is associated with the poorest prognosis?
    A. Rheumatoid factor antibodies
    B. Anti-CCP antibodies
    C. Male sex
    D. Age <50 at onset
    E. Speed of onset

6. A 72-year-old woman is referred to the emergency unit with severe unilateral (left-sided) headache. She described no eye symptoms or visual signs. The left temporal artery is tender to palpitation. Pulse is 60 bpm and the blood pressure 160/85 mmHg. The ESR is at 90 mm/h. What is your next immediate action?
    A. Obtain temporal artery biopsy before any treatment is started
    B. Prescribe prednisolone at 40 mg orally
    C. Request radiographs of the left temporomandibular joint
    D. Give intravenous methylprednisolone
    E. Arrange an urgent CT scan of the brain

7. **A young man presents with back pain, and has been diagnosed with ankylosing spondylitis. Which of the following is not associated with this condition?**
    A. Aortic regurgitation
    B. Enthesitis
    C. Lung fibrosis
    D. Retinitis
    E. HLA B27

8. **A 55-year-old woman on long-term prednisolone has a dual X-ray energy absorptiometry (DXA) with a T-score of minus 1.0. What is the most appropriate course of action? Select the single most appropriate response:**
    A. Commence alendronic acid 70 mg weekly
    B. Arrange DXA scanning
    C. Recommend lifestyle measures and calcium and vitamin D. supplementation
    D. Prescribe calcium and vitamin D. supplementation (e.g. Adcal D3)
    E. No action required

9. **A 64-year-old woman with a history of rheumatoid arthritis has failed to respond to a number of second-line agents to control her disease activity. She comes to the clinic complaining of continued pain in the small joints of her hands, her feet, wrists, and knees. Her ESR is elevated at 45, consistent with continued disease activity. You decide to commence etanercept. Which of the following scenarios would prompt caution with respect to its use?**
    A. Iron deficiency anaemia
    B. Concomitant methotrexate
    C. Concomitant sulphasalazine
    D. History of psoriasis
    E. History of inflammatory bowel disease

10. **A 27-year-old woman is being investigated for possible antiphospholipid syndrome. Which of the following blood test results is not associated with this syndrome?**
    A. Lupus anticoagulant positive
    B. Thrombocytopaenia
    C. Positive antibodies to beta-2 glycoprotein-1
    D. Antibodies to voltage-gated potassium channels
    E. Lymphopaenia

11. **A 25-year-old woman is referred to you with a photosensitive malar rash, oral ulcers, and joint pain. You think she may have systemic lupus erythematosus (SLE) and carry out some immunological tests. Which of the following antibodies, if they came back positive, would NOT increase your confidence in the diagnosis of SLE?**

    A. Antinuclear antibodies (ANA)
    B. Anti-Smith antibody
    C. Anti-cardiolipin antibody
    D. Anti-proteinase 3 antibody (c-ANCA)
    E Anti double-stranded DNA antibody

12. **A patient presents with symptoms suggestive of Reynaud's phenomenon, and on further questioning you suspect she may have systemic sclerosis. What feature of this condition is used to differentiate the limited form of this disease from the diffuse?**

    A. If any symptoms other than the 'CREST' symptoms (calcinosis, Raynaud's, oesophageal dysmotility, sclerodactyly, telangiectasia) are present, it is classified as diffuse disease
    B. If it extends above the knees or elbows, or below the neck, it is classified as diffuse disease
    C. If any organ apart from the skin is affected, it is classified as diffuse disease
    D. The presence of lung disease makes it classified as diffuse disease
    E. The presence of renal disease makes it classified as diffuse disease

13. **In clinic, you see a 45-year-old woman with severe rheumatoid arthritis. You are considering treatment with an anti-TNF such as infliximab. Which of these statements most closely reflects the NICE guidelines for its use?**

    A. Treatment has failed with two disease-modifying agents including methotrexate
    B. It should be the first treatment given after diagnosis to prevent joint damage
    C. Severe disease at onset i.e. disease activity score (DAS 28) greater than 5.1
    D. More than five joints involved at the time of treatment initiation
    E. NICE does not recommend its use in rheumatoid arthritis

14. **You are looking after a patient with a flare of her rheumatoid arthritis, and treating her with intravenous rituximab. What is the mechanism of action of this drug?**

    A. Suppression of T and B cells
    B. Suppression of T cells
    C. Suppression of B cells
    D. Inhibition of macrophage degranulation
    E. Inhibition of macrophage migration

15. **You are looking after a patient with Sjögren's syndrome, who is positive for anti-Ro antibody. She is 15 weeks into her first pregnancy. What complication in the foetus/neonate should you be aware of that is associated with this antibody?**
    A. Foetal cardiac valve defects
    B. Foetal renal dysgenesis
    C. Foetal limb malformations
    D. Foetal heart block
    E. Neonatal hypoglycaemia

16. **Which one of the following medications has been shown to accelerate bone loss/osteoporosis in some patients?**
    A. Atypical antipsychotics (such as olanzapine)
    B. Non-dihydropyridine calcium channel antagonists (verapamil, diltiazem)
    C. Phenytoin
    D. Beta-blockers
    E. NSAIDs

17. **A 42-year-old woman presents with a three-week history of painful, stiff, swollen right knee. In the last month, there were two episodes of swelling involving the entire left index finger. These lasted for 5–7 days and resolved completely. She has had psoriasis on her scalp for the last year. On examination, there is right knee effusion and a mildly tender, swollen distal inter-phalangeal joint on the right side. What is the next step in her long-term management?**
    A. Diclofenac
    B. Etanercept
    C. Methotrexate
    D. Intra-articular corticosteroid
    E. Oral corticosteroid

18. **A 54-year-old man comes to the clinic complaining of acute pain and swelling over the first MTP joint which has come on acutely over the past 24 hours. He has hypertension for which he is prescribed ramipril and indapamide and his BP in the clinic is 145/82. There is redness and swelling over the first MTP consistent with gout. His creatinine is 129 micromol/l and his urate is 0.55 mmol/l (2.5–6.7). Which of the following is the most appropriate treatment for him?**
    A. Prednisolone
    B. Diclofenac
    C. Colchicine
    D. Rasburicase
    E. Allopurinol

19. **Which of the following T-score results from dual X-ray energy absorptiometry (DXA) scanning falls into the category of osteopaenia?**

A. −0.9

B. −2.5

C. −2

D. 1

E. −1.7

20. **A 49-year-old woman complains that she is having increasing problems getting up out of a low chair and climbing the stairs. She also has a lot of pain over her thighs and the upper part of her shoulders. There is shortness of breath on fairly minimal exercise and on lying flat in bed. On examination she is obese with signs of interstitial lung disease. CK is elevated at 650, ESR is elevated at 62, and anti-Jo1 antibodies are positive. What diagnosis fits best with this picture?**

A. Polymyositis

B. Dermatomyositis

C. Polymyalgia rheumatica

D. Cushing's disease

E. Temporal arteritis

21. **A 45-year-old woman has recently been diagnosed with TB, and has started a variety of new medications. She now presents with joint pains and a rash in a 'butterfly' distribution. She has positive ANA with anti-histone antibody positive. Which of her following medications is likely to be the culprit?**

A. Rifampicin

B. Isoniazid

C. Pyrazinamide

D. Ethambutol

E. Pyridoxine

22. **A 44-year-old woman presents with a two-week history of a painful, stiff, swollen right knee. In the last month, there were two episodes of swelling involving the entire left index finger. These lasted for 5–7 days and resolved completely. Her younger sister suffers from psoriasis. On examination, there is right knee effusion and a mildly tender, swollen distal inter-phalangeal joint on the right side. You notice evidence of nail pitting. What is the diagnosis?**

A. Acute gout

B. Acute rheumatic fever

C. Psoriatic arthritis

D. Reactive arthritis

E. Rheumatoid arthritis

23. A 32-year-old woman is referred to the clinic for recurrent miscarriage. She has suffered three miscarriages over the past four years. Other past history of note includes a deep vein thrombosis which occured after a flight from Australia. On examination her BP is 135/80, her pulse is 72 and regular. She has a skin rash consistent with livedo reticularis. Which of the following is the most likely diagnosis?

A. Anti-phospholipid antibody syndrome
B. SLE
C. Mixed connective tissue disease
D. Rheumatoid arthritis
E. Systemic sclerosis

24. A 35-year-old woman presents with a painful swollen left knee and difficulty in walking for the last three days. She was treated for a sexually transmitted infection two months ago with complete resolution of symptoms. She rarely drinks alcohol and there is no significant past or family history. On examination she has a temperature of 36.1°C. There is a right knee effusion. Knee flexion is painful and restricted to 90°. Which of the following is the most appropriate investigation for this patient?

A. Aspirate right knee, send synovial fluid for culture and microscopy
B. High vaginal swab
C. HLA-B27
D. Urine microscopy and culture
E. X-ray knee

25. A 22-year-old woman has been on minocycline for the last three months for resistant acne. Over the last two weeks she has developed arthralgia in her hands, puffy and swollen knuckles, fatigue, myalgia, fevers, and Raynaud's phenomenon. There are oral ulcers, and widespread papular erythematous rash. Recent blood tests are as follows: Hb 12.1 g/dl, WBC 9 x 10³/microlitre, neutrophils 87%, eosinophils <1%, platelets 176 x 10³/microlitre, ESR 46 mm/h, urea, electrolytes and creatinine: normal, CK 120 IU/ml, alkaline phosphatase 135 IU/ml, ALT 80 IU/ml, AST 95 IU/ml, bilirubin 47 mmol/ml, gamma GT 215 IU/ml, CRP 31 mg/l, anti-nuclear antibody positive 1:6400 (homogeneous pattern), anti-dsDNA antibody negative, anti-ssDNA antibody positive, anti-histone antibody positive, anti-Ro antibody negative, anti-La antibody negative. What is the diagnosis?

A. Behçet's disease
B. Discoid lupus erythematosus
C. Drug-induced systemic lupus
D. Drug hypersensitivity
E. Systemic lupus erythematosus

26. **A 69-year-old woman tripped and fell while walking her dog. She has a long history of rheumatoid arthritis, which is well controlled on sulfasalazine (2 g/day). A DEXA scan report is as follows: bone mineral density (BMD) at femoral neck: T score –3.5, Z score +0.3; bone mineral density (BMD) at lumbar spine: T score –2.0, Z score +0.5. What is the diagnosis?**
    A. Osteopenia
    B. Osteoporosis
    C. Osteopetrosis
    D. Pathological fracture
    E. None of the above

27. **A 60-year-old woman has knee pain due to knee osteoarthritis. She is currently on co-codamol, ibuprofen gel, and takes occasional naproxen tablets for pain relief. She has recently seen a physiotherapist, and is doing all her knee exercises. Her body weight is normal. Which of the following interventions as recommended by the NICE guidelines should be the next step for treatment of her knee pain?**
    A. Acupuncture
    B. Chondroitin
    C. Glucosamine
    D. Intra-articular hyaluronic acid injections
    E. Transcutaneous electrical nerve stimulation

28. **A 45-year-old woman with limited cutaneous systemic sclerosis has developed a gradually worsening cough and shortness of breath. On examination, the pulse is 90/min, BP 120/80 mmHg, and respiratory rate is 22/min. There is no oedema, and the JVP is normal. On auscultation, S1 is normal, S2 is loud. There is a faint pansystolic murmur at the left sternal edge. The examination of the respiratory system is normal. A chest X-ray is normal, and the ECG shows tall R waves in V1–V4. What is the likely diagnosis?**
    A. Interstitial lung disease
    B. Pericardial effusion
    C. Pulmonary arterial hypertension
    D. Pulmonary embolism
    E. Pulmonary venous hypertension

29. **A 70-year-old man presents to his GP with left-sided headache, and jaw pain on eating for one week. On examination he has tender left temporal artery pulsations. Here are the results of his blood tests: Hb 12.1 g/dl, WBC 8x10³/microlitre, neutrophils 80%, platelets 290x10³/microlitre, ESR 100 mm/h, urea, electrolytes and creatinine normal, alkaline phosphatase 235 IU/ml, ALT 40 IU/ml, AST 35 IU/ml, bilirubin 17 mmol/ml, gamma GT 85 IU/ml, calcium 2.4 g/dl, albumin 42 g/l, CRP 75 mg/l. What is the most likely diagnosis?**

    A. Giant cell arteritis
    B. Microscopic polyangitis
    C. Polymyalgia rheumatica
    D. Takayasu's arteritis
    E. Wagener's granulomatosis

30. **A 36-year-old Caucasian housewife with sero-positive rheumatoid arthritis presents with a one-week history of fever, malaise, dry cough, and exertional breathlessness. She was commenced on methotrexate and folic acid three months ago. She is currently on methotrexate (25 mg/week) and folic acid (5 mg/week). A full blood count, liver and kidney function tests are normal. Chest X-ray reveals both peripheral airspace and interstitial shadowing at the right lower lobe. After 48 hours of intravenous augmentin and oral clarithromycin there is no improvement in her symptoms. What is the likely diagnosis?**

    A. Atypical pneumonia
    B. Fibrosing alveolitis
    C. Methotrexate pneumonitis
    D. Pneumocystis jiroveci pneumonia
    E. Tuberculosis

31. **A 62-year-old man presents with left knee pain, redness, and swelling for three days. In the last year, he has had four episodes of pain, redness, and swelling affecting the first metatarso phalangeal joint. These resolved with ibuprofen (400 mg t.d.s.). A knee aspirate was performed, and the synovial fluid shows negatively birefringent crystals on polarized light microscopy. The serum urate is 440 micromol/l. The left knee was injected with corticosteroids to control the acute attack. Which of the following drugs should he be started on, 1–2 weeks after the acute attack has resolved?**

    A. Allopurinol
    B. Allopurinol and colchicine
    C. Colchicine
    D. Febuxostat and colchicine
    E. Febuxostat

32. A 34-year-old woman with a ten-year history of Raynaud's phenomenon has developed tight, thick skin over her hands and forearm. She has also noticed difficulty in opening her mouth, and has developed facial telangiectasias. Recent blood tests are as follows: Hb 12.1 g/dl, WBC 8x10³/microlitre, neutrophils 80%, platelet 190x10³/microlitre, ESR 20 mm/h, urea, electrolytes, and creatinine normal, CRP <5 mg/l, anti-nuclear antibody positive 1:6400, anti-centromere antibody positive. What is the diagnosis?

    A. Diffuse cutaneous systemic sclerosis
    B. Limited cutaneous systemic sclerosis
    C. Mixed connective tissue disease
    D. Sjögren's syndrome
    E. Systemic lupus erythematosus

33. A 30-year-old housewife presents with an eight-hour history of sudden onset weakness of the left arm, left leg, and left lower facial muscles. On examination, the power is 4/5, the left plantar is upgoing, and there is no sensory loss. She is a non-smoker, and has no significant past or family history. The results of her investigations show thrombocytopenia (platelet count 100x10³/microlitre), normal inflammatory markers (ESR 10 mm/h, CRP <5 mg/dl), normal INR, and prolonged APTT (42 seconds (normal 24–38 seconds)). An ECG is normal, CT head shows a small hypodense area in the right internal capsule area. Anti-cardiolipin antibodies and lupus anticoagulant are positive. What is the next step in her management?

    A. Aspirin (75 mg/day)
    B. Corticosteroids
    C. Cyclophosphamide
    D. Plasma exchange
    E. Warfarin

34. A 30-year-old housewife presents with an eight-hour history of sudden onset weakness of the left arm, left leg, and left lower facial muscles. On examination, the power is 4/5, the left plantar is upgoing, and there is no sensory loss. She is a non-smoker, and has no significant past or family history. The results of her investigations are as follows: Hb 13.1 g/dl, WBC 9 x10³/microlitre, neutrophils 85%, platelets 100x10³/microlitre, blood film: thrombocytopenia, no schistocytes, ESR 10 mm/h, INR 1.0, aPTT 42 seconds (normal 24–38 seconds), urea, electrolytes, and creatinine normal, CRP <5 mg/l, ECG normal sinus rhythm. CT head shows a small hypodense area in the right internal capsule area. What is the most likely cause for her symptoms?

    A. Anti-phospholipid antibody syndrome
    B. Disseminated intra-vascular coagulation
    C. Idiopathic thrombocytopenic purpura
    D. Takayasu's arteritis
    E. Thrombotic thrombocytopenic purpura

35. **A 55-year-old lady attends a rheumatology clinic, complaining of a several-year history of painful joints. She has an X-ray of both hands. Which of the following associations is most likely to be found?**

    A. Osteoarthritis and loss of joint space confined to the MCP joints
    B. Psoriatic arthropathy with calcification of the soft tissues
    C. SLE and subarticular erosions
    D. Rheumatoid arthritis and periarticular osteopenia
    E. Osteoarthritis and extensive sub-articular erosions that involve the carpals

36. **A 70-year-old woman complains of a one-week history of right temporal headache, with localized scalp tenderness, and jaw pain on chewing. On examination you find tender temporal artery pulsations on the right side. The visual fields are normal. Blood tests done by her GP shows a haemoglobin 10 g/dl, WBC. count 6.8 x 1000/cm^3, platelets 520 x 10,000,000/cm^3, ESR 60 mm/h, normal UEC and liver function tests. What should be the next step in her management?**

    A. Arrange PET scan, and start prednisolone only if giant cell arteritis likely
    B. Arrange temporal artery biopsy, and start prednisolone only if giant cell arteritis confirmed
    C. Arrange vascular Doppler, and start prednisolone only if giant cell arteritis likely
    D. Start prednisolone 40 mg/day, and arrange temporal artery biopsy within the next week
    E. Start prednisolone 40 mg/day, and monitor response to trial of corticosteroids

37. **A 49-year-old woman with insulin-dependent diabetes mellitus and osteoarthritis presents with a painful right knee and inability to weight bear for the previous 24 hours. There is no history of injury, excessive alcohol intake, past or family history of skin disorders. On examination, the heart rate is 110/min, blood pressure is 120/70 mm Hg, and temperature is 37.0°C. The knee is held in a flexed attitude and both active and passive movements are extremely painful. What is the investigation of choice?**

    A. Blood culture
    B. C-reactive protein
    C. Knee X-ray
    D. Knee synovial fluid aspiration and Gram stain, microscopy, and culture
    E. Serum urate

38. **Which of the following conditions is associated with hepatitis C infection?**

    A. Mixed cryoglobulinemia
    B. Polyarteritis nodosa
    C. Psoriatic arthritis
    D. Rheumatoid arthritis
    E. Systemic lupus erythematosus

39. **Which of the following is a common side effect of bisphosphonate drugs (e.g. alendronic acid)? Select the single most appropriate answer.**

A. Oesophagitis and oesophageal ulceration

B. Derangement of liver function

C. Psychosis

D. Postural hypotension

E. Osteonecrosis of the jaw

40. **Which of the following drugs causes hyperuricaemia, and has the potential for inducing gout?**

A. Cyclosporin

B. Losartan

C. Mycophenolate mofetil

D. NSAIDs

E. Probenecid

41. **A 62-year-old woman with dry mouth and dry eyes was found to have a positive Schirmer's test. Which of the following antibodies when positive are highly suggestive of Sjögren's syndrome?**

A. Anti-Ro antibodies

B. Rheumatoid factor

C. Anti-CCP antibodies

D. Anti-mitochondrial antibodies

E. Anti-nuclear antibodies

42. **A 29-year-old man presents with left ankle pain, swelling, and difficulty in walking for one month. He also has ongoing urinary frequency and dysuria. He had an episode of diarrhoea lasting five days about three months ago. This resolved on its own. On examination, there is a painless rash on the glans penis and a red left eye. There are no oro-genital ulcers. Recent blood tests, FBC, UEC, and LFTs are normal. CRP is 56 mg/l. A chest X-ray and radiograph of the affected ankle is normal. What is the diagnosis?**

A. Behçet's disease.

B. Inflammatory bowel disease.

C. Reiter's syndrome.

D. Sarcoidosis.

E. Whipple's disease.

43. **A 28-year-old woman presents with a one-year history of Raynaud's phenomenon, diffuse skin thickening, and puffy hands. Over the last three months she has noticed exertional shortness of breath, and difficulty in climbing stairs, due to weakness of the thigh muscles. On examination, she has sclerodactyly and extensive skin thickening. On auscultation, there is bi-basal coarse crepitation. Power is 4/5 for hip flexion. Recent blood tests are as follows: Hb 11.1 g/dl, WBC 8 x 10³/microlitre, neutrophils 80%, platelets 170 x 10³/microlitre, ESR 46 mm/h, urea, electrolytes and creatinine: normal, CK 2000 IU/ml, CRP 35 mg/l, anti-nuclear antibody: positive 1:6400, anti-centromere antibody: negative, anti-Scl70 antibody: negative, anti-U1RNP: positive, anti-Ro antibody: negative, anti-La antibody: negative. What is the diagnosis?**

A. Dermatomyositis

B. Mixed connective tissue disease

C. Polymyositis

D. Scleroderma

E. Sjögren's syndrome

44. **An 80-year-old man with a one-week history of right temporal headache and scalp tenderness is referred to the MAU for urgent assessment of intermittent episodes of visual loss in the right eye. On examination he has a tender, beaded, right temporal artery. Initial investigations reveal: haemoglobin of 11 g/dl, normal WBC count, normal U&E, and normal liver function tests. The ESR is 50 mm/h and the CRP is 68 mg/l. What should be the initial step in his management?**

A. IV cyclophosphamide 500 mg every two weeks for six weeks

B. IV cyclophosphamide every two weeks for six weeks and IV methylprednisolone 1 g/day for three days

C. IV methylprednisolone 1 g/day for three days

D. Prednisolone 60 mg/day

E. Prednisolone 40 mg/day

45. **A 52-year-old man presents to the emergency department complaining of pain over his left knee. He says that the joint has become acutely red and painful over the past 12 hours. Past history of note includes one episode of renal colic. On examination he is pyrexial 37.6°C and his left knee is hot, swollen, and tender. His uric acid is raised at 0.6 mmol/l, his creatinine is normal at 90 micromol/l. Which of the following is the most appropriate initial treatment for him?**

A. Allopurinol

B. Ibuprofen

C. Prednisolone

D. Colchicine

E. Flucloxacillin

46. A 22-year-old man presents to the clinic for review; he has been suffering from morning stiffness and lower back pain for the past six or more months. He has some minor shortness of breath and has had pain on flexion for the past 2–3 months. On examination there is evidence of sacroilitis which is also suggested by a lumbar spine and pelvis X-ray. Which of the following is the most likely diagnosis?

    A. Rheumatoid arthritis
    B. Osteoarthritis
    C. Ankylosing spondylitis
    D. Enteropathic arthritis
    E. Sciatica

47. You suspect one of your patients to have rheumatoid arthritis clinically, but her Rh factor is negative. Which of these further blood tests may help you the most in confirming the diagnosis?

    A. Anti Jo-1 antibody
    B. Anti-nuclear antibodies (ANA)
    C. Voltage-gated potassium channel (VGKC) antibodies
    D. Anti-cyclic citrullinated peptide (CCP) antibody
    E. Anti-Ro antibodies

48. A 60-year-old man presents to the clinic for review, some six weeks after an acute attack of gout. Unfortunately he has not tolerated allopurinol and is now on prophylaxis against further attacks of gout. Past medical history of note includes hypertension, for which he is treated with ramipril 10mg. His creatinine is normal and his urate is 600 mmol/L. Which of the following is the most appropriate therapeutic intervention?

    A. Diclofenac
    B. Colchicine
    C. Febuxistat
    D. Rasburicase
    E. Continue on no medication

49. A 54 year old man who takes allopurinol for prophylaxis against acute attacks of gout presents to the Emergency department with a flare. His serum urate is measured at 580 micromol/L. Apart from urate crystals, which cytokine is thought to be primarily involved in driving flares of gout?

    A. IL-6
    B. IL-10
    C. IL-1 beta
    D. IL-18
    E. Interferon gamma

50. **A 29-year-old woman presents to the general medical clinic for review. She has suffered a left leg DVT, for which she took warfarin for six months, a few years earlier, but has otherwise been relatively well. Other past history of note includes three miscarriages which have occurred since she and her partner began trying for a baby some two years earlier; all three occurred between 12 and 14 weeks gestation. On examination her BP is 122/72, pulse is 75 and regular. She has livedo reticularis visible on both her upper and lower limbs. Which of the following is likely to point most to the underlying diagnosis?**
   A. Pelvic ultrasound scan
   B. Hysteroscopy
   C. Thrombophilia screen
   D. Autoantibody screen
   E. Folate assay

51. **A 60-year-old man with psoriatic arthritis presents for review. He has recently returned from a holiday to Egypt and complains of a worsening rash on his face and upper chest in addition to his usual psoriasis. On examination he has a rash on his face and upper body. Medication includes ramipril and amlodipine for hypertension, and sulfasalzine for arthritis. Blood testing reveals positive anti-nuclear antibodies, positive anti-histone antibodies; C3/C4 levels are in the normal range. What diagnosis fits best with this clinical picture?**
   A. SLE
   B. Drug-induced lupus
   C. Mixed connective tissue disease
   D. Drug-induced photosensitivity
   E. Worsening psoriasis

52. **A 32-year-old man comes to the rheumatology clinic for review. He has suffered from recurrent shoulder dislocation affecting both the left and the right, and knee cap dislocation on the left. Otherwise he is completely well. He tells you that other members of the family have had problems with hypermobility but have had a normal lifespan and no major problems apart from joint troubles. On examination his BP is 115/72, pulse is 70 and regular. You notice he has blue sclerae, and a few bruises on his legs which he puts down to playing for the local pub soccer team. He has moderate skin elasticity but no obvious scarring. His height is 6ft 2 in and his BMI is 25. Which of the following is the most likely diagnosis?**
   A. Osteogenesis imperfecta
   B. Classic Ehlers–Danlos syndrome
   C. Vascular Ehlers–Danlos syndrome
   D. Benign hypermobile syndrome
   E. Kyphoscoliosis type Ehlers–Danlos syndrome

53. **A 35-year-old woman presents with an acutely swollen, tender left knee. She has a long history of Crohn's disease, for which she underwent a small bowel resection one year earlier. On examination she is apyrexial, her left knee is swollen and tender, and flexion is limited to 35 degrees. Aspiration reveals positively birefringent, bipyramidal crystals on microscopy. Which of the following is the most likely diagnosis?**
   A. Oxalate arthropathy
   B. Pyrophosphate arthropathy
   C. Urate arthropathy
   D. Septic arthritis
   E. Osteoarthritis

54. **A 54-year-old man with a history of haemochromatosis comes to the emergency room for review with an acutely swollen, tender right knee. He has a history of type 2 diabetes controlled with diet, hypertension, and early hepatic fibrosis. On examination the right knee is swollen, tender, and flexion is limited to 30 degrees by pain. A serum urate is measured at 3.8mg/dl (226 micromol/l) and is in the normal range. A CRP is 28. Which of the following is the most likely diagnosis?**
   A. Osteoarthritis
   B. Septic arthritis
   C. Gout
   D. Pseudogout
   E. Inflammatory arthritis

55. **A 35-year-old Caucasian male describes a three-month history of worsening dyspnoea, with a dry, non-productive cough. He also has noticed a loss in weight, along with joint pain. He has not recently travelled abroad, has no pets and works as an accountant. He has become increasingly breathless at rest and was reviewed in the chest clinic. Plain chest radiograph suggested possible upper zone interstitial shadowing. Sputum investigations showed no obvious findings. Mantoux test was was negative. Spirometry revealed a restrictive picture with a reduced transfer co-efficient. HIV test was negative. He went to have a high resolution CT scan of his chest which revealed bilateral upper lobe fibrosis. Which of the following is the most likely diagnosis?**
   A. Histiocytosis-X
   B. Silicosis
   C. Extrinsic allergic alveolitis
   D. Bronchopulmonary aspergillosis
   E. Cryptogenic fibrosing alveolitis

56. **A 29-year-old man is investigated for dyspnoea. He describes a six-month history of joint pain, particularly in the morning, and easing off towards the end of the day. Plain chest radiograph shows upper lobe fibrosis. Which is the most likely underlying cause?**
    A. Cryptogenic fibrosing alveolitis
    B. Rheumatoid arthritis
    C. Asbestosis
    D. Ankylosing spondylitis
    E. Systemic lupus erythematosus

1. E. Reactive arthritis

Reactive arthritis usually presents 2–6 weeks after an antecedent infection. Acute gout presents initially with first meta-tarso phalangeal joint involvement. There are no risk factors for gout like excess alcohol intake, age > 40 years, male gender, diuretic use, and renal impairment. Gonococcal arthritis (*Neisseria gonorrhoeae*) presents with fever, asymmetric migratory or additive polyarthralgia, tenosynovitis, pustular rash or dermatitis, and mono- or oligo-arthritis. Upper limb joints and small joints are frequently affected. Pseudogout is caused by shedding of intra-articular calcium pyrophosphate (CPP) crystals. CPP deposition (CPPD) is common in patients >60 years old and frequently co-exists with osteoarthritis (OA). Pseudogout is unlikely in someone in the fourth decade of their life, and in the absence of other risk factors. Metabolic conditions like hyperparathyroidism, haemochromatosis, hypomagnesemia, and hypophosphatasia predispose to CPPD. Intra-articular CPPD commonly occurs at the knee, wrist, and hips, and may be seen as linear calcification of either fibro- or hyaline articular cartilage (chondrocalcinosis). CPP crystals are weakly positively bi-refringent under polarized light microscopy. There is no family or past history of psoriasis making psoriatic arthritis unlikely. However, psoriatic arthritis may precede skin involvement in 10–15% of patients.

Doherty M et al., *Davidson's Principles and Practice of Medicine*, Elsevier Health Sciences, 2006, pp. 1065–1144.

2. A. X-linked HPRT deficiency (Lesch–Nyhan)

X-linked HPRT deficiency (Lesch–Nyhan) is an X-linked HPRT (hypoxanthine-guanine phosphoribosyltransferase) deficiency. A deficiency in this enzyme causes a build-up in the levels of uric acid, and predisposes the individual to gout and renal damage. Other features include hypotonia, movement disorders, mental retardation, and behavioural disorders including self-harm. Treatment involves allopurinol and treatment of complications. The prognosis is poor, with renal failure or complications from hypotonia leading to death before the age of 20. Von Hippel–Lindau: this autosomal dominant condition is associated with haemangioblastomas, retinal angiomas, renal cell carcinoma, and renal, pancreatic, and epididymal cysts, as well as phaeochromocytoma. Lambert–Eaton syndrome (often known as Lambert–Eaton myasthenic syndrome) is a paraneoplastic condition, usually associated with small cell lung cancer. It causes a syndrome similar to myasthenia gravis (there are some differences) and is associated with antibodies to voltage-gated calcium channels on the pre-synaptic membrane of the neuromuscular junction. Prader–Willi syndrome is a genetic disorder caused by an abnormality on chromosome 15. It is associated with hypotonia, short stature, hypogonadism, and learning difficulties. It can also cause a chronic feeling of hunger and decreased calorific requirement that can lead to severe obesity. Reye's syndrome is usually a childhood illness that has been linked with aspirin use and recent viral illness. It causes liver and brain damage, which is progressive. Even when treated, the mortality is high, and many children are left with permanent neurological disability.

Hakim A et al., *Oxford Handbook of Rheumatology*, Third Edition, Oxford University Press, 2011, Chapter 7, The crystal arthropathies, Gout and hyperuricaemia

3. D. Fibromyalgia

The pain over multiple areas of the axial skeleton without evidence of an inflammatory disorder, coupled with low mood and lethargy fits well with fibromyalgia. The condition appears to occur more commonly in women of lower socio-economic status or with learning difficulties. Education, including cognitive behavioural therapy, is important in its management, and tricyclic anti-depressants or pregabalin may also be of value in pain control.

Longmore M et al., *Oxford Handbook of Clinical Medicine*, Eighth Edition, Oxford University Press, 2010, Chapter 12, Rheumatology, Fibromyalgia and chronic fatigue syndrome.

4. E. In rheumatoid arthritis it is more specific than the rheumatoid factor (RF)

Anti-CCP antibodies are potentially important surrogate markers for diagnosis and prognosis in rheumatoid arthritis (RA), because they are as sensitive as, and more specific than, rheumatoid factors (RF) in early and fully established disease. They may predict the eventual development into RA when found in undifferentiated arthritis. They are markers of erosive disease in RA and may be detected in healthy individuals years before onset of clinical RA. The use of anti-CCP antibodies may allow the clinical rheumatologist to better predict the diagnosis and prognosis of individual patients with RA. In general, the sensitivity of anti-CCP has been comparable to RF (50–75%) with a much higher specificity than RF at (90–95%). The RF is positive in about 70–90% of cases of Sjögren's syndrome. However anti-CCP antibodies are only positive in a minority of patients. Anti-CCP antibody levels do not fluctuate with disease activity and levels would not improve when clinical remission is achieved.

Lee DM, Schur PH, Clinical utility of the anti-CCP assay in patients with rheumatic diseases, *Annals of the Rheumatic Diseases* 2003;62(9):870–874.

5. B. Anti-CCP antibodies

Anti-CCP antibodies are now recognized as being associated with a worse prognosis from the point of view of joint erosions and deformity. Acute onset and earlier age at onset is associated with a better prognosis. Male sex is associated with a worse prognosis in rheumatoid arthritis. Out of the two antibodies (rheumatoid factor and anti-CCP) it is anti-CCP which carries the worse prognosis.

Hakim A et al., *Oxford Handbook of Rheumatology*, Third Edition, Oxford University Press, 2011, Chapter 5, Rheumatoid arthritis, The evaluation and treatment of rheumatoid arthritis.

6. B. Prescribe prednisolone at 40 mg orally

The patient's symptoms are typical of temporal arteritis (TA). Oral steroid should be started immediately to control the disease and prevent sudden loss of vision, which is a recognized complication of untreated disease. Steroid should be given even before the diagnosis is confirmed by biopsy. Temporal artery biopsy should be obtained in all cases, although the diagnostic yield of the biopsy diminishes with the initiation of corticosteroid therapy. Hence, biopsy should be performed as quickly as practical (within seven days), but treatment should not be delayed to allow scheduling of the procedure. Intravenous methylprednisolone treatment is usually reserved for cases presenting with visual loss. CT scan of the brain is usually normal in uncomplicated cases of TA and is not generally indicated. It should, however, be considered when the clinical scenario is not typical and intracerebral pathology needs to be ruled out. Temporomandibular arthritis should not be confused with TA, as pressure on the joint line produces localized tenderness. This is more prominent when the patient is asked to open and close their mouth while firm pressure is applied to the joint line anterior to the tragus of the ear.

Mukhtyar C et al., Eular recommendations for the management of primary small and medium vessel vasculitis, *Annals of the Rheumatic Diseases* 2009;68:310–317.

7. D. Retinitis

Ankylosing spondylitis is an inflammatory arthritis. It is one of the HLA-B27-associated arthritides, and characteristically affects the spine and sacroiliac joints. There are a host of associated features, including enthesitis, Achilles tendonitis and dactylitis. There are also extra-articular complications that can occur, including aortic root dilatation and regurgitation, and lung fibrosis. Uveitis is seen in 20–30% at some point, and can recur. Retinitis is not associated with this condition.

Rajesh K et al., Spondyloarthropathies, *American Academy of Family Physicians* 2004;15;69(12):2853–2860. http://www.aafp.org/afp/2004/0615/p2853.html

8. C. Recommend lifestyle measures and calcium and vitamin D supplementation

In accordance with RCP guidelines, those aged younger than 65 years are considered to be at lower risk of steroid-induced osteoporosis and fractures. Therefore it is recommended that bone density is measured in these patients and only those with a T score of –1.5 or less (osteopaenia) should be offered bisphosphonate therapy. However, those under 65 years with a previous fragility fracture should be considered for treatment with a bisphosphonate without the need for DXA scanning.

Glucocorticoid-induced osteoporosis: A concise guide to prevention and treatment; Royal College of Physicians and National Osteoporosis Society, 2003. https://www.nos.org.uk/NetCommunity/Document.Doc?id=423

9. C. Concomitant sulphasalazine

Specifically in combination with sulphasalazine, etanercept has been shown to result in significant decreases in white blood cell count. As such, use in combination should be avoided, or significant caution exercised with respect to frequent monitoring of full blood count. Caution and close monitoring should take place in patients with active viral hepatitis or multiple sclerosis. There is also a high risk of re-activation of tuberculosis in patients using anti-TNF agents.

emc+, Enbrel 25 mg powder and solvent for solution for injection, last updated December 2015, http://emc.medicines.org.uk/medicine/3343/SPC/Enbrel+25+mg+powder+and+solvent+for+solutio n+for+injection/

10. D. Antibodies to voltage-gated potassium channels

Antiphospholipid syndrome is a condition most commonly found in young women. It may occur as a primary disorder or may be secondary to other diseases such as systemic lupus erythematosus. Patients may suffer from venous and arterial thrombosis, migraine, recurrent spontaneous abortion, and other obstetric complications such as pre-eclampsia. Blood tests are often abnormal, and thrombocytopaenia is common. Antiphospholipid antibodies may be detected, and the most common one to test is anticardiolipin. However, anti beta-2 glycoprotein1 can also be tested for. Lupus anti-coagulant may also be positive. The criteria for diagnosis include one of the clinical criteria (proven vascular thrombosis or obstetric complications) and one of the laboratory criteria (anticardiolipin, anti beta-2 glycoprotein1 antibody, lupus anticoagulant). The mnemonic 'CLOTS' may be helpful in recalling some of the manifestations of the syndrome: C—Clots (venous and arterial thromboses), L—Livedo reticularis, O—Obstetric complications, T—Thrombocytopaenia.

In this question, all the abnormalities may be seen in this syndrome except anti-VGKC. These are seen in antibody-mediated neurological disease such as limbic encephalitis.

Cohen D, Clinical Review. Diagnosis and management of the antiphospholipid syndrome, *British Medical Journal* 2010;340:c2541. http://www.bmj.com/content/340/bmj.c2541.long?ath_user=nhslkent012&ath_ttok=%3CTNFwZaPl4gvysWIStA%3E

11. D. Anti-proteinase 3 antibody (c-ANCA)

The American Rheumatism Association (ARA, now the American College of Rheumatology or ACR) developed some criteria that are often used to help in the diagnosis of SLE (see Box 5.1). In terms of immunological profile, there are a number of antibodies that may be found in this condition. Anti-nuclear antibodies are found most often (in about 98% of patients or more). Anti-ds-DNA antibody is also found in more than half of patients. Other antibodies that may be found include anti-Smith, -Ro, -La and cardiolipin. The further reading below shows a table of potential antibodies and their prevalence. c-ANCA is not associated with SLE, and is most often found in granulomatosis with polyangiitis (previously known as Wegener's granulomatosis).

Box 5.1 Revised criteria (serial or simultaneous) for diagnosing SLE

Dianose SLE in an appropriate clinical setting if ≥4 out of 11 criteria are present:

Malar rash (butterfly rash)

Discoid rash

Photosensitivity

Oral ulcers

Non-erosive arthritis

Serositis

Renal disorder

CNS disorder

Haematological disorder

Immunoogical disorder

Antinuclear antibodd (ANA)

Adapted from Longmore M et al., *Oxford Handbook of Clinical Medicine*, Ninth Edition, 2014 with permission from Oxford University Press.

Hakim A et al., *Oxford Handbook of Rheumatology*, Third Edition, Oxford University Press, 2011, Chapter 10, Systemic lupus erythematosus: Diagnosis and investigation of systemic lupus erythematosus.

12. B. If it extends above the knees or elbows, or below the neck, it is classified as diffuse disease

Scleroderma is a connective tissue disease which affects the skin and internal organs. The classification of this condition has changed over the years, and there is still some confusion. The first differentiation is between localized and systemic disease. Localized scleroderma only affects the skin, and the internal organs are not affected. In systemic sclerosis, the internal organs are affected. Here, there is a further subdivision based on the extent that the skin is involved. In limited systemic sclerosis, skin thickening does not extend above the elbows or knees, or below the neck. This category is similar to the old 'CREST' syndrome, but is classified as above rather than by

CREST symptoms. In diffuse disease, the skin involvement does extend to involve the more central body areas.

Hakim A et al., *Oxford Handbook of Rheumatology*, Third Edition, Oxford University Press, 2011, Chapter 13, Systemic sclerosis and related disorders: Epidemiology and diagnostic criteria.

13. A. Treatment has failed with two disease-modifying agents including methotrexate

The NICE guidelines are specific about their recommendations for the use of anti-TNF therapy in rheumatoid arthritis, which covers adalimumab, etanercept, and infliximab. They state that for one of these medications to be used, the disease must be active, with a disease activity score (DAS28) greater than 5.1. This should be checked twice, a month apart. They also state that the patient should have tried two disease-modifying anti-rheumatic drugs including methotrexate (unless contraindicated). Other recommendations include the fact that they should normally be used with methotrexate unless contraindicated. The response should be monitored, and treatment should only be continued if the DAS28 score falls by 1.2 points or more after six months.

NICE guidance on rheumatoid arthritis, 2009 (Full guidance: section 10, p. 203). http://guidance.nice.org.uk/CG79/Guidance/pdf/English

14. C. Suppression of B cells

Rituximab is a relatively new therapy classed as a biologic. It is a monoclonal antibody against the antigen CD20, a protein that is mainly found on the surface of B cells. By binding to this protein, the antibody activates a series of mechanisms, leading to a reduction in B cells. This drug is effective in rheumatological disease, particularly rheumatoid arthritis. In this case, it is the immunosuppressive action that is important. It is also used in other conditions, such as haematological disorders, other autoimmune diseases, and anti-rejection after transplant. As it is a fairly new therapy, it is likely that the full extent of its benefits is yet to be discovered. In addition to this, there are increasing numbers of other biologics being developed, with a range of different mechanisms of action.

Arthritis Care website. Section on medication. Note particularly the links to the 'factsheets' near the bottom of the page. http://www.arthritiscare.org.uk/AboutArthritis/Treatments/taking-medication

15. D. Foetal heart block

Patients with SLE can have antibodies against a variety of nuclear antigens, including ds-DNA, smith, Ro, and La. The anti-Ro and anti-La antibodies in particular are associated with congenital heart block. About 1% of babies born to mothers with these antibodies (either or both) are likely to have this condition. It is therefore worth being aware of this if a patient with SLE is planning a pregnancy.

Tunaoglu FS et al., Isolated congenital heart block, *Texas Heart Institute Journal* 2010;37(5):579–583. http://www.ncbi.nlm.nih.gov/pmc/articles/PMC2953227/?tool=pubmed

16. C. Phenytoin

It is established that phenytoin can be a cause of accelerated bone loss, although this is not the case for the other listed medications. Alongside other anti-convulsants (carbamazepine, barbiturates), phenytoin can cause bone loss through the mechanism of treatment-induced vitamin D deficiency.

emc+, Phenytoin Injection BP, last updated Novebmer 2014. http://www.medicines.org.uk/emc/medicine/650/SPC/phenytoin%20injection%20bp/

17. C. Methotrexate

Erosive and deforming arthritis occurs in 40–60% of psoriatic arthritis patients. A Cochrane systematic review supports the use of sulphasalazine and methotrexate to prevent joint damage in psoriatic arthritis. Psoriatic arthritis is an inflammatory arthritis which leads to deformities if not adequately treated. The appropriate treatment is to commence the patient on a disease-modifying anti-rheumatic drug to prevent joint damage. Non steroidal anti-inflammatory drugs (NSAIDs) may be used for short term symptom control only. Etanercept is one of the three anti-tumour necrosis factor alpha antibodies available in the UK. It is more effective than methotrexate. However, in the UK, in order to begin treatment with anti-tumour necrosis factor alpha antibody therapies when patients have failed to respond to at least two traditional disease modifying drugs. Intra-articular corticosteroid injection may be used for short-term symptom control only, not for long-term management. The long-term use of oral corticosteroids is associated with significant side effects, like osteoporosis, diabetes, hypertension, myopathy, weight gain, psychiatric disturbances, and skin thinning. Also, avoid long-term corticosteroid use as their discontinuation is often followed by a flare of cutaneous psoriasis or the development of severe pustular psoriasis.

Kyle S et al., Guideline for anti-TNF-alpha therapy in psoriatic arthritis, *Rheumatology* 2005;44(3): 390–397. http://rheumatology.oxfordjournals.org/content/44/3/390.full.pdf

18. B. Diclofenac

Given that this patient's blood pressure is relatively well controlled, a short course of non-steroidals is the most appropriate initial therapy. Any more prolonged therapy, however, is likely to be detrimental with respect to salt and water retention. Allopurinol may precipitate worsening of the acute attack of gout and should not be started until a few days after non-steroidals have been initiated. If non-steroidals are unsuitable then colchicine or a short course of prednisolone are both potential options. Rasburicase is an IV therapy that can be used as prophylaxis against acute urate nephropathy in chemotherapy.

Ramrakha P et al., *Oxford Handbook of Acute Medicine*, Third Edition, Oxford University Press, 2010.

19. E. –1.7

The results of a bone density measurement (DXA scan) are reported in two ways: as T scores and as Z scores. The T score represents the bone mineral density as compared to the optimal peak bone density for gender: >–1.0 = normal, –1.0 to –2.5 = osteopaenia, <–2.5 = osteoporosis. Scores <–2.5 represent osteoporotic bone. The Z score provides age- and gender-matched bone mineral density measurement.

Royal College of Physicians, Glucocorticoid-induced osteoporosis: guidelines for prevention and treatment, Royal College of Physicians, 2002.

20. A. Polymyositis

The symptoms of proximal myopathy and raised CK are consistent with polymyositis, with the shortness of breath possibly due to respiratory muscle weakness. We are not told of any skin rash/discolouration, so this makes dermatomyositis unlikely. CK levels may be between five and 50 times the upper limit of normal. The presence of anti-Jo antibodies further supports the diagnosis. Five-year survival rates are 80% or more, and the majority of patients show a favourable response to oral corticosteroids. In those who require high doses for a prolonged period, steroid-sparing second-line agents may be added.

Dalakas MC, Immunotherapy of myositis: issues, concerns and future prospects, *Nature Reviews Rheumatology* 2010;6:129–137. http://www.nature.com/nrrheum/journal/v6/n3/abs/nrrheum.2010.2.html

21. B. Isoniazid

This lady presents with symptoms suggestive of an SLE-like illness. She also has antibodies that are strongly associated with drug-induced lupus. The more common medications associated with this condition include: minocycline, hydralazine, procainamide, isoniazid, quinidine, methyldopa, chlorpromazine, salazopyrine (sulfasalazine). Therefore, out of the list given, isoniazid is most likely to be associated with drug-induced lupus.

Hakim A et al., *Oxford Handbook of Rheumatology*, Third Edition, Oxford University Press, 2011, Chapter 10, Systemic lupus erythematosus, Drug-induced lupus erythematosus.

22. C. Psoriatic arthritis

Psoriatic arthritis is likely as there is a history of dactylitis (sausage finger), asymmetric oligo-arthritis, and distal inter-phalangeal joint inflammation, a distinctive feature of psoriatic arthritis. In the absence of psoriasis, a history of psoriasis in a first-degree relative supports the diagnosis of psoriatic arthritis in this patient. Distal inter-phalangeal joint involvement in psoriatic arthritis commonly co-exists with nail dystrophy due to psoriasis (nail pitting and onycholysis—separation of nail plate from the nail bed). Acute gout presents initially with first meta-tarso phalangeal joint involvement (podagra). Moreover, there are no risk factors for gout-like excess alcohol intake, male gender, diuretic use, and renal impairment. Acute rheumatic fever, an immunological reaction to a preceding beta haemolytic streptococcus infection is rare in the western world. The arthritis in acute rheumatic fever is migratory, transient, non-erosive, and affects one joint area for hours to a few weeks. Reactive arthritis usually presents 2–6 weeks after an antecedent infection. The absence of a preceding infection makes reactive arthritis less likely. Although dactylitis (sausage finger) can occur in reactive arthritis, distal-interphalangeal joint involvement is uncommon in reactive arthritis. Rheumatoid arthritis (RA) presents with symmetric inflammatory arthritis, predominantly involving the wrists, meta-carpo phalangeal joints, and proximal inter-phalangeal joints. It rarely affects the distal inter-phalangeal joints alone. However, up to 5% of patients with psoriatic arthritis have symmetric arthropathy, indistinguishable from RA at disease onset.

Burden AD et al., Diagnosis and management of psoriasis and psoriatic arthritis in adults: summary of SIGN guidance, *British Medical Journal* 2010;341:c5623.

23. A. Anti-phospholipid antibody syndrome

The clinical history given is consistent with a diagnosis of anti-phospholipid antibody syndrome. The absence of joint involvement or other features of SLE such as a photosensitive rash make this the more likely diagnosis. There are no other features suggesting mixed connective tissue disease such as joint pain, respiratory or renal pathology, and absence of joint pain and morning stiffness counts against rheumatoid. Systemic sclerosis is associated with pulmonary fibrosis, reflux oesophagitis, and subcutaneous calcinosis. Rather than warfarinizing her for her disease, because of the risks associated with warfarin in pregnancy, aspirin and low molecular weight heparin would be the treatment of choice after pregnancy is confirmed.

Hakim A et al., *Oxford Handbook of Rheumatology*, Third Edition, Oxford University Press, 2011, Chapter 11, The antiphospholipid (antibody) syndrome, Clinical features of antiphospholipid syndrome.

24. A. Aspirate right knee, send synovial fluid for culture and microscopy

This patient has reactive arthritis. However, septic arthritis needs to be excluded, as in any individual with acute mono-arthritis. Septic arthritis is a serious illness with a mortality of 11%. Joint aspiration, followed by microscopy and culture of the synovial fluid is critical to its diagnosis. Examination of joint fluid under polarized microscope may show mono sodium urate (negatively birefringent) or CPP (weakly positively birefringent) crystals. Negatively birefringent crystals suggest acute gout, while positively birefringent crystals suggest acute CPP crystal arthritis (pseudogout). Knee radiograph is likely to be normal in someone with inflammatory joint symptoms of such short duration. In most individuals, the infection that triggers reactive arthritis has been treated by the time of onset of reactive arthritis. If not, then appropriate microbiological investigations may be undertaken. Although reactive arthritis associates with HLA-B27, 50% of individuals with reactive arthritis are negative for HLA-B27. This test is therefore of limited diagnostic value. However, HLA-B27 may be used as a prognostic test in individuals with reactive arthritis. This is because individuals with reactive arthritis who are HLA-B27 positive are more likely to develop severe, aggressive, and long-lasting reactive arthritis. These patients are also more likely to develop sacro-ilitis (note: HLA-B 27 associates with ankylosing spondylitis). Knee X-ray is likely to be normal in a young person with a short clinical history.

Hamdulay SS et al., When is arthritis reactive? *Postgraduate Medical Journal* 2006;82(969):446–453.

25. C. Drug-induced systemic lupus

This patient has drug-induced lupus. Procainamide, hydralazine, sulfasalazine, carbamazepine, phenytoin, minocycline, isoniazide, interferons, and anti-TNFα agents have been shown to cause drug-induced lupus. These patients have a purpuric, erythematous, papular rash, and do not have a malar or discoid rash. They have anti-nuclear antibody (homogeneous pattern), are positive for anti-ssDNA antibody, anti-histone antibody, and classically are negative for anti-dsDNA antibody. However drug-induced lupus due to interferon and due to anti-TNFα agents, presents with malar and discoid rash, and these patients are frequently anti-dsDNA antibody positive. The deranged LFT may be a result of reactive metabolites produced by the liver. Drug-induced lupus remits after stopping treatment with the incriminating drug. Pattern of ANA and disease association: homogenous: non-pathological, SLE, autoimmune chronic active hepatitis (CAH), drug-induced SLE; peripheral: SLE, CAH; Speckled (coarse): SLE, MCTD; speckled (fine): SLE, SCLE, scleroderma, Sjögren's syndrome; speckled (centromere): primary Raynaud's phenomenon, scleroderma, SLE. Behçet's disease is a systemic vasculitis of unknown cause, associated with HLA-B51. It is most commonly found in Turkey, the Mediterranean, and Japan. It manifests as recurrent oral and genital ulceration, ocular inflammation (e.g. anterior or posterior uveitis), skin lesions (e.g. erythema nodosum, papulopustular lesions), neurological involvement (e.g. aseptic meningitis, encephalitis, CN palsies, confusion), vasculitis, non-erosive large joint oligoarthropathy, diarrhoea, and colitis. The presence of chronic erythematous, papular, or plaque-like skin lesions with scarring and/or central atrophy constitutes discoid lupus erythematosus. This may be isolated, or co-exist with systemic lupus erythematosus. Drug hypersensitivity syndrome is a severe, multi-organ system adverse drug reaction characterized by cutaneous eruptions, fever, lymphadenopathy, eosinophilia, hepatitis, and less frequent involvement of the kidneys, lungs, and heart. It is unlikely in the absence of eosinophilia, and in the presence of ANA antibodies. Systemic lupus erythematosus manifests as a photosensitive malar or discoid rash, sparing of nasolabial folds, oral ulcers, serositis, arthralgia, Raynaud's phenomenon, usually in the presence of a positive ANA antibody. Typically the anti-dsDNA antibodies are positive as well. SLE patients are usually negative for anti-ssDNA and anti-histone antibodies.

Camacho ID et al., Drug-induced lupus erythematosus, *eMedicine*, 2012.

http://emedicine.medscape.com/article/1065086-overview

26. B. Osteoporosis

This patient has established osteoporosis. Risk factors for low BMD are: increasing age, female gender, low body mass index (BMI) (<22 kg/m^2), medical conditions such as ankylosing spondylitis,

Crohn's disease, and conditions that result in prolonged immobility. This woman has osteoporosis, not osteopenia. The World Health Organization (WHO) has established diagnostic criteria for osteoporosis based on the measurement of BMD, expressed as the T score, which is the number of standard deviations (SD) below the mean BMD of young adults at their peak bone mass. Osteopetrosis variably referred to as 'marble bone disease' and 'Albers-Schönberg disease', comprises a clinically heterogeneous group of conditions that share the hallmark of increased bone density. The increase in bone density results from abnormalities in osteoclast differentiation or function. The more severe forms tend to have autosomal-recessive inheritance, while the mildest forms are observed in adults and are inherited in an autosomal-dominant manner. The main complications are fractures, scoliosis, osteoarthritis, and osteomyelitis. In the presence of osteoporosis, and other risk factors for fracture, pathological fracture is less likely.

Kumar P, Clark M, *Clinical Medicine*, Seventh Edition, Saunders Elsevier, 2009, Chapter 10, Rheumatology and bone disease.

27. E. Transcutaneous electrical nerve stimulation

Transcutaneous electrical nerve stimulation (TENS) can be used for pain relief in OA. It works by blocking the transmission of painful stimuli in the spinal cord (neural gating). There is not enough consistent evidence that acupuncture is clinically effective, or cost-effective for pain in osteoarthritis. Chondroitin sulphate is not recommended by NICE for the treatment of osteoarthritis. Glucosamine is not recommended for the treatment of osteoarthritis. The use of intra-articular hyaluronic acid is not supported by NICE guidelines for the treatment of OA, mainly due to its limited efficacy.

NICE Guidance [CG 117], Osteoarthritis: care and management, 2014. https://www.nice.org.uk/guidance/cg177

28. C. Pulmonary arterial hypertension

Pulmonary arterial hypertension is the most likely diagnosis. The murmur is due to tricuspid regurgitation. This and tall R waves in right-sided ECG leads point to the presence of right ventricular strain. Patients with limited cutaneous systemic sclerosis are at a high risk of developing pulmonary arterial hypertension. These patients should be screened by annual echocardiogram (to measure their estimated systolic pulmonary artery pressure) and annual lung function tests. A reduction in DLCO, in the absence of a reduction in FVC or TLC, suggests the presence of pulmonary hypertension. Patients with diffuse cutaneous systemic sclerosis are at a high risk of developing ILD. They have bi-basal crackles. On lung function tests, the FVC and TLC are reduced more than the DLCO. However, occasionally patients with limited cutaneous systemic sclerosis may develop interstitial lung disease. Pericardial effusion may occur in limited cutaneous systemic sclerosis. However, loud heart sounds, presence of a murmur, normal JVP, and tall R waves in the ECG all point against it. Small recurrent pulmonary embolism can present as pulmonary arterial hypertension. However, patients with limited cutaneous systemic sclerosis are not at any more risk of pulmonary embolism than the general population. Pulmonary venous hypertension occurs due to left heart failure, as a result of backflow from an overloaded left atrium/ventricle. There is no clinical evidence of left-sided heart failure (e.g. bibasal crepitations) in this patient.

National Pulmonary Hypertension Centres of the UK and Ireland, Consensus statement on the management of pulmonary hypertension in clinical practice in the UK and Ireland, *Thorax* 2008;63(Suppl II):ii1–ii41.

29. A. Giant cell arteritis

Giant cell arteritis (cranial or temporal arteritis) is common in the elderly. It is rare in those under 55 years. The symptoms include headache, temporal artery and scalp tenderness (e.g.

when combing hair), jaw claudication, amaurosis fugax, or sudden blindness, typically in one eye. Extracranial symptoms may include dyspnoea, morning stiffness, and unequal or weak pulses. Polymyalgia rheumatica is not a true vasculitis, but shares the same demographic characteristics as giant cell arteritis, and the two conditions often co-exist in the same patient. There is usually subacute onset (< 2 weeks) of symmetrical aching, tender. Takayasu's arteritis (aortic arch syndrome, pulseless disease) is a systemic vasculitis and affects the aorta and its major branches, causing stenosis, thrombosis and aneurysms. It often affects women 20–40 years old. Cerebral, ophthalmological, and upper limb symptoms (e.g. dizziness, visual changes, and weak arm pulses) are common. Systemic features such as fever, weight loss, and malaise are common. Hypertension is often a feature, due to reno-vascular involvement. Localized temporal artery tenderness is uncommon in Takayasu's arteritis. Microscopic polyangitis is a necrotizing vasculitis affecting small and medium-sized vessels. The symptoms include rapidly progressive glomerulonephritis and pulmonary haemorrhage. Wagener's granulomatosis is a necrotizing granulomatous inflammation and vasculitis of small and medium vessels. It has a predilection for the upper respiratory tract, lungs, and kidneys. Upper airways disease is common, with nasal obstruction, ulcers, epistaxis, or destruction of the nasal septum causing a characteristic 'saddle-nose' deformity. Sinusitis is often a feature. Renal disease causes rapidly progressive glomerulonephritis with crescent formation, proteinuria or haematuria. Pulmonary involvement may cause cough, haemoptysis (severe if pulmonary haemorrhage) or pleuritis.

Longmore M et al., *Oxford Handbook of Clinical Medicine*, Eighth Edition, Oxford University Press, 2010, Chapter 12, Rheumatology, vasculitis.

30. C. Methotrexate pneumonitis

This patient has methotrexate pneumonitis (MP), a rare idiosyncratic hypersensitivity reaction. It is most frequently but not exclusively seen within the first year of treatment. Many studies suggest that it is more common in individuals with pre-existing lung disease. It presents as a flu-like illness, with fever, cough, and breathlessness. There is a high mortality, with some patients responding to drug cessation, and moderate- to high-dose corticosteroids. Atypical pneumonia would be expected to show some improvement after 48 hours of treatment with macrolides. Fibrosing alveolitis occurs in RA, predominantly affects the lower lobes, and presents with gradually worsening shortness of breath over weeks to months. There are only a few reports of *Pneumocystis jiroveci* pneumonia in patients on low-dose methotrexate for RA. Most patients are also on prednisolone. A retrospective audit from Christchurch, New Zealand reported that the annual incidence of *Pneumocystis jiroveci* pneumonia was 0.17% in RA patients treated with methotrexate. The short duration of symptoms and the location of radiographic changes make pulmonary tuberculosis unlikely. Tubercular infiltrates and cavities predominantly affect the upper lobe.

Hargreaves MR et al., Acute pneumonitis associated with low dose methotrexate treatment for rheumatoid arthritis: report of five cases and review of published reports, *Thorax* 1992;47:628–633. http://thorax.bmj.com/content/47/8/628.full.pdf+html

31. B. Allopurinol and colchicine

Allopurinol should always be started at a low dose (100 mg/day) in combination with colchicine or NSAIDs. Of these colchicine (500 micrograms, BD) is preferred, as it is potentially less toxic, and may be continued for up to six months. NSAIDs may be used. Allopurinol, a xanthine oxidase inhibitor, prevents the oxidation of xanthine and hypoxanthine to urate. Although xanthine and hypoxanthine are less soluble than urate, crystal formation is inhibited as the total purine excretion is spread over the three metabolites. Allopurinol also reduces total purine concentration. Allopurinol is itself metabolized by xanthine oxidase to oxypurinol, its active metabolite. While colchicine is used in treatment and prophylaxis of acute gout, it does not reduce the serum urate levels. Febuxostat is a non-purine xanthine oxidase inhibitor which is currently licensed for use in individuals who are intolerant or allergic to allopurinol. Allopurinol hypersensitivity is rare and potentially life-threatening with a mortality of 25%. It manifests as fever, erythematous skin rash, toxic epidermal necrolysis, Stevens–Johnson syndrome, eosinophilia, acute interstitial nephritis, and hepatitis. It is more common in individuals with renal impairment. This patient meets the criteria to start urate-lowering therapy. Drug treatment of hyperuricaemia is indicated in patients with gout if a second attack or further attacks occur within one year; and in all patients with gouty tophi or renal insufficiency or uric acid stones and gout, and in those who need to continue treatment with diuretics. Treatment of asymptomatic hyperuricaemia in the absence of gout is not indicated.

Jordan KM et al., British Society for Rheumatology and British Health Professionals in Rheumatology guideline for the management of gout, *Rheumatology* 2007;46(8):1372–1374.

32. B. Limited cutaneous systemic sclerosis

This patient has limited cutaneous systemic sclerosis. The skin involvement in limited cutaneous systemic sclerosis is restricted to the face, and to areas distal to the elbow and knee. The skin involvement in diffuse cutaneous systemic sclerosis is not restricted to any part of the body. Facial involvement occurs in both limited and diffuse subtypes. Most patients with diffuse cutaneous systemic sclerosis have positive anti-Scl 70 antibody (also called anti-topoisomerase III antibody). Patients with diffuse cutaneous systemic sclerosis have Raynaud's phenomenon for <1–2 years before the onset of skin thickening. Mixed connective tissue disease combines features of systemic sclerosis, SLE, and polymyositis. It usually associates with a positive anti U1-RNP antibody. Sjögren's syndrome presents with dry eyes, dry mouth, and Raynaud's phenomenon. It may be primary (occurring on its own) or secondary to other autoimmune conditions like RA, SLE, or systemic sclerosis. It usually associates with a positive anti-Ro and anti-La antibodies. SLE patients do not have skin thickening and telangiectasias.

Doherty M et al., *Davidson's Principles and Practice of Medicine*, Elsevier Health Sciences, 2006, pp. 1065–1144.

33. E. Warfarin

Due to the high risk of recurrence of stroke, warfarin is recommended thromboprophylaxis for someone with antiphospholipid syndrome and arterial or venous thrombosis. Aspirin (75 mg/day) is insufficient thromboprophylaxis for someone with antiphospholipid syndrome, and history of a thrombosis, as there is a high risk of recurrence of stroke. Corticosteroids may be used for the treatment of thrombocytopenia (usually <50 x10³/microlitre) in antiphospholipid syndrome, usually in consultation with a haematologist. There is no role of cyclophosphamide in the treatment of antiphospholipid syndrome. Plasma exchange may be used in individuals with catastrophic antiphospholipid syndrome, which presents with thromboses in multiple organ systems like the lungs, bowel, kidney, and skin.

Doherty M et al., *Davidson's Principles and Practice of Medicine*, Elsevier Health Sciences, 2006, pp. 1065–1144.

34. A. Anti-phospholipid antibody syndrome

This patient has antiphospholipid syndrome, a non-inflammatory pro-thrombotic state in vivo, in the presence of laboratory tests suggesting an anti-coagulant state. Antiphospholipid syndrome may be primary (more common) or may associate with SLE (20–30%). The antiphospholipid antibodies (anti-cardiolipin and lupus anti-coagulant) cause coagulation defects in vitro (raised aPTT, dilute Russell's viper venom time), livedo reticularis, recurrent miscarriage, and thrombocytopenia (↓platelets). However, despite the coagulation defects and thrombocytopenia, the lupus anticoagulant causes arterial and venous thromboses in vivo. The thromboses may affect vessels of any size. Antiphospholipid syndrome does not cause micro-angiopathic haemolytic anaemia. Disseminated intra-vascular clotting is a severe systemic illness, where bleeding may occur due to consumption of clotting factors and platelets by an overactive clotting cascade. It is a consumptive coagulopathy. Idiopathic thrombocytopenic purpura does not cause thromboses. It is caused by antiplatelet autoantibodies. It is acute (usually in children, two weeks after infection with sudden self-limiting purpura) or chronic (seen mainly in women). Chronic ITP runs a fluctuating course of bleeding, purpura (especially dependent pressure areas), epistaxis and menorrhagia. There is no splenomegaly. The diagnosis of Takayasu's arteritis is unlikely in the presence of a normal ESR and CRP. Takayasu's arteritis (aortic arch syndrome, pulseless disease) is a systemic vasculitis and would be expected to associate with thrombocytosis, and not thrombocytopenia. It affects the aorta and its major branches, causing stenosis, thrombosis, and aneurysms. It often affects women aged 20–40 years old. Cerebral, ophthalmological and upper limb symptoms (e.g. dizziness, visual changes, and weak arm pulses) are common. Systemic features such as fever, weight loss, and malaise are common. Hypertension is often a feature, due to reno-vascular involvement. Thrombotic thrombocytopenic purpura is unlikely. It is a serious illness with fever, fluctuating CNS signs (e.g. seizures, hemiparesis, low consciousness, poor vision), micro-angiopathic haemolytic anaemia (schistocytes on blood film), thrombocytopenia, jaundice, and renal failure. It has a high mortality, and affects adult women. There is a genetic or acquired deficiency of a protease that normally cleaves multimers of von Willebrand factor (vWf). As a result, large vWf multimers form, cause platelet aggregation, fibrin deposition in small vessels, and lead to microthrombi. As it is a consumptive coagulopathy, the fibrinogen levels are normal, or reduced, and fibrinogen degradation products are elevated.

Doherty M et al., *Davidson's Principles and Practice of Medicine*, Elsevier Health Sciences, 2006, pp. 1065–1144.

35. D. Rheumatoid arthritis and periarticular osteopenia

Osteoarthritis predominantly affects the inter-phalangeal joints, as well as the first carpo-metacarpal joint. Erosions are sometimes seen, but not involving the carpals. Psoriatic arthropathy is not usually associated with soft tissue calcification. SLE does not typically cause erosions. The hallmarks of rheumatoid arthritis are erosions, subluxation, and juxta-articular osteopenia.

Grainger RG et al., *Diagnostic Radiology*, Fourth Edition, Churchill Livingstone, 2001, Joint Disease, pp. 1195–2026.

36. D. Start prednisolone 40 mg/day, and arrange temporal artery biopsy within the next week

This patient has giant cell (temporal) arteritis, a chronic vasculitis of large and medium vessels. It leads to granulomatous inflammation histologically, and predominantly affects the cranial branches of arteries arising from the arch of the aorta. Temporal artery biopsy is the most established investigation for the diagnosis of temporal arteritis. PET scans and Doppler ultrasound findings cannot be relied upon to establish the diagnosis of giant cell (temporal) arteritis on their own. Prompt institution of corticosteroid treatment is necessary to prevent visual complications—this patient has jaw claudication, a risk factor for visual involvement in giant cell (temporal) arteritis. Symptoms usually begin to resolve within a few days to a week of starting corticosteroids, but this cannot be used as a diagnostic test. Giant cell arteritis may present with a normal temporal artery biopsy, and therefore a negative temporal artery biopsy does not rule it out. As explained in the British Society for Rheumatology guidelines, symptoms and signs of giant cell (temporal) arteritis include: abrupt-onset headache (usually unilateral in the temporal area and occasionally diffuse or bilateral), scalp pain (diffuse or localized), difficulty in combing hair, jaw, and tongue claudication, visual symptoms (amaurosis fugax, blurring, and diplopia), systemic symptoms of fever, weight loss, loss of appetite, depression, and tiredness. There may be polymyalgic symptoms, limb claudication, fever, weight loss, and other constitutional symptoms. Examination may reveal abnormal superficial temporal artery, tender, thickened or beaded with reduced or absent pulsation, scalp tenderness, transient or permanent reduction in visual acuity (partial or complete), visual field defect, relative afferent papillary defect on the swinging flashlight test, pale, swollen optic disc with haemorrhages on fundoscopy (anterior ischaemic optic neuritis), unilateral or bilateral central retinal artery occlusion, upper cranial nerve palsies.

Dasgupta B et al., BSR and BHPR Guidelines for the management of giant cell arteritis. http://www. rheumatology.org.uk/includes/documents/cm_docs/2010/m/2_management_of_giant_cell_arteritis.pdf

37. D. Knee synovial fluid aspiration and gram stain, microscopy, and culture

This is the investigation of choice, and should be performed prior to administering antibiotics, unless the patient is in shock. Septic arthritis is most commonly caused by *Staphylococcus aureus*. Once synovial fluid is aspirated, the patient may be commenced on intravenous flucloxacillin, with or without gentamicin (depending on local policy). Second- or third-generation cephalosporins or clindamycin may be used in individuals with penicillin allergy. Blood culture: this person should be assumed to have septic arthritis unless proven otherwise. The risk factors for septic arthritis are pre-existing joint disease, prosthetic joints, low socio-economic status, intravenous drug abuse, alcoholism, diabetes, previous intra-articular corticosteroid injection, and ulcerated skin. Although a blood culture should be taken, it is not the investigation of choice as half of patients with septic arthritis have a positive blood culture. C-reactive protein is elevated in acute monoarthritis of any cause. It does not help in the differential diagnosis of this individual. There is no history of injury. Articular chondrocalcinosis may be visualized on plain knee X-ray, suggesting CPPD, and a diagnosis of pseudogout in this context. However, pseudogout and septic arthritis may co-exist, and the visualization of chondrocalcinosis on plain knee X-ray does not exclude septic arthritis. Serum urate is elevated in individuals with gout, and is not indicated in this patient. However, a high serum urate may occur in a large number of conditions, and is not specific to gout.

Coakley G et al., BSR & BHPR, BOA, RCGP and BSAC guidelines for management of the hot swollen joint in adults, *Rheumatology* 2006;45(8):1039–1041. http://www.ncbi.nlm.nih.gov/pubmed/16829534

38. A. Mixed cryoglobulinemia

Mixed cryoglobulinemia which manifests as purpura, cutaneous ulcers, polyneuropathy, membranoproliferative glomerulonephritis, and non-erosive polyarthralgias is associated with hepatitis C. HCV infection can also lead to a non-erosive symmetric arthropathy, and the interferon? used to treat hepatitis C can also lead to drug-induced lupus. Laboratory investigations show positive rheumatoid factor, low C4, active urine sediments, and type II or III serum cryoglobulins. There may be axonal polyneuropathy, and active urinary sediment in those with polyneuropathy, and membranoproliferative glomerulonephritis respectively.

Doherty M et al., *Davidson's Principles and Practice of Medicine*, Elsevier Health Sciences, 2006, pp. 1065–1144.

39. A. Oesophagitis and oesophageal ulceration

Bisphosphonates are generally well tolerated, but have been associated with oesophageal reactions including oesophagitis, erosions, ulcers, and strictures. This can largely be avoided by advising patients to take them on an empty stomach, 30 minutes before breakfast with plenty of water and remain upright for about 30 minutes afterwards. Osteonecrosis of the jaw has been reported as an infrequent side effect of intravenous and, very occasionally, oral bisphosphonates. The risk can be decreased by maintenance of adequate oral hygiene during and after treatment. Bisphosphonates are contraindicated in patients with pre-existing oesophageal abnormalities such as achalasia or strictures.

Royal College of Physicians, Glucocorticoid-induced osteoporosis: guidelines for prevention and treatment, Royal College of Physicians, 2002.

40. A. Cyclosporin

Causes of drug-induced hyperuricaemia and subsequent gout include aspirin (low dose), thiazide diuretics, cyclosporine, tacrolimus, cytotoxic chemotherapeutic agents, nicotinamide, ethambutol, pyrazinamide, and levodopa. Losartan, fenofibrate, vitamin C, oestrogens, and calcium channel blockers reduce serum urate, and have the potential to reduce gout.

Jordan KM et al., British Society for Rheumatology and British Health Professionals in Rheumatology guideline for the management of gout, *Rheumatology* 2007;46(8):1372–1374.

41. A. Anti-Ro antibodies

The presence of objective evidence for dry mouth and/or dry eyes in a patient presenting with sicca symptoms and positive anti-Ro antibodies is highly suggestive of Sjögren's syndrome (SS). This is a chronic inflammatory disorder characterized primarily by diminished lacrimal and salivary gland secretions resulting in symptoms of dry eyes and dry mouth. SS is characterized by polyclonal B-cell activation as well as lymphocytic infiltration of the exocrine glands. In patients with SS there is an increased incidence of primary biliary cirrhosis and its related anti-mitochondrial antibodies. Rheumatoid factor is positive in the majority of cases of SS but it is not specific for this disorder. Anti-CCP antibodies are highly specific for rheumatoid arthritis and are often negative in SS. Anti-nuclear antibodies are highly sensitive for connective tissue disorders such as systemic lupus erythematosus but lack specificity with high positive results especially at low titres. Anti-Ro and Anti-La antibodies are most often seen in primary SS (70% and 60% respectively), less frequently in SLE and least frequently in secondary SS. Anti-Ro and Anti-La antibodies are strongly associated with subacute cutaneous LE, neonatal lupus dermatitis, congenital complete heart block and rarely in lupus nephritis.

Delaleu N et al., Biomarker profiles in serum and saliva of experimental Sjögren's syndrome: associations with specific autoimmune manifestations, *Arthritis Research & Therapy* 2008;10(1):R22.

42. C. Reiter's syndrome

Reiter's syndrome is a form of reactive arthritis where there is concurrence of arthritis and non-infective urethritis. This patient has all features of Reiter's syndrome, i.e. urethritis, arthritis, and conjunctivitis. Other muco-cutaneous manifestations of reactive arthritis are: psoriasiform skin, nail, and mucosal lesions, keratoderma blenorrhagica (palmo-plantar pustulosis), and circinate balanitis. Behçet's disease presents with oral aphthous ulcers, genital ulcers, and panuveitis. Genital ulceration affects the scrotum in men and labia in women. Cervical or urethral ulcers are rare. Urethritis does not occur unless there is urethral meatal ulceration. Peripheral arthropathy in inflammatory bowel disease (IBD) is oligo-articular, asymmetric, and predominantly involves the lower limbs. Sacroilitis, spondylitis, enthesopathy (inflammation of bony insertion of tendons and ligaments), uveitis, and conjunctivitis. Sarcoidosis leads to acute, chronic arthropathy, and uveitis, but does not lead to urethritis. Whipple's disease is a rare disease which results from infection with *Tropheryma whippelii*. It manifests as polyarticular symmetrical arthropathy. Diarrhoea, weight loss, lymphadenopathy, and fever are common manifestations. It can be diagnosed using polymerase chain reaction for *T. whippelii*, and is treated by a one-year course of oral tetracyclines.

Colledge NR et al., *Davidson's Principles and Practice of Medicine*, Twenty-first Edition, Churchill Livingstone Elsevier, pp. 1065–1144.

43. B. Mixed connective tissue disease

This patient has mixed connective tissue disease (MCTD). MCTD is characterized by positive anti-RNP antibody, oedema of hands, arthritis, myositis, Raynaud's phenomenon, and acrosclerosis. Pulmonary arterial hypertension may also occur in MCTD. She does not have a rash. Dermatomyosisits is associated with Gottron's papules on the hands, and a periorbital heliotrope rash. This patient has symptoms, signs, and laboratory findings suggestive of an inflammatory myositis. However, she also has features of scleroderma, SLE, and pulmonary fibrosis. The co-existence of these features suggests the presence of an overlap syndrome (i.e. when clinical features of two or more connective tissue diseases are present in an individual). This patient is negative for scleroderma-specific antibodies. Some individuals with anti-Pm/Scl antibodies have features of inflammatory myositis and scleroderma. They are considered to have scleroderma/myositis overlap syndrome. They do not develop pulmonary fibrosis. Both myositis and fibrosing alveolitis can occur in Sjögren's syndrome. However, Sjögren's syndrome is unlikely in the absence of symptoms of dry eyes, dry mouth, anti-Ro, and anti-La antibody.

Greidinger EL, Mixed connective tissue disease, *eMedicine*, March 2015. http://emedicine.medscape.com/article/335815-overview

44. C. IV methylprednisolone 1 g/day for three days

This patient has giant cell (temporal) arteritis, a chronic vasculitis of large and medium vessels. It leads to granulomatous inflammation histologically, and predominantly affects the cranial branches of arteries arising from the arch of the aorta. As explained in the British Society for Rheumatology guidelines, complications of giant cell (temporal) arteritis include neuro-ophthalmic complications, such as vision loss and stroke. If one eye is affected there is a high risk (20–50%) of bilateral vision loss and total blindness with any delay or stoppage of treatment. This is usually early in the course of giant cell (temporal) arteritis. In those with evolving visual loss or history of amaurosis fugax, IV methylprednisolone 500 mg to 1 g daily for three days should be administered. There is no role for IV cyclophosphamide in the early treatment of neuro-ophthalmic complications in giant cell (temporal) arteritis. Suggested tapering regimens vary, and depend on the clinical presentation, but most patients need to remain on 40–60 mg prednisolone for 3–4 weeks.

Dasgupta B et al., BSR and BHPR guidelines for management of giant cell arteritis. *Rheumatology* 2010;49(8):1594–1597. http://www.rheumatology.org.uk/includes/documents/cm_docs/2010/m/2_management_of_giant_cell_arteritis.pdf

45. B. Ibuprofen

This patient has acute gout, as evidenced by the mono arthritis and raised uric acid. It is likely that his episode of renal colic may have been due to the formation of urate stones. Initial therapy of choice is non-steroidal-based. In a patient with abnormal renal function, corticosteroids or colchicine may be potential options. Rasburicase is an IV option to prevent acute urate nephropathy in patients undergoing chemotherapy. In practice, in patients with a mono-arthritis, infection should be at least excluded as a possibility, with a white count and crp as a minimum, +/– joint aspiration.

Khanna D et al., 2012 American College of Rheumatology Guidelines for Management of Gout Part II: therapy and anti-inflammatory prophylaxis of acute gouty arthritis, *Arthritis Care & Research (Hoboken)* 2012;64(10):1431–1446.

46. C. Ankylosing spondylitis

The evidence of sacroilitis, back pain, and morning stiffness over the past six months is entirely consistent with a diagnosis of ankylosing spondylitis. Ankylosing spondylitis usually starts in the sacroiliac joints and begins as buttock pain, extending to involve other parts of the axial skeleton.

Peripheral arthritis occurs in approximately one-third of patients, and may even involve the temporomandibular joints in some individuals. Anterior uveitis occurs in 20–30% of patients, cardiac involvement in less than 10%, with aortic regurgitation the commonest manifestation. Pulmonary fibrosis is also recognized. Initial therapy of choice is a combination of non-steroidals and physiotherapy designed to maintain flexibility. Sulphasalazine and methotrexate are potential second-line agents, infliximab is reserved under NICE guidance for patients who have failed conventional therapies.

Hakim A et al., *Oxford Handbook of Rheumatology*, Third Edition, Oxford University Press, 2011, Chapter 8, The spondyloarthropathies, Ankylosing spondylitis.

47. D. Anti-cyclic citrullinated peptide (CCP) antibody

This is the correct answer. Anti-CCP antibodies are found in about 60% of patients with RA. However, this test is very specific as it is rarely seen in other conditions. It is therefore helpful in confirming the diagnosis if positive. It is usually the next test to do after rheumatoid factor when RA is suspected. Anti Jo-1 antibodies are a type of anti-nuclear antibodies ANA, mostly associated with polymyositis/dermatomyositis. ANA are antibodies against contents of the cell nucleus. They are present in a variety of autoimmune conditions such as SLE. They are sometimes positive in RA, but are not specific for this condition and are therefore not likely to help in confirming the diagnosis. VGKC antibodies are seen in immune CNS disorders such as limbic encephalitis. Anti-Ro antibodies are also a type of ANA. They are positive particularly in Sjögren's syndrome and SLE.

National Rheumatoid Arthritis Society website. Section on laboratory tests. http://www.nras.org.uk/laboratory-tests-used-in-the-diagnosis-and-monitoring-of-rheumatoid-arthritis

48. C. Febuxistat

Febuxistat is now available as an alternative xanthine oxidase inhibitor, and in this case would be the next choice medication for prophylaxis. Its use is endorsed by NICE guidance for patients who cannot tolerate allopurinol as first-line therapy. In this case NSAIDs are best avoided because of their risk of worsening hypertension, and colchicine is associated with diarrhoea. Rasburicase is used IV as prophylaxis against acute urate nephropathy. Leaving him without medication puts him at significant risk of a further acute episode.

NICE Guidance [TA 164], Febuxostat for the management of hyperuricaemia in people with gout. http://guidance.nice.org.uk/TA164

49. C. IL-1 beta

Over recent years the pathophysiology which drives acute flares of gout has become clear. It is well known in the classic works of fiction, that binge eaters suffer acute gout attacks, and the pathway as to why that occurs is now described. The presence of both urate crystals and elevated free fatty acids drives up regulation of IL-1 beta. This then precipitates the acute inflammatory arthritis which underlines an acute gout attack. For these reason agents which impact both on free fatty acids and are uricosuric, such as fenofibrate are thought to reduce the frequency of attacks, and IL-1 beta antagonists such as canakinumab or XOMA-52 are effective in reducing inflammation at the time of an acute flare.

Dinarello CA, How interleukin-1ß induces gouty arthritis, *Arthritis & Rheumatism* 2010;62:3140–3144. http://onlinelibrary.wiley.com/doi/10.1002/art.27663/pdf

50. C. Thrombophilia screen

Either an inherited disorder leading to increased risk of clotting, such as Factor V Leiden, Protein C or S deficiency, or an acquired one, such as anti-phospholipid antibody syndrome is the most likely cause of the presentation seen here. The livedo reticularis is also suggestive of anti-phospholipid antibody syndrome. All of the other options listed, such as pelvic ultrasound, and hysteroscopy, are reasonable next steps if initial blood testing is unhelpful.

Provan D et al., *Oxford Handbook of Clinical Haematology*, Third Edition. Oxford University Press, 2009, Chapter 10.

51. B. Drug-induced lupus

The average age at onset for drug induced lupus is 50–70 years, with an equal male and female sex ratio. Antihistone antibodies are positive in more patients with drug-induced lupus than systemic lupus erythematosis; C3/C4 levels are normal, whereas complement levels are usually decreased in active SLE. Drugs associated with drug-induced lupus include hydralazine, procainamide, minocycline and quinidine, captopril and sulfasalzine Discontinuation of the suspected agent is the mainstay of therapy; low-dose corticosteroids may speed recovery in patients who do not show rapid improvement.

Hakim A et al., *Oxford Handbook of Rheumatology*, Third Edition, Oxford University Press, 2011.

52. D. Benign hypermobile syndrome

The picture of marked joint hypermobility with no significant scarring and blue sclerae raises the possibility of benign hypermobile syndrome (formerly known as Ehlers–Danlos Type III). In particular the lack of significant sequalae apart from musculoskeletal disorders supports this diagnosis. Other forms of Ehlers–Danlos are summarized below. Classic (formerly known as Type I and II): classical features include soft, doughy, hyperelastic skin with atrophic scars; multiple bruises are seen, especially on the legs, and easy skin-splitting shows in childhood over the forehead, elbows, knees, and chin. Vascular type (formally known as Type IV): appears as thin skin with venous patterns readily visible, ecchymoses over the knees and shins, premature ageing of the skin on the dorsum of the hands, feet, and shins. There is a characteristic facial appearance with large eyes, nasal thinning, and small ear lobes. The main problem is spontaneous rupture of medium/large arteries at any age from mid-adolescence to late adult life. Arterial aneurysms are also common. Death results from arterial rupture but rupture of the sigmoid colon is also common. Overall median lifespan is reduced to 48 years. Kyphoscoliosis type (formally known as Type VI): severe main features include early progressive fibrosis and severe motor delay. Arthrochalasia type (formally known as Types VII A and B): severe main features include short stature, hip dislocation, dentinogenesis imperfecta. Dermatosparaxis type (formally known as Type VII C): main features are variable, early tooth loss with severe periodontitis is seen in the majority of patients. Of note is the fact that osteogenesis imperfecta also presents with blue sclerae; it is, however, associated with multiple fractures which occur from a young age.

Hakim A et al., *Oxford Handbook of Rheumatology*, Third Edition, Oxford University Press, 2010.

53. A. Oxalate arthropathy

Patients with Crohn's disease affecting their small bowel, will have fat malabsorption. Fat binds to calcium, leaving oxalate (a type of salt) free to be absorbed and deposited in the kidney, where it can form into stones. Calcium oxalate arthritis is an unusual form of arthritis. The crystals are positively birefringent and bipyramidal on polarized light microscopy. Treatment is the same as that for pyrophosphate disease with NSAIDs or low-dose colchicine. In some cases dietary oxalate restriction or vitamin supplementation may also be of benefit. It is associated with a number of conditions including: end-stage renal disease on dialysis; short bowel syndrome; diet rich in rhubarb, spinach, ascorbic acid; thiamine deficiency; pyridoxine deficiency; primary oxalosis.

Hakim A et al., *Oxford Handbook of Rheumatology*, Third Edition, Oxford University Press, 2011, Chapter 7, The crystal arthopathies.

54. D. Pseudogout

Whilst it is not impossible that this patient has gout, the fact that his urate is well within the normal range makes it somewhat unlikely. The non-elevated CRP also reduces the likelihood that this is either rheumatoid arthritis or a septic episode. Osteoarthritis would also not usually be associated with an acute presentation in one joint. This leaves us with pseudogout or pyrophosphate arthropathy, which is well known to be associated with haemochromatosis. It is the second most common crystal arthropathy after gout itself, and is usually managed with NSAIDs, although low-dose colchicine may reduce the frequency of acute episodes.

Hakim A et al., *Oxford Handbook of Rheumatology*, Third Edition, Oxford University Press, 2011, Chapter 7, The crystal arthopathies.

55. E. Cryptogenic fibrosing alveolitis

This patient has features of cryptogenic fibrosing alveolitis (also known as idiopathic fibrosing alveolitis). The clinical picture of progressive shortness of breath includes a wide differential. Additional features of weight loss and arthralgia are not always present, but may be associated with this condition. It is important to perform spirometry in these patients, along with an HIV test. The radiological features on a HRCT will help to confirm the diagnosis. The following describes the different causes of upper versus lower lobe fibrosis. Causes for upper lobe fibrosis: BREAST X; bronchopulmonary aspergillosis; radiotherapy; extrinsic allergic alveolitis; ankylosing spondylitis; sarcoidosis/silicosis; tuberculosis; histiocytosis X. Causes for lower lobe fibrosis: CRABSS; cryptogenic fibrosing alveolitis; rheumatoid arthritis; asbestosis; bleomycin; systemic lupus erythematous; scleroderma.

Longmore M et al., *Oxford Handbook of Clinical Medicine*, Eighth Edition, Oxford University Press, 2010, Chapter 4, Lung disease, Interstitial lung disease.

56. D. Ankylosing spondylitis

Ankylosing spondylitis is the option most in keeping with upper lobe changes on a plain chest X-ray. In addition, the history of joint pain, supports this diagnosis. Typically, the joint pain in ankylosing spondylitis is more prominent early, easing off throughout the course of the day. The mnemonics 'TAXERS' and 'CARDS' help to differentiate the causes between upper and lower zone fibrosis. Causes of upper lobe fibrosis can be remembered by using the mnemonic 'TAXERS':

Tuberculosis
Ankylosing spondylitis
Histiocytosis X
Extrinsic allergic alveolitis
Radiotherapy
Sarcoidosis, Silicosis.

Causes of lower lobe fibrosis can be remembered by using the mnemonic 'CARDS':

Cryptogenic fibrosing alveolitis
Asbestosis
Rheumatoid arthritis
Drugs—bleomycin
Systemic lupus erythematosus, Scleroderma.

Longmore M et al., *Oxford Handbook of Clinical Medicine*, Eighth Edition, Oxford University Press, 2010, Chapter 4, Lung disease, Interstitial lung disease.

INDEX

Note: Page numbers in *q* refer to Question and *a* refer to Answer. References to figures, tables, and boxes are indicated by '*f*', '*t*', and '*b*' following the page number, for example 14*af* refers to a figure on page 14.

hepatopulmonary syndrome 165q, 191a
hepatorenal syndrome 9q, 28a
hereditary motor and sensory neuropathy (HMSN) 42q, 82a
 see also Charcot–Marie–Tooth disease
heroin dependence 122q, 132a
herpes simplex encephalitis 66q, 80a, 104a
herpes simplex meningitis 39q, 80a
hilar lymphadenopathy 164q, 183a, 190a
HIV infection, presentation 102a
HLA B27 219a
Horner's syndrome 96a
Huntington's disease 109a
hydrocephalus, normal pressure 49q, 50q–51q, 54q,
 90a–91a, 92a–93a, 95a
hypercalcaemia 12q, 149q
 in chronic renal failure 1q, 22a
 familial hypocalciuric hypercalcaemia (FHH) 30a
 management 178a
 sarcoidosis 25a
hyperemesis gravidarum 64q, 103a
hyperkalaemia 11q, 29a
hypermobility 209q, 228a
hyperosmolar non-ketotic coma (HONK) 68q, 106a
hyperparathyroidism 11q, 18q, 30a
 secondary 35a
hyperphosphataemia 6q
 management in chronic kidney disease 11q, 26a, 30a
hyperprolactinaemia 68q
hypersensitivity pneumonitis 153q, 181a
hypertension, management in chronic kidney
 disease 6q, 26a
hypertrophic pulmonary osteoarthropathy (HPOA) 171a,
 173a, 176a
hyperuricaemia 26a
 drug-induced 206q, 225a
 indications for treatment 222a
 see also gout
hypoalbuminaemia, causes 8q
hypocalcaemia, secondary hypoparathyroidism 18q
hypoglycaemia, in alcohol abuse 107a
hypomagnesaemia 133a
hyponatraemia 2q, 4q, 12q, 24q, 133a
 management 30a–31a

I

idiopathic fibrosing alveolitis (cryptogenic fibrosing
 alveolitis) 229a
idiopathic interstitial pneumonias, prognosis 160q, 187a
idiopathic intracranial hypertension 47q, 88a–89a
idiopathic pulmonary fibrosis 156q, 161q, 184a, 187a
 lung transplantation 144q, 174a
idiopathic thrombocytopenic purpura 223a
IgA nephropathy (Berger's disease) 16q, 22a, 25a, 34a
inclusion bodies, causes 135a
inclusion body myositis 55q, 96a
inflammatory bowel disease, peripheral arthropathy 225a
interferon gamma test for TB 191a

interleukin 1 beta (IL-1 beta), role in acute gout 227a
internuclear ophthalmoplegia 81a

J

jaw claudication, temporal arteritis 203q, 205q, 223a
jaw osteonecrosis 224a
JC virus 60q, 101a
joint aspiration 218a–219a, 224a

K

Kaposi's sarcoma 103a
ketamine, acute intoxication 130a
kidney stones see renal stones
knife-edge atrophy 135a

L

lacunar stroke 72q, 82a, 110a
Lambert–Eaton myasthenic syndrome 65q, 71q, 104a,
 108a, 212a
lamotrigine 93a
 use during pregnancy 106a
lateral medullary syndrome 44q, 84a–85a
latex fruit syndrome 158q, 186a
Legionnaire's disease 175a
Lesch–Nyhan syndrome 212a
levetiracetam 93a
levodopa 138a
Lewy body dementia 97a, 99a, 125q, 134a, 135a, 138a
 histological findings 135a
Lhermitte's sign 97a, 116a, 117a
liberty cap mushroom 33a
limbic encephalitis 46q, 86a, 101a
limited cutaneous systemic sclerosis 204q, 222a
 pulmonary hypertension 220a
Listeria meningitis 107a
lithium
 toxicity 135a
 withdrawal symptoms 131a
livedo reticularis 201q, 209q, 214q, 222a, 228a
liver disease, alcoholic 130a–131a
lofexidine 132a
loin pain
 in amyloidosis 9q
 papillary necrosis 2q
 pelvi-ureteric junction obstruction 18q, 35a
 polycystic kidney disease 4q, 14q, 24a, 32a
long-term oxygen therapy (LTOT) 141q
 indications for 156q, 159q, 171a, 184a, 186a
lorazepam, for rapid tranquillization 130a
lumbar puncture tap test 93a
lung carcinoma 189a–190a
 adrenal metastases 163q, 189a
 contraindications to surgery 162q, 188a–189a
 non-small cell 147q, 176a
 Pancoast tumours 152q, 180a
 paraneoplastic syndromes 140q, 143q, 171a,
 173a, 176a